Progress in
Cancer Research and Therapy
Volume 19

MEDIATION OF CELLULAR IMMUNITY IN CANCER BY IMMUNE MODIFIERS

Progress in Cancer Research and Therapy

Progress in
Cancer Research and Therapy
Volume 19

Mediation of Cellular Immunity in Cancer by Immune Modifiers

Editors

Michael A. Chirigos
*Chief, Virus and Disease
Modification Section
National Cancer Institute
National Institutes of Health
Bethesda, Maryland*

Malcolm Mitchell
*Departments of Medicine and
Microbiology
University of Southern California
Medical Center
Los Angeles, California*

Michael J. Mastrangelo
*Director, Melanoma Unit
Fox Chase Cancer Center
Philadelphia, Pennsylvania*

Mathilde Krim
*Sloan-Kettering Institute
New York, New York*

Raven Press ■ New York

Raven Press, 1140 Avenue of the Americas, New York, New York 10036

Made in the United States of America

International Standard Book Number (0-89004-628-y)
Library of Congress Catalog Number (80-5877)

Preface

A considerable amount of new and pertinent information is presented concerning the characteristics of cytotoxicity against a variety of tumor cells (animal and human) by macrophages, natural killer cells (NK cells), and antibody dependent cellular cytotoxicity (ADCC). Of particular importance is the evidence presented for the role of biological response modifiers on these effector cells.

Kinetics of macrophage activation and tumor cell killing are discussed in view of one step or multistep mechanisms. The interrelationships of interferon and interferon inducers to enhance macrophage, NK cell, and ADCC tumorlytic effect on animal and human tumors are discussed. The relationship of prostaglandins and other immunoregulating agents on feedback inhibition mechanisms and suppressor cells which can modify the immune response is discussed in detail. Several new test systems are described for measuring macrophage, NK cell, and ADCC.

This volume will be of interest to clinical and experimental oncologists, chemotherapists, immunologists, and immunopharmacologists.

Michael A. Chirigos

Acknowledgments

The editors of this volume wish to express their gratitude to Dr. V. T. DeVita, Jr., Director of the Division of Cancer Treatment, Dr. R. K. Oldham, Associate Director, Biological Response Modifiers Program, Office of the Director, Division of Cancer Treatment, National Cancer Institute, and his staff for their invaluable support that made this Workshop possible, and to the members of the Biological Response Modifiers Subcommittee: Drs. E. Mihich, A. Fefer, E. Hersh, M. J. Mastrangelo, M. A. Chirigos, H. Oettgen, M. Krim, A. Goldstein, M. Mitchell, J. Whisnant, J. Betram, and A. Goldin for their encouragement and suggestions.

Contents

vii

Contributors

P. Allavena
Istituto di Ricerche Farmacologiche "Mario Negri"
62-20157 Milan, Italy

Anthony C. Allison
International Laboratory for Research on Animal Diseases
Nairobi, Kenya

Anna Bartocci
Viruses and Disease Modification Section
Division of Cancer Treatment
National Cancer Institute
National Institutes of Health
Bethesda, Maryland 20205

James A. Bennett
The Departments of Surgery and Physiology
Albany Medical College
Albany, New York 12208

H. Blomgren
Radiumhemmet
Karolinksa Hospital
Department of Immunology
University of Stockholm
Stockholm, Sweden

Robert J. Bonney
Departments of Immunology and Biochemistry
Merck Institute for Therapeutic Research
Rahway, New Jersey 07065

Michael A. Chirigos
Viruses and Disease Modification Section
Division of Cancer Treatment
National Cancer Institute
National Institutes of Health
Bethesda, Maryland 20205

James L. Cook
Veterans Administration Medical Center
and Department of Medicine
Division of Infectious Diseases
University of Utah Medical Center
Salt Lake City, Utah 84148

P. Davies
Departments of Immunology and Biochemistry

Merck Institute for Therapeutic Research
Rahway, New Jersey 07065

Gunther Dennert
Department of Cancer Biology
The Salk Institute for Biological Studies
San Diego, California 92138

J. Y. Djeu
Food and Drug Administration
Bureau of Biologics
Division of Virology
Bethesda, Maryland 20205

Beth-Ellen Drysdale
Department of Microbiology
Johns Hopkins University School of Medicine
Baltimore, Maryland 21205

S. Einhorn
Radiumhemmet
Karolinska Hospital
Department of Immunology
University of Stockholm
Stockholm, Sweden

Sandra L. Emmons
Division of Tumor Immunology
Fred Hutchinson Cancer Research Center
and the Department of Microbiology and Immunology
University of Washington
Seattle, Washington 98104

D. M. Garagiola
Simpson Memorial Research Institute
University of Michigan Medical Center
Ann Arbor, Michigan 48109

Ronald B. Herberman
Laboratory of Immunodiagnosis
National Cancer Institute
Bethesda, Maryland 20205

John B. Hibbs, Jr.
Veterans Administration Medical Center
and Department of Medicine
Division of Infectious Diseases
University of Utah Medical Center
Salt Lake City, Utah 84148

T. K. Huard
Simpson Memorial Research Institute
University of Michigan Medical Center
Ann Arbor, Michigan 48109

J. L. Humes
Departments of Immunology and
 Biochemistry
Merck Institute for Therapeutic Research
Rahway, New Jersey 07065

M. Introna
Istituto di Ricerche Farmacologiche
 "Mario Negri"
62-20157 Milan, Italy

William T. Jackson
Lilly Research Laboratories
Eli Lilly and Company
Indianapolis, Indiana 46285

Eugenie S. Kleinerman
Cellular Immunology Section
Metabolism Branch
Division of Cancer Biology and Diagnosis
National Cancer Institute
National Institutes of Health
Bethesda, Maryland 20205

Janis K. Lazdins
Immunopathology Section
Laboratory of Immunobiology
Division of Cancer Biology and Diagnosis
National Cancer Institute
National Institutes of Health
Bethesda, Maryland 20205

Edward J. Leonard
Immunopathology Section
Laboratory of Immunobiology
Division of Cancer Biology and Diagnosis
National Cancer Institute
National Institutes of Health
Bethesda, Maryland 20205

Andrew M. Lewis, Jr.
National Institute of Allergy and
 Infectious Diseases
National Institutes of Health
Bethesda, Maryland 20205

Albert F. LoBuglio
Simpson Memorial Research Institute
University of Michigan Medical Center
Ann Arbor, Michigan 48109

C. Mangioni
Clinica Ostetrica e Ginecologica
Universita di Milano
Milan, Italy

A. Mantovani
Istituto di Ricerche Farmacologiche
 "Mario Negri"
62-20157 Milan, Italy

John C. Marsh
The Departments of Medicine and
 Pharmacology
Yale University School of Medicine
New Haven, Connecticut 06510

Monte S. Meltzer
Immunopathology Section
Laboratory of Immunobiology
Division of Cancer Biology and Diagnosis
National Cancer Institute
National Institutes of Health
Bethesda, Maryland 20205

Malcolm S. Mitchell
The Departments of Medicine and
 Microbiology
University of Southern California
Los Angeles, California 90033

Robert N. Moore
Cellular Immunology Section
Laboratory of Microbiology and
 Immunology
National Institute of Dental Research
National Institutes of Health
Bethesda, Maryland 20205

Andrew V. Muchmore
Cellular Immunology Section
Metabolism Branch
Division of Cancer Biology and Diagnosis
National Cancer Institute
National Institutes of Health
Bethesda, Maryland 20205

Joost J. Oppenheim
Cellular Immunology Section
Laboratory of Microbiology and
 Immunology
National Institute of Dental Research
National Institutes of Health
Bethesda, Maryland 20205

John R. Ortaldo
Laboratory of Immunodiagnosis
National Cancer Institute
Bethesda, Maryland 20205

Judith L. Pace
Division of Comparative Pathology
Colleges of Veterinary Medicine and
 Medicine
University of Florida
Gainesville, Florida 32610

V. Papdademetriou
Virus and Disease Modification Section
Laboratory of Chemical Pharmacology
National Cancer Institute
National Institutes of Health
Bethesda, Maryland 20205

G. Peri
Istituto di Ricerche Farmacologiche
"Mario Negri"
62-20157 Milan, Italy

B. Perussia
The Wistar Institute of Anatomy and
Biology
Philadelphia, Pennsylvania 19104

N. Polentarutti
Istituto di Ricerche Farmacologiche
"Mario Negri"
62-20157 Milan, Italy

Sylvia B. Pollack
Division of Tumor Immunology
Fred Hutchinson Cancer Research Center
and the Department of Microbiology and
Immunology
University of Washington
Seattle, Washington 98104

Elizabeth Read
Viruses and Disease Modification Section
Division of Cancer Treatment
National Cancer Institute
National Institutes of Health
Bethesda, Maryland 20205

Perry Robinson
Simpson Memorial Research Institute
University of Michigan Medical Center
Ann Arbor, Michigan 48109

Luigi P. Ruco
Immunopathology Section
Laboratory of Immunobiology
Division of Cancer Biology and Diagnosis
National Cancer Institute
National Institutes of Health
Bethesda, Maryland 20205

Stephen W. Russell
Division of Comparative Pathology
Colleges of Veterinary Medicine and
Medicine
University of Florida
Gainesville, Florida 32610

D. Santoli
The Wistar Institute of Anatomy and
Biology
Philadelphia, Pennsylvania 19104

Richard M. Schultz
Lilly Research Laboratories
Eli Lilly and Company
Indianapolis, Indiana 46285

C. Sessa
Clinica Ostetrica e Ginecologica
Universita di Milano
Milan, Italy

W. Shih
University of California at Los Angeles
and the Department of Microbiology and
Immunology
School of Medicine
The Center for the Health Sciences
Los Angeles, California 90024

Hyun S. Shin
Department of Microbiology
Johns Hopkins University School of
Medicine
Baltimore, Maryland 21205

Patricia S. Steeg
Cellular Immunology Section
Laboratory of Microbiology and
Immunology
National Institute of Dental Research
National Institutes of Health
Bethesda, Maryland 20205

L. K. Steel
Laboratory of Clinical Investigation
National Institute of Allergy and
Infectious Diseases
National Institutes of Health
Bethesda, Maryland 20205

Maxine Solvay
Simpson Memorial Research Institute
University of Michigan Medical Center
Ann Arbor, Michigan 48109

Carleton C. Stewart
Section of Cancer Biology
Division of Radiation Oncology
Washington University School of Medicine
St. Louis, Missouri 63110

H. Strander
Radiumhemmet
Karolinska Hospital
Department of Immunology
University of Stockholm
Stockholm, Sweden

Steven M. Taffet
Department of Bacteriology and
  Immunology
University of North Carolina
School of Medicine
Chapel Hill, North Carolina 27514

David L. Thomasson
Section of Cancer Biology
Division of Radiation Oncology
Washington University School of Medicine
St. Louis, Missouri 63110

T. Timonen
National Cancer Institute
Laboratory of Immunodiagnosis
Bethesda, Maryland 20205

G. Trinchieri
The Wistar Institute of Anatomy and
  Biology
Philadelphia, Pennsylvania 19104

M. Troye
Radiumhemmet
Karolinska Hospital
Department of Immunology
University of Stockholm
Stockholm, Sweden

Stefanie N. Vogel
Cellular Immunology Section
Laboratory of Microbiology and
  Immunology
National Institute of Dental Research
National Institutes of Health
Bethesda, Maryland 20205

Joyce M. Zarling
Immunobiology Research Center
Department of Laboratory Medicine and
  Pathology
University of Minnesota
Minneapolis, Minnesota 55455

J. Zighelboim
University of California at Los Angeles
  and the Department of Microbiology and
  Immunology
School of Medicine
The Center for the Health Sciences
Los Angeles, California 90024

Mediation of Cellular Immunity in Cancer by Immune Modifiers, edited by M. A. Chirigos et al., Raven Press, New York © 1981.

Macrophage Tumoricidal Activity: Activation and Killing Kinetics

David L. Thomasson and Carleton C. Stewart

Section of Cancer Biology, Division of Radiation Oncology, Washington University School of Medicine, St. Louis, Missouri 63110

INTRODUCTION

In recent years, macrophages have received considerable interest with regard to their ability to kill tumor cells. Several investigators have shown that murine peritoneal macrophages obtained from animals previously injected with facultative intracellular bacteria such as Mycobacterium bovis strain Bacillus Calmette Guerin (BCG), will inhibit the growth of neoplastic cells in vitro but not normal cells (5,6). This inhibitory action was interpreted as the net result of macrophage-induced cytocidal and cytostatic effects upon the neoplastic target cells. Further, this activity was apparently nonspecific since these macrophage-mediated actions were seen to occur with several immunologically different tumor cell lines (4).

More recently, attention has focused on the in vitro activation of non-inhibitory macrophages to a state which renders them inhibitory for neoplastic cells (3,7,8,10,11). This can be easily accomplished by incubating the macrophages in a lymphokine-rich medium (LKRM), prepared by stimulating specifically sensitized spleen cells with antigen or normal spleen cells with a nonspecific mitogen such as concanavalin A (con-A).

In spite of the numerous studies which have focused on this essential component of cellular defense against neoplasia, little is known regarding the time required for the in vitro development of inhibitory macrophages after addition of LKRM, how long they remain tumoricidal after removal of LKRM, and how long macrophages must interact with tumor cells before they are lethally damaged. We examined these time-related actions in detail.

MATERIALS AND METHODS

Animals

Adult female C3Hf/An and C57Bl/6 mice, 20 to 25 g, were used. These were obtained from the Radiation Oncology Breeding Facility, Washington University School of Medicine, St. Louis, Missouri.

Medium

The medium used for cell preparation and production of LKRM was α-Minimal Essential Medium (αMEM). Culture medium was αMEM supplemented with 10% fetal calf serum (FCS). All media contained 100 units/ml penicillin and 100 µg/ml streptomycin and were buffered with sodium bicarbonate.

1

Cell Counting

All cell counts were performed on an electronic particle counter according to the method of Stewart et al. (13). The counting solution consisted of 30.0 g cetyltrimethylammonium bromide (cetrimide), 8.5 g NaCl and 0.37 g EDTA to a final volume of 1000 ml with water (the pH was adjusted to 5.0 with HCl). Since cetrimide completely lyses the cell cytoplasm, liberating individual nuclei adherent cells can easily be removed for counting.

Peritoneal Macrophages

Tumoricidal peritoneal macrophages were obtained from mice which were intraperitoneally (ip) injected with 10^7 viable units of Mycobacterium bovis strain Bacillus Calmette Guerin (BCG) (Pasteur substrain, supplied by Trudeau Institute, Saranac Lake, New York). Non-tumoricidal macrophages were obtained from mice which received 1.5 ml of Brewer's thioglycollate medium (Difco Laboratories, Detroit, Michigan) 3 days previously. To harvest peritoneal exudate cells (PEC) from these animals, they were killed by cervical dislocation and their peritoneal cavities infused with 5 ml of αMEM containing heparin sodium (5 units/ml, Abbott Laboratories, Chicago, Illinois). Following surgical exposure of the peritoneum, the exudate fluids were withdrawn through the lateral peritoneal wall using a 20-guage needle. Peritoneal fluids from several mice were then pooled, and a small sample was removed for counting. The remainder was centrifuged at 200 xg for 10 min. at 4°C. Afterwards, the cell-free supernatant was decanted and discarded, and the cell pellet was gently resuspended in αMEM. To obtain macrophages from the cell suspension, aliquots were pipetted into plastic tissue culture dishes (Falcon Product, Oxnard, California) which were incubated for one hour at 37°C in 5% CO_2-humidified air. The nonadherent cells (mostly lymphocytes) were removed using several rinses with αMEM. The adherent macrophages (consistently 95% of the total plated cells) were identified by morpho-logical criteria and by their ability to phagocytose yeast as described previously (14). The numbers of adherent cells were removed with cetrimide.

Preparation of Lymphokine-rich Medium (LRM)

Spleens from 10-15 untreated mice were removed, minced and passed through a sterile 120-mesh stainless steel screen into a 100 mm culture dish containing 25 ml of α MEM. This cell suspension was centrifuged at 300 xg for 10 min at 4°C and the medium discarded. The cell pellet was then resuspended in α MEM to 10^7 cells per ml, and 25 ml of this suspension were added to 75-cm^2 plastic tissue culture flasks (Falcon Products). To stimulate production of lymphokines, concanavalin A (con A, 5 μ g/ml), prepared by the Sephadex adsorption method of Agrawal and Goldstein (1), was added to the flasks which were incubated at 37°C in a 5% CO_2-humidified air atmosphere for 24 hr. The culture medium and cells were separated by centrifugation at 800 xg for 15 min at 4°C. This LKRM was sterilized by filtration and stored at 4°C until use. Control medium (CM) was prepared by the same method but without con A.

Target Cells

The EMT6 mammary adenocarcinoma, originally derived from BALB/c mice (9), was maintained in 75-cm^2 tissue culture flasks (Falcon Products, Oxnard, California) at 37°C in a 5% CO_2-humidified air atmosphere. To prepare the tumor cells for use in our experiments, we decanted and discarded the culture medium. The adherent tumor cell monolayer was then rinsed once with 5 ml of α MEM, followed by 5 ml of calcium- and magnesium-free Hank's balanced salt solution containing 0.25% tryspin, which also was immediately discarded. Following a 5 minute incubation at room temperature, the tumor cells were resuspended in culture medium, and a small sample was removed for counting.

Assay for Inhibition of Target Cells

Two assays were used to evaluate macrophage antitumor activity. A qualitative assay (5,12), was used to screen for conditions which resulted in positive antitumor activity. Briefly, cells were adjusted to 2 x 10^6 cells per ml for thioglycollate medium elicited or 4 x 10^6 cells per ml for BCG elicited peritoneal exudate cells; 80 and 40% respectively of the cells from the two groups were adherent macrophages. The cells in 0.1 ml were plated in the center of 35mm culture dishes. Following incubation of the macrophages for 45 min., the supernatants were removed, and the cells were washed two times with fresh medium. The cells were then treated in various ways as described under results. The cultures then received 3 ml of *in vitro* passaged EMT-6 tumor cells at 4 x 10^4 cells/ml in complete α-MEM. After incubation for 3 days at 37°C, all cultures were rinsed with phosphate-buffered saline (PBS) and stained with a 3% methylene blue-10% formaldehyde solution. An antitumor effect upon EMT-6 cells was recognized by a cleared plaque in the center of the culture dish where the macrophages were spotted. Lack of tumor cell inhibition was indicated with a complete overgrowth by neoplastic cells.

For those conditions which yielded a positive antitumor effect, the inhibition of tumor cell growth was quantified by a clonogenic assay (15). Briefly, macrophages were prepared as just described except that 1.0 ml of a 1/10 dilution in α MEM of peritoneal exudate cells was added to 16 mm-24 well cluster dishes (Falcon Products) to produce a monolayer over the entire 2 cm^2 surface. After rinsing, a final density of about 1.6 x 10^5 cells/cm^2 remained. These adherent cells were incubated for 18 to 24 hours in LKRM and rinsed. EMT-6 tumor cells were then added to give 1.2 x 10^4 cells/cm^2. Forty-eight hours later, the tumor cells were removed with 0.25% trypsin (Grand Island Biological Company, Grand Island, N.Y.). For the most part, macrophages, which are resistant to trypsin (2), remained attached to the wells. Several tenfold dilutions were added to 60 mm tissue culture dishes and cultured at 37°C in humified CO_2-in-air for 7 days. The surviving tumor cells formed colonies which were stained with methyylene blue-formaldehyde and counted. Previous studies indicated that any macrophages removed from the wells with tumor cells failed to express additional inhibitory actions (15).

RESULTS

Time for Activation

We determined the optimal time requirement for the conversion of non-inhibitory macrophages to an inhibitory, or activated, state. To examine this, peritoneal macrophages were collected from thioglycollate-injected C3Hf/An mice and seeded as described. After elimination of the nonadherent cells, one replicate set of cultures received 3 ml of LKRM (diluted 1:4 with culture medium). The remaining cultures received only culture medium. All cultures were incubated at 37°C. As a function of time, the culture medium on replicate cultures was replaced with LKRM. At 24 hr after the macrophages were initially plated, all cultures were rinsed several times with fresh α MEM and received 3 ml of culture medium containing 10^5 EMT6 cells (10^4 cells/cm^2). Seventy-two hours later, all cultures were stained and examined for evidence of macrophage-induced inhibitory activity. As Table 1 indicates, when the qualitative spot-stain assay method was used, inhibitory activity by macrophages toward tumor cell targets could be demonstrated only when the macrophages were preincubated for 12-16 hr with LKRM.

TABLE 1. Activation of non-tumoricidal macrophage to a tumoricidal state.

Preincubation time (HR)	Inhibitory action against target cells[a]
0 (no LKRM)	−
4	−
8	−
12	±
16	+
20	+
24	+

[a] − complete overgrowth of macrophages by EMT6 cells; + cleared plaque-like area in center (macrophage-rich) of dish.

This effect was quantified between 10 and 16 hrs using the clonogenic assay and the results are shown in Table 2. We observed that the number of EMT6 clonogenic survivors decreased to 43%, i.e., 57% of tumor cells were inhibited when macrophages were incubated for 16 hrs with MAF.

TABLE 2. Quantitative clonogenic assay of macrophage-mediated inhibitory activity.

Preincubation time (HK)	Fraction of Surviving EMT6 clonogenic cells
0 (no LKRM)	1.00
10	0.90
11	0.75
12	0.71
13	0.62
14	0.43
15	0.46
16	0.43

Preincubating the macrophages for longer than 16 hr did not improve inhibitory activity as macrophages were actually slightly less inhibitory than when the preincubation interval was shorter (14-16 hr).

In another series of experiments, we examined the loss of antitumor capacity from inhibitory macrophages. In these studies, the peritoneal macrophages were activated in vivo with BCG. After collection and plating, these cells were incubated at 37°C in growth medium and, as a function of time, received EMT6 tumor cell targets. At 72 hr after the targets were added, the cultures were stained and examined for evidence of macrophage antitumor activity. Also, cell counts were done on duplicate macrophage cultures as a function of time since a loss of effector cells due to death might reduce the cell density (cells/cm^2) to a point where the assay would appear negative. Table 3 indicates that when the spot-stain method was used, a strong inhibitory action was displayed by macrophages when the targets were added immediately. Further, no waning of the antitumor effects was noted when the macrophages were preincubated in culture medium (prior to addition of tumor cells) for up to 12 hr. At 16 hr, however, a decline in the inhibitory effect was seen and by 20 hr, macrophages had totally lost their ability to kill. When these results were quantified using the clonogenic assay (Table 3) however we noted that a continuous decline in antitumor capacity was actually occuring which was evident at the first observation time at 4 hr after culture initiation. All antitumor activity was lost by 24 hrs. When we examined the total number of viable adherent macrophages as a function of time, we noted only a slight decrease in cell survival over the 24-hr incubation period (Table 3).

TABLE 3. <u>Loss of inhibitory activity by BCG-macrophages.</u>

Incubation Time (HR)	Inhibitory Activity on EMT6 Target Cells[a]		
	spot assay[a]	clonogenic assay[b]	fraction macrophage remaining[c]
0	+	0.39	1.00
4	+	0.50	0.98
8	+	0.53	0.94
12	+	0.65	0.90
16	±	0.80	0.89
20	−	0.92	0.86
24	−	1.00	0.82

[a] For evaluation of results, see legend to Table 1.
[b] fraction of surviving tumor cell colonies.
[c] fraction of macrophages surviving after same culture period except no tumor cells were added to them. Number of macrophages at time zero was 132,000.

In a third set of experiments, we sought to determine how long
activated macrophages had to interact with target cells to produce an
irreversible lethal event. Heat-killed yeast cells, after being
phagocytosed by macrophages will inhibit their tumorcidal activity. By
adding the yeast at different times after adding tumor target cells,
further tumoricidal activity will be inhibited. These studies are
important because the expression of tumor cell death maybe at a different
time than the acquisition of the lethal damage. For the present study,
EMT6 cells were added to BCG elicited macrophages at time 0. As a
function of time, yeast cells were added to the cultures. In Table 4, we
see that when yeast were added at 0, 2 hr or 4 hr, macrophage-mediated
tumoricidal activity was inhibited. However, when yeast cells were added
to macrophage-tumor cell cultures which had previously incubated for 6 hr
Using time lapse cinemicrography we determined the time tumor cells
died. After interacting with BCG activated macrophages. The first tumor
cell died 16 hrs after initiation of the interaction. The greatest number
of tumor cells died after 30 hrs of incubation. Tumor cell death was
characterized by a rounding of the tumor cell followed by rapid lysis.
This process took from 60 to 90 minutes. Up to the time of lysis tumor
cells remained well spread on the dish even though they did not divide.

TABLE 4. Effects of heat-killed yeast cells on macrophage-mediated
              inhibitory activity on EMT6 cells.

Time^a (Hr)	Fraction of Surviving EMT6 lonogenic Cells
0	1.0
2	0.91
4	0.79
6	0.44
No yeast	0.56

^{a} Time the yeast was added to the macrophages.

DISCUSSION

This study shows that macrophages are activated to the tumor inhibitory
state after incubation with LKRF. The time to reach this inhibitory level
may vary with the tumor target used (4). Once activated to this
inhibitory state, macrophages loose this activity with time. Indeed the
time to maximum activation is about the same length as the time for them
to loose the activity.

The most important finding was that macrophages do not have to
continuously interact with the target to impart lethal damage. Rather, it
would seem that the macrophage must interact during the first 12 hrs after
activation before it looses this activity.

Once the macrophage has lost its activated state for whatever reasons
this occurs it can no longer kill. The target cell, however, does not die
during the time of meaningful interaction. Rather, it remains in a
nonproliferative state up to two days before it dies. Thus, the lethal
damage imposed by macrophages is displaced in time from the phenotypic
expression of cell death. In this respect, the kinetics are similar to

those on radiation induced lethality wherein few if any cells die while being irradiated, death occurs hours or days later.

REFERENCES

1. Agrawal, B.B.L. and Goldstein, I.J. (1967) Biochim. Biophys. Aca. 147:262.
2. Evans, R. (1973) J. Natl. Cancer Inst. 50:271.
3. Fidler, I.J. (1975) J. Natl. Cancer Inst. 55:1159.
4. Fidler, I.J. (1978) Israel J. Med. Sci. 14:177.
5. Hibbs, J.B., Jr. (1974) J. Natl. Cancer Inst. 53:1487.
6. Keller, R. (1976) J. Natl. Cancer Inst. 56:369.
7. Leonard, E.J., Ruco, L.P., and Meltzer, M.S. (1978) Cellular Immunol. 41:347.
8. Lohmann-Matthes, M.-L., Kolb, B., and Meerpohl, H.G. (1978) Cell Immunol. 41:231.
9. Rockwell, S.C., Kallman, R.F., and Fajardo, L.F. (1972) J. Natl. Cancer Inst. 49:735.
10. Ruco, L.P. and Meltzer, M.S. (1978) Cell Immunol. 41:35.
11. Sharma, S.D. and Piessens, W.F. (1978) Cellular Immunol. 37:20.
12. Stewart, C.C., Adles, C., and Hibbs, J.B., Jr. (1976) In: The Reticuloendothelial System in Health and Disease: Immunologic and Pathologic Aspects, edited by H. Friedman, M. R. Escobar, and S. M. Reichard, p. 423. Plenum Publishing Co., NY.
13. Stewart, C.C., Cramer, S.F., and Steward, P.G. (1975) Cell Immunol. 16:237.
14. Stewart, C.C., Lin, H.S., and Adler, C. (1975) J. Exp. Med. 141:1114.
15. Thomasson, D.L. and Stewart, C.C. (1981) J. Immunol. Methods (in press).

Mediation of Cellular Immunity in Cancer by Immune Modifiers, edited by M. A. Chirigos et al., Raven Press, New York © 1981.

Suppressor Macrophages: Their Induction, ·Characterization, and Regulation

*James A. Bennett, **John C. Marsh, and †Malcolm S. Mitchell

*The Departments of Surgery and Physiology, Albany Medical College, Albany, New York 12208; **The Departments of Medicine and Pharmacology, Yale University School of Medicine, New Haven, Connecticut 06510; †The Departments of Medicine and Microbiology, University of Southern California, Los Angeles, California 90033*

Macrophages are an essential component of the immune system. They comprise part of the framework within which lymphocytes recognize and respond to antigens (30,21). Immunologically programmed lymphocytes can in turn elicit the services of macrophages by releasing appropriate chemical stimuli (31,24). This is a tightly regulated mutually responsive interrelationship that enables the host to process, respond to, and eliminate foreign substances with exquisite specificity and minimal toxicity to the host. This interrelationship is for the most part controlled by the macrophages and lymphocytes themselves, and any breakdown in this control through either hyper- or hypo-activity on the part of either macrophages or lymphocytes can result in pathological consequences (20). One may be willing or forced to accept some of the toxicity of these pathological consequences in order to achieve a particular end result. For instance non specific stimulation of the lymphoreticular system with microbial preparations like Bacillus Calmette-Guerin (BCG) can result in the induction of inflammation and ulceration at the injection site (15,11), or in systemic problems such as hepatic dysfunction (27) but BCG usually primes the lymphoreticular system for increased immunological reactivity to subsequently administered antigens (19). However, the undesired end result of immunosuppression can occur when an excessive amount (12,32) of the microbial preparation is used or when its route (7) of administration or schedule (25,22) of administration in relation to the specific antigen is inappropriate. One idea that has been offered to explain the mechanism of this immunosuppression is the induction of a toxic environment resulting from the excessive activation of macrophages that is deleterious for the specific immunization of lymphocytes (1,13). In this context these macrophages have been described as suppressor macrophages. In this report the tissue distribution, phenotypic characteristics, and pharmacological regulation of suppressor cells that are induced by systemic administration of a large dose of BCG will be described. Parts of this report have been described in detail elsewhere (1,2,3).

MATERIALS AND METHODS

Animals

C57Bl/6 (H-2^b) female mice were obtained from Charles River Laborator-(Wilmington, Mass., U.S.A.). Experimental mice were 8-12 weeks old and weighed 19-23 grams.

BCG

Mycobacterium bovis, Tice substrain, was obtained as a freeze-dried product from the University of Illinois. Each ampule containing $5 \pm 3 \times 10^8$ viable units was reconstituted by adding 1.0 ml of sterile water immediately before use. Except for those experiments reported in Table 1, mice that received BCG were given 2×10^7 viable units intravenously.

Drugs

Indomethacin (Sigma, St. Louis, Mo.), generic aspirin, and salicylic acid were each dissolved in 70% ethanol at 10^{-2}M and further diluted in Hank's Balanced Salt Solution (BSS) (calcium and magnesium free). Ro3-1314 (a gift from Dr. W.E. Scott of Hoffmann, La Roche Inc., Nutley, N.J.) was dissolved in 10% NaHCO$_3$ at 10^{-3}M and diluted in BSS. Prostaglandin E$_1$ (PGE$_1$) (a gift from Dr. John Pike of the Upjohn Company, Kalamazoo, Mich.) was dissolved in 95% ethanol at 3×10^{-2}M and diluted in BSS.

Cell Separation Techniques

(a) Nylon Wool Column.
Fractionation of cells over nylon wool columns was performed as previously described (2). Adherent cells were freed from the nylon wool by agitation with forceps in cold phosphate buffered saline. With this procedure we routinely recovered approximately 75% of the total number of cells added to the columns.

(b) Treatment of Spleen Cells with Antisera.
Rabbit anti-mouse thymocyte serum was purchased from Microbiological Associates, Bethesda, Md. Rabbit anti-mouse immunoglobulin serum was raised by injecting mouse gamma globulin emulsified in complete Freund's adjuvant into rabbits and repeating the injections at 10 day intervals. After the third injection rabbits were bled and their serum was obtained. Anti Ly5.1 serum was kindly supplied by Dr. Harvey Cantor, Harvard Medical School.
Spleen cells at a final concentration of 10^7 cells/ml were added to antithymocyte serum (final dilution 1/15), antiimmunoglobulin serum (final dilution 1/8 in the presence of 0.2% sodium azide), or anti Ly5.1 serum (final dilution 1/20) and mixed slowly for 30 minutes at 4^0 C. Cells were centrifuged, then resuspended at a concentration of 10^7 cells/ml in rabbit complement (final dilution 1/15) and incubated at 37^0 C for another 30 minutes. Cells were again centrifuged, resuspended, and the number of trypan blue-excluding cells was adjusted to the desired concentration.

(c) Density Gradient Centrifugation.

Discontinuous density gradients were obtained by layering different concentrations of Ficoll-400 (Pharmacia, Piscataway, N.J.) into polycarbonate centrifuge tubes (34). In 4 ml aliquots, 25%, 21%, 16%, and 12% Ficoll were layered into the tubes. Spleen cells at a concentration of 2.5×10^7 cells/ml were contained in the 21% fraction. Cells were centrifuged at 20,000 g for 60 minures at 4^0 C. Four cell fractions were obtained, washed, and counted.

Immunization In Vitro

Spleen cells were immunized in vitro according to a modification of the procedure originally described by Mishell and Dutton (18). Briefly, 2×10^7 viable C57B1/6 spleen cells (H-2b) were cultured with 2×10^5 irradiated (4000r) P815 mastocytoma cells (H-2d) in 35 X 10 mm plastic dishes in a total volume of 1 ml.. The culture medium was RPMI supplemented with heat inactivated, dialyzed fetal calf serum (5%), glutamine (2mM), sodium pyruvate (1mM), 100X non-essential amino acids (1%), penicillin (100 units/ml), streptomycin (100 µg/ml), and 2 mercaptoethanol (5×10^{-5}M). Cultures were incubated for 4 days at 37^0 C in an atmosphere of 5% CO_2 in air, and were fed daily with 0.1 ml of RPMI 1640 medium supplemented as previously described (1). At the end of culture, cells were agitated with a rubber policeman, collected, washed and counted. After viability was assessed by trypan blue dye exclusion, cells were adjusted to appropriate concentrations in fresh culture medium.

Assays for Cell-Mediated Immunity (CMI)

CMI against.P815Y target cells was measured using both the 4hr ^{51}Cr release assay (5) and the 48hr growth inhibition assay (4). The percent ^{51}Cr released and the percent growth inhibition were calculated in the following ways:

1) % ^{51}Cr release= $\dfrac{\text{CPM in supernatant}}{\text{CPM in pellet + CPM in supernatant}}$ X 100%

2) % growth inhibition = (1 - T/N) X 100%

where T = number of target cells remaining in the presence of test lymphocytes and N = number of target cells remaining in the presence of normal lymphocytes. The values reported in this manuscript were obtained using an effector to target cell ratio of 100:1 for the ^{51}Cr release assay and 10:1 for the growth inhibition assay.

Suppressor Cells

The suppressive influence of cells in the spleen or bone marrow was determined by cocultivating 6×10^6 cells with 2×10^7 normal spleen cells being immunized against allogeneic P815Y cells in vitro. Unless otherwise indicated, cells from BCG treated mice were obtained 14 days after intravenous inoculation of .2 $\times 10^7$ viable units of BCG.

CFU Assay

Macrophage-granulocyte colony-forming units were measured by a modification (17) of the technique of Gordon (10). This method does not require an added source of colony-stimulating factor. Marrow or spleen cells were mixed with medium (Fischer's medium with 20% horse serum) and 0.3% molten Noble agar (Difco Laboratories, Detroit, Mich.). Bone marrow (1.5 to 5 X 10^4) or spleen cells (5 to 10 X 10^4) in a total volume of 0.35 ml were placed in a diffusion chamber (composed of a Lucite ring, a circular coverslip, and a 0.22-µm Millipore filter), and the orifice was sealed with paraffin. After the gelling of the agar, the chamber was implanted in the peritoneal cavity of a mouse under light ether anesthesia. Four chambers were used for each experimental point. At the end of 7 days, the chambers were removed, the Millipore filters were removed, and the colonies were counted under a dissecting microscope. Both small (8 to 50 cells) and large (>50 cells) colonies were counted. The mean ± S.E. of the colony numbers for each experimental point were calculated.

RESULTS

Effect of Dose and Schedule of BCG on the Development of Suppressor Cells

As shown in Table 1, an increase in weight of the spleen was found in mice that had received BCG intravenously eight days earlier. The increase was manifested in mice receiving 1 X 10^7 viable units of BCG and

TABLE 1. Effect of i.v. treatment of mice with BCG on the in vitro generation of an immune response by their spleen cells

No. of BCG Organisms	Spleen Wt. (grams)	% Specific ^{51}Cr Release	% Specific Growth Inhibition
Control	0.08 ± .01	65	80
1 X 10^6	0.07 ± .01	66	75
5 X 10^6	0.08 ± .01	63	76
1 X 10^7	0.19 ± .05	15	26
2 X 10^7	0.31 ± .04	5	0
5 X 10^7	(Lethal Dose)		

appeared to be proportional to the amount of BCG given up to the lethal dose, which was 5 X 10^7 viable units of BCG. When cell suspensions were prepared from these BCG-treated spleens, the ability of the cells to be immunized against alloantigens in vitro was markedly reduced. In fact, no significant CMI developed after attempts to immunize spleen cells from mice that had received 2 X 10^7 viable units of BCG as assayed by both ^{51}Cr release and growth inhibition assays. In mice receiving 2 X 10^7 BCG, splenomegaly was apparent at day 7 after treatment and continued to increase until day 14, at which point it reached its maximum but remained apparent 50 days after treatment (Table 2). When 2 X 10^7 normal spleen cells were immunized in the presence of 6 X 10^6 spleen cells from BCG-treated mice, the inhibitory activity in spleen from BCG-

TABLE 2. Effect of spleen cells from BCG-treated mice on the immunization of normal spleen cells against alloantigen in vitro

Days After BCG	Spleen Wt. (grams)	% Specific ^{51}Cr Release	% Specific Growth Inhibition
2	0.08 ± .01	64	88
5	0.07 ± .01	66	83
7	0.25 ± .05	45	60
11	0.41 ± .04	33	37
14	0.67 ± .05	29	25
16	0.73 ± .08	31	31
50	0.63 ± .06	40	36

C57Bl/6 mice were given 2 X 10^7 viable units of BCG intravenously. At
various times after treatment their spleens were excised, weighed, and
teased into single cell suspension. Six million of these spleen cells
were added to 2 X 10^7 normal C57Bl/6 spleen cells, and this mixture was
cultured for 4 days with 2 X 10^5 killed P815 cells. At the end of the
culture period the CMI of the sensitized spleen cells was determined
using an effector to target cell ratio of 100:1 in the ^{51}Cr release
assay and 10:1 in the growth inhibition assay.

treated mice increased as splenomegaly developed.

In data not shown 2 X 10^5 BCG organisms were identified among
6 X 10^6 spleen cells obtained from BCG-treated mice. However, the
organism itself played no direct role in suppression, since addition
of 2 X 10^5 organisms to 2 X 10^7 normal spleen cells did not affect the
ability of these cells to be immunized in vitro.

BCG also had a marked influence on the number of cells in the bone
marrow and thymus (Figure 1). Within 2 days after the administration of
BCG, there was a 40% decrease in the number of bone marrow cells and a
90% decrease in the number of thymus cells. The decrease in bone marrow cells persisted and was still apparent 16 days after BCG, whereas
in the thymus a gradual recovery in cellularity began 5 days after BCG,
but cellularity did not return to normal levels until 16 days after BCG.
In contrast, in the spleen there was no reduction in the number of cells
as a result of BCG administration. Rather, a 2-fold, 3-fold, and 6-fold
increase in spleen cell number was found respectively on days 7, 11 and
16 after BCG.

The suppressive influence of cells in the spleen, bone marrow, or
thymus was determined by adding them to cultures of normal spleen and
immunizing this mixture against P815. As shown in Table 3, significant
suppression of CMI occurred as a result of adding 6 X 10^6 normal syngeneic bone marrow cells to splenic lymphocytes before immunization in
vitro. No suppression resulted from the addition of normal spleen or
normal thymus cells. Treatment of mice with BCG markedly enhanced the
suppressive activity in bone marrow and induced suppressive activity in
spleen. Enhanced suppression by bone marrow cells occurred two days
after administration of BCG, and this enhancement was still apparent 14
days later. However in spleen, suppression was not apparent until 7
days after BCG, and was further increased 11 and 16 days after BCG.

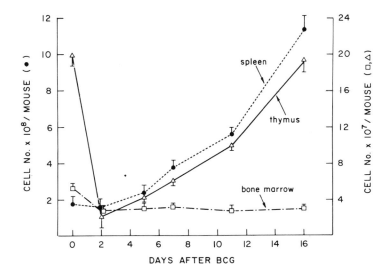

FIG. 1. The effect of BCG on the number of cells in mouse spleen, bone marrow, and thymus.

TABLE 3. Effect of spleen, bone marrow, and thymus cells from BCG-
          treated mice on the immunization of normal spleen cells
                      against alloantigen in vitro

Days After BCG	% Specific ^{51}Cr Release with sensitized spleen cells immunized in presence of:			% Growth Inhibition with sensitized spleen cells immunized in presence of:		
	Spleen	Bone Marrow	Thymus	Spleen	Bone Marrow	Thymus
No BCG	66	38	62	82	45	74
2	64	9	66	88	10	70
7	45	5	59	60	8	79
11	33	7	67	37	19	85
16	31	3	64	31	12	80

Unlike bone marrow and spleen, thymus cells from BCG treated mice did not suppress the immunization of normal spleen cells.

Identification of the BCG-Induced Suppressor Cell by Nylon Wool Fractionation

When nylon wool nonadherent and adherent spleen cells from normal mice were mixed in various proportions and then immunized in vitro, optimal immunization developed when 80% adherent cells were mixed with 20% nonadherent cells. This was apparent in the CMI produced by T cells as well as that produced by T and non T cells as measured by the ^{51}Cr

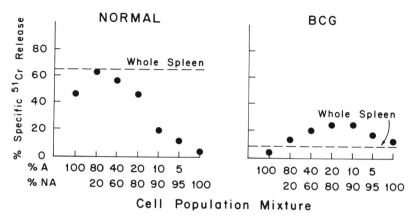

FIG. 2. The effect of BCG treatment on the subsequent immunization of mouse spleen cell populations in culture. Suppressor cells were obtained approximately 2 weeks after treatment of mice with BCG in this figure and in all subsequent figures and tables, except figure 4.

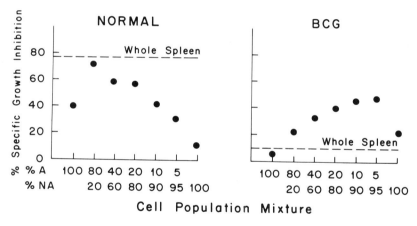

FIG. 3. The effect of BCG treatment on the subsequent immunization of mouse spleen cell populations in culture.

release and growth inhibition assays respectively (Figs. 2 and 3). The degree of immunity developed was similar at this ratio to that obtained with unfractionated spleen cells, which contain approximately 70% adherent and 30% nonadherent cells. As the percent of adherent cells was decreased, the level of immunity which was generated also diminished. Exactly the opposite pattern was found with spleen cells from BCG-treated mice; that is, a predominance of nonadherent over adherent cells in the mixture improved the development of an immune response. However, the response never recovered to the level found after immunization of normal whole spleen, as long as both the adherent and nonadherent spleen cells were derived from BCG-treated animals.

TABLE 4. In vitro immunization of mixtures of nylon wool fractionated
Spleen cells from normal and BCG-treated mice

Cell Population(s)	% Specific ^{51}Cr Release	% Specific Growth Inhibition
Normal Whole	69	83
BCG Whole	4	0
Norm N.A. + Norm A.	62	80
Norm N.A. + BCG A.	9	12
BCG N.A. + BCG A.	5	0
BCG N.A. + Norm A.	54	70

When adherent and non-adherent cells from normal and BCG mice were
mixed in the 70%:30% proportion found in normal spleen and then immunized, dramatic suppression in the development of CMI occurred when adherent cells from BCG mice were mixed with nonadherent cells from normal
mice (Table 4). In contrast, no deficit in the ability to be immunized
was noted when nonadherent cells from BCG mice were mixed with adherent
cells from normal mice. Thus, suppressor cell activity was concentrated
in the adherent fraction of spleen from BCG-treated mice. However, it
should be mentioned here that suppressor cell activity was limited to
the process of sensitization, for addition of adherent spleen cells from
BCG mice to already sensitized effector cells did not affect the expression of CMI (data not shown).

Investigation of the Involvement of T Cells in Suppression

Suppression of the immunization of normal spleen cells by adherent
spleen cells from BCG mice was proportional to the number of the suppressor adherent cells added to the mixture (Table 5). Pretreatment of
the adherent cells with anti T cell serum and complement killed 23% of
the cells but did not reduce their suppressive activity (Table 5).
Although these data indicated that the suppressor cells were not T cells,
it was possible that T cells were required for the development of suppressor activity. To test this point, mice that had been thymectomized,
irradiated and protected with syngeneic bone marrow ("B" mice) were
treated with BCG. It is apparent from Table 6 that admixture of adherent
spleen cells from these mice significantly inhibited the immunization of
normal lymphocytes. It should be pointed out, however, that the suppressor cells in "B" mice did not develop until 10 days after treatment with
BCG, whereas in normal mice suppressive activity was detected 7 days
after treatment with BCG. Interestingly, splenic suppressor cells were
evident in the bone marrow-repopulated "B" mice that were not treated
with BCG, but only when 10 million of these cells were added to the 20
million normal spleen cells being immunized against alloantigen. There
was no evidence of suppressor cells in an equivalent number of cells
from the spleen of normal mice.

TABLE 5. The effect of rabbit anti mouse T cell serum treatment of
nylon wool adherent spleen cells from BCG mice on their ability
to suppress the in vitro immunization of normal spleen cells

Additional Adherent Cells	% Specific ^{51}Cr Release	% Specific Growth Inhibition
None	60	80
Normal Spleen (6×10^6)	61	78
BCG Spleen (2×10^6)	50	43
BCG Spleen (6×10^6)	28	14
BCG Spleen + Anti T + C[1] (2×10^6)	48	38
BCG Spleen + Anti T + C[1] (6×10^6)	24	11

TABLE 6. Effect of nylon wool adherent spleen cells from untreated or
BCG-treated "B" mice on the in vitro immunization of spleen
cells from normal mice against alloantigen

Additional Adherent Cells	% Specific ^{51}Cr Release	% Specific Growth Inhibition
None	64	84
Normal Spleen (1×10^7)	63	80
"B" Spleen (6×10^6)	67	78
"B" Spleen (1×10^7)	51	60
BCG "B" Spleen (6×10^6)	15	30
BCG "B" Spleen (1×10^7)	7	0

Activity of BCG-Induced Suppressor Cells
Following Treatment with Anti Mouse Immunoglobulin Serum Plus Complement

Pretreatment of adherent spleen cells from BCG mice with anti-mouse
Ig serum and complement reduced the viability of that population from
85% to 67% but did not diminish its capacity to inhibit the immunization
of normal spleen cells (Table 7).

Activity of BCG-Induced Splenic Suppressor Cells
Following Treatment with Anti Ly5.1 Serum Plus Complement

Glimcher et al. (9) had shown that natural killer cell activity in the
spleen of C57Bl/6 mice could be eliminated by treatment with anti Ly 5.1
serum plus complement. Pretreatment of spleen cells from C57Bl/6 mice
that had received i.v. BCG with anti Ly 5.1 serum plus complement killed
15% of the cells but did not diminish the capacity of the remaining cells
to inhibit the immunization of normal splenic lymphocytes in vitro
(Table 8).

TABLE 7. The effect of anti Ig serum treatment of nylon wool adherent
          spleen cells from BCG mice on their ability to suppress the
          in vitro immunization of normal spleen cells

Additional Adherent Cells	% Specific [51]Cr Release	% Specific Growth Inhibition
None	61	81
Normal Spleen	60	82
BCG Spleen	29	36
BCG Spleen + Anti Ig	31	29
BCG Spleen + Anti Ig + C[1]	28	33

Further Separation of Suppressor Activity in Adherent Spleen Cells from BCG Mice by Centrifugation through a Discontinuous Ficoll Density Gradient

Four cell fractions were obtained following density gradient centrifugation of adherent spleen cells. The two lighter fractions found near
the top of the gradient had very few cells in each fraction and thus
were pooled. When this pooled population was stained with Wright's
stain and examined microscopically, 17% of the population were of the
monocyte-macrophage lineage, 50% were lymphocytes, 18% were nucleated
red blood cells and 13% were cells in mitosis. The third fraction from
the top of the gradient consisted of 22% monocyte-macrophages, but these
were smaller than those found in the pooled "light" fractions, 67%
lymphocytes, 6% nucleated red blood cells, and 3% were mitotic figures.
The fourth fraction which was the cell pellet contained 11% monocyte-
macrophages, 74% lymphocytes, 10% nucleated red blood cells, and no
mitotic figures. The effects of these fractions on the immunization of
normal spleen cells are shown in Table 9. Suppressor activity was found
in all the cell fractions, but was greatest in the "medium", slightly
less in the "dense", and least in the "light" fraction.

TABLE 8. The effect of treating spleen cells from BCG mice with anti
          Ly 5.1 serum plus complement on their ability to suppress
          the in vitro immunization of normal spleen cells

Additional Cells	% Specific [51]Cr Release
None	65
Normal Spleen	62
BCG Spleen	40
BCG Spleen + C[1]	38
BCG Spleen + Anti Ly 5.1 + C[1]	43

TABLE 9. Effect of nylon wool adherent spleen cells of various densities from BCG mice on the in vitro immunization of normal spleen cells

Additional Adherent Cells	% Specific ^{51}Cr Release	% Specific Growth Inhibition
None	65	79
BCG Spleen	32	20
BCG Spleen "Light"	53	47
BCG Spleen "Medium"	34	22
BCG Spleen "Dense"	40	30

Relationship of BCG-Induced Suppressor Cells to Granulocyte-Macrophage Colony Forming Unit Cells (CFU)

The relationship of these suppressor cells to CFU was investigated by comparing CFU concentration and suppressor cell activity in marrow and spleen of normal and BCG-treated mice. Typical values of CFU and suppressor cell activity are shown in Table 10.

TABLE 10. CFU concentration and suppressor cell activity in bone marrow and spleen of normal and BCG-treated mice

MARROW

	CFU/10^4 cells	Cells/leg	CFU/leg	% Specific ^{51}Cr Release	% Suppression of Immunization
Normal	44.5 ± 5.9	37.2 x 10^6	16.6 x 10^4	38	42
BCG	83.5 ± 12.2	15.8 x 10^6	13.5 x 10^4	4	94

SPLEEN

	CFU/10^4 cells	Cells/Spleen	CFU/Spleen	% Specific ^{51}Cr Release	% Suppression of Immunization
Normal	3.2 ± 1.5	226.5 x 10^6	7.2 x 10^4	66	0
BCG	47.1 ± 6.9	602.5 x 10^6	283.9 x 10^4	33	49

The kinetics of the changes induced by BCG are shown in Figure 4. The data are expressed as % of control because the CFU in a given number of normal bone marrow or spleen cells as determined by their growth in agar varied from experiment to experiment. A 40% increase in marrow CFU concentration occurred as early as 2 days after treatment with BCG, and further increases in this activity were apparent by day 13. Similarly a 40% increase in marrow suppressor cell activity also occurred 2 days after BCG. Further increases in this activity were seen on days 7 and 13, but these were not significant. No significant increase in splenic CFU concentration was apparent until 7 days after BCG, and an enormous increase occurred between days 7 and 13. Similarly, BCG induced no

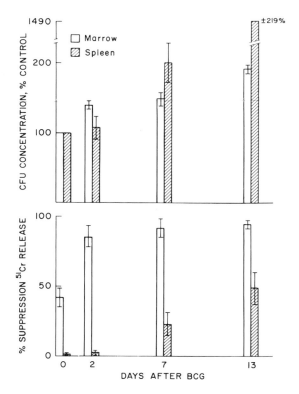

FIG. 4 Changes in CFU concentration and suppressor cell activity in bone marrow and spleen after treatment of mice with BCG.

splenic suppressor cell activity until day 7, and by day 13 a further large increase was observed. Both CFU concentration and suppressor cell activity were measured at additional time points out to Day 25, and these values were not significantly different from those found on Day 13.

Spleen cell suspensions from BCG-treated mice were fractionated by various procedures in an attempt to compare CFU's and suppressor activity in the resulting fractions. In the adherent population of nylon wool separated spleen cells there was a four-fold increase in CFU concentration compared to the non-adherent fraction (Table 11). Likewise, there was 3 times more suppressor activity in the adherent spleen cell fraction from BCG treated mice than in the non-adherent fraction.

TABLE 11. Nylon wool fractionation of post BCG spleen

	CFU/5x10⁴ Cells	% Suppression of Immunization
Unfractionated	42.0 ± 15.0	49 ± 2
Non-adherent	9.8 ± 3.0	17 ± 4
Adherent	41.0 ± 10.0	52 ± 2

TABLE 12. Density gradient centrifugation of post BCG spleen

	CFU/2.5x10^4 Cells	% Suppression of Immunization
Unfractionated	38.3 ± 4.8	51
Light fraction	5.5 ± 0.5	8
Medium fraction	31.8 ± 4.8	52
Heavy fraction	34.5 ± 6.8	63

Following centrifugation of cells through discontinuous density gradients, the light fraction contained little CFU or suppressor activity (Table 12). On the other hand the medium and heavy fractions had approximately 6 to 7 times more CFU and suppressor activity than the light fraction (Table 12). Thus by several experimental criteria, there were quantitative kinetic, and qualitative parallels in the biological response of CFU and suppressor cells to Tice BCG.

Prostaglandins and BCG-Induced Suppressor Cells

Indomethacin, salicylate, aspirin, or the experimental drug Ro3-1314 added at the initiation of coculture of BCG-induced splenic suppressor cells and normal lymphocytes almost completely blocked the inhibition of alloimmunization produced by these suppressor cells (Table 13). All of the above drugs inhibit prostaglandin synthesis, and the compound Ro3-1314 has this as its only known site of action. Indomethacin appeared to be the most active drug among the group that was tested and was thus selected for further study.

TABLE 13. Effect of different inhibitors of prostaglandin synthesis on the suppression of normal spleen cell immunization by BCG-induced splenic suppressor cells

Immunization of:	% Specific ^{51}Cr Release	% Suppression of Immunization
Normal spleen	66	-
Normal Spleen + BCG Spleen	35	47
Normal Spleen + BCG Spleen:		
+ 10^{-5}M Indomethacin	64	3
+ 10^{-5}M Salicylate	53	20
+ 10^{-5}M Aspirin	56	15
+ 10^{-5}M Ro3-1314	50	24

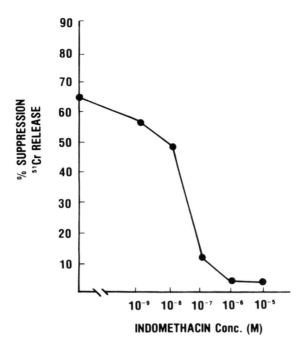

FIG. 5. Effect of different concentrations of indomethacin on the
suppression of normal spleen cell immunization by BCG-induced splenic
suppressor cells.

As shown in Figure 5, indomethacin, at concentrations of 10^{-5}M to
10^{-7}M, was active in blocking the inhibitory activity of BCG-induced
splenic suppressor cells. Indomethacin was not active at concentrations
lower than 10^{-7}M (Fig. 5), and at concentrations higher than 10^{-5}M
indomethacin was found to be immunosuppressive by itself (data not
shown). Addition of equivalent amounts of the indomethacin diluent had
no effect on the immunization of normal spleen cells or on the activity
of suppressor cells (data not shown). Also indomethacin did not poten-
tiate the immunization of normal spleen cells cultured in the absence
of suppressor cells (data not shown).

As described earlier, the inhibitory activity of BCG-induced splenic
suppressor cells resided primarily in the adherent portion of nylon
wool fractionated spleen cells. Indomethacin was as effective in blocking suppressor cell activity in this adherent fraction of cells as it
was in blocking suppressor cell activity generated by unfractionated
spleen cells (Fig. 6).

Bone marrow cells were also investigated for the presence of suppressor cells sensitive to indomethacin. 10^{-6}M indomethacin only partially
blocked the suppressor activity generated by marrow from either normal
or BCG-treated mice (Fig. 7). Concentrations of indomethacin one log
higher or lower than 10^{-6}M were not effective in blocking this activity.
This was quite unlike the suppressor cell population in the spleen that
was highly sensitive to indomethacin. When marrow from BCG-treated mice

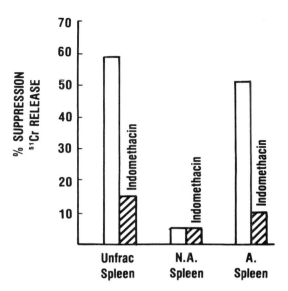

FIG. 6. Effect of indomethacin on the suppression of normal spleen cell immunization by unfractionated, non-adherent (N.A.) and adherent (A.) spleen cells from BCG-treated mice.

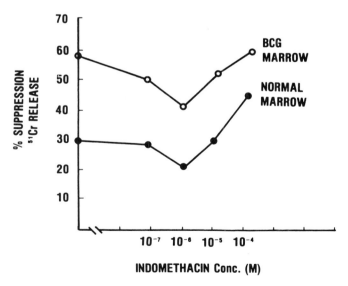

FIG. 7. Effect of different concentrations of indomethacin on the suppression of normal spleen cell immunization by normal bone marrow or by bone marrow from BCG-treated mice.

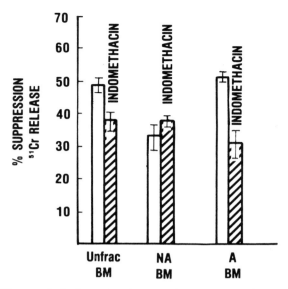

FIG. 8. Effect of indomethacin on the suppression of normal spleen
cell immunization by unfractionated, N.A., and A. bone marrow from
BCG-treated mice.

was fractionated over nylon wool, suppressor cell activity was found in
both the adherent and non-adherent populations. Suppression by the adherent population was partially blocked by indomethacin whereas that in
the non-adherent population was completely insensitive to indomethacin
(Fig. 8).

DISCUSSION

The above results indicate that systemic administration of Tice BCG
induced hematological changes that resulted in the production of suppressor cells. BCG induced a rapid and persistent decrease in bone
marrow cellularity and a gradual increase in spleen cellularity. This
paralleled a rapid and persistent activation of existing suppressor
cells in the bone marrow and a gradual development of suppressor cells
in the spleen. This pattern coupled with the fact that suppressor
cells were found in the spleen of bone marrow-reconstituted mice suggested that splenic suppressor cells stemmed from natural suppressor
cells in the bone marrow that were activated by BCG to emigrate from
the marrow and colonize the spleen.

Treatment with BCG has been shown to increase the number and or
activity of T cells (16,6), B cells (28,29), natural killer cells (33)
and macrophages (8,23). In the present study there was an increase in
the number of all of these cell types in the spleen of BCG-treated mice
(3). Incubation of these spleen cells with antisera specific for T
cells, B cells, or natural killer cells followed by complement mediated
lysis of these cell types did not reduce suppressor cell activity.
However, increases in suppressor cell activity coincided with increases

in the concentration of granulocyte-macrophage progenitor cells (CFU), and these two activities were inseparable following fractionation of cells into several subpopulations. It thus seems reasonable to deduce that the BCG-induced splenic suppressor cells were immature macrophages.

Kurland et al. (14) have shown that macrophage development is controlled by the feedback of mediators secreted by the mature macrophage end product; that is, mature macrophages release colony stimulating factor and prostaglandins which respectively stimulate and inhibit the proliferation of macrophage progenitor cells. The results of the present study support this control mechanism. We found a very significant increase in the proliferation of macrophage progenitor cells following systemic administration of BCG. This increase was most likely mediated by CSF released from BCG stimulated macrophages. That BCG can stimulate the production of CSF has been shown by the studies of Singer et al. (26). There is also evidence in our study that in response to BCG, macrophages increased their production of prostaglandins. This is suggested by the block of splenic suppressor cell activity by indomethacin. According to the hypothesis put forth by Kurland et al. (14), the increased production of prostaglandins is meant to control the proliferation of macrophage progenitors. However in our study it appears that an additional effect of increased prostaglandin levels is the inhibition of lymphocyte proliferation. In fact the increased production of prostaglandins inhibited lymphocytes more than macrophage progenitors since the proliferation of macrophage progenitors occurred within the same cell population that completely inhibited the alloantigen induced proliferation and immunization of T lymphocytes. The immunization of these lymphocytes was inhibited by other mediators as well since suppressor cell populations insensitive to indomethacin were found in the bone marrow.

In summary, in our study the activation and production of macrophages by BCG created an environment that inhibited the specific immunization of T lymphocytes. At first glance such an effect would appear to be self defeating since functional macrophages and lymphocytes are both required for an intact immune system. However, this may simply be an exaggeration of the normal control mechanisms regulating the activities of lymphocytes. Such a regulation may be essential for self preservation, preventing the development of T cell mediated autoimmunity within tissues where there is active production or concentration of macrophages reacting against foreign cells.

REFERENCES

1. Bennett, J.A., Rao, S.V., and Mitchell, M.S. (1978): Proc. Natl. Acad. Sci., 75:5142-5144.
2. Bennett, J.A., and Marsh, J.C. (1980): Cancer Res.,40:80-85.
3. Bennett, J.A., and Mitchell, M.S. (1980): In: Neoplasm Immunity: Experimental and Clinical, edited by R.G. Crispen, pp. 397-412. Elsevier/North Holland, New York.
4. Brunner, K.T., Mauel, J., and Schindler, R. (1966): Immunol., 11: 499-506.
5. Brunner, K.T., Mauel, J., Cerottini, J.C., and Chaupis, B. (1968): Immunol., 14:181-196.
6. Davies, M., and Sabbadini, E. (1978): J. Natl. Cancer Inst. 60: 1059-1073.

7. Doft, B.H., Merchant, B., Johannessen, L., Chaparas, S.D., and Sher, N.A. (1976): J. Immunol., 117:1638-1643.
8. Fisher, B., Taylor, S., Levine, M., Saffer, E., and Fisher, E.R. (1974): Cancer Res., 34:1668-1670.
9. Glimcher, L., Shen, F.W. and Cantor, H. (1977): J. Exp. Med., 145: 1-9.
10. Gordon, M.Y. (1974): Br. J. Cancer, 30:421-428.
11. Hanna, M.G., and Bucana, C. (1981): Cancer Res., in press.
12. Kaledin, V.I., Kurunov, Y.N., Matienko, N.A., and Nikolin, V.P. (1978): J. Natl. Cancer Inst., 61:1393-1396.
13. Klimpel, G.R. and Henney, C.S. (1978): J. Immunol., 120:563-569.
14. Kurland, J., and Moore, M.A.S. (1977): Exp. Hemat., 5:357-373.
15. Mackaness, G.B., Auclair, D.J., and LaGrange, P.H. (1973): J. Natl. Cancer Inst., 51:1669-1676.
16. Mackaness, G.B., LaGrange, P.H., and Ishibashi, T. (1974): J. Exp. Med., 139:1540-1552.
17. Marsh, J.C. (1979): Cancer Res., 39:360-364.
18. Mishell, R.I., and Dutton, R.W. (1967): J. Exp. Med., 126:423-442.
19. Mitchell, M.S., and Murahata, R.I. (1979): Pharmac. Ther. 4:329-353.
20. Oehler, J.R., Herberman, R.B., and Holden, H.T. (1978): Pharmac. Ther., 2:551-593.
21. Oppenheim, J.J., and Seeger, R.C. (1976): In: Immunobiology of the Macrophage, edited by D.S. Nelson, pp. 111-130. Academic Press, New York.
22. Peters, L.C., Hanna, M.G., Gutterman, J.V., Mavligit, G.M., and Hersh, E.M. (1974): Proc. Soc. Exp. Biol. Med., 147:344-349.
23. Poplack, D.G., Sher, N.A., Chaparas, S.D., and Blaese, R.M. (1976): Cancer Res., 36:1233-1237.
24. Rocklin, R.E., Bendtzen, K., and Greineder, D. (1980): Adv. Immunol. 29:55-136.
25. Schaedler, R.W., and Dubos, R.J. (1957): J. Exp. Med., 106:719-726.
26. Singer, J.W., and Bernstein, I.D. (1978): Exp. Hemat., 6:760-766.
27. Sparks, F.C., Silverstein, M.J., Hunt, J.S., Haskell, C.M., Pilch, Y.H., and Morton, D.L. (1973): New Eng. J. Med., 289:827-830.
28. Stjernsward, J. (1966): Cancer Res., 26:1591-1594.
29. Sultzer, B.M. (1978): J. Immunol. 120:254-261.
30. Unanue, E.R. (1972): Adv. Immunol. 15:95-157.
31. Waksman, B.H. (1978): Pharmac. Ther., 2:623-672.
32. Wile, A.G., and Sparks, F.C. (1977): Cancer 39:570-574.
33. Wolfe, S.A., Tracey, D.E., and Henney, C.S. (1976): Nature 262: 584-586.
34. Zembala, M., and Asherson, G.L. (1970): Immunol. 19:677-682.

Mediation of Cellular Immunity in Cancer by Immune Modifiers, edited by M. A. Chirigos et al., Raven Press, New York © 1981.

Activated Macrophage-Induced Modification of Transformed Cell Energy Metabolism: Identification of Lytic and Nonlytic Phenotypic Responses to Inhibition of Mitochondrial Respiration

John B. Hibbs, Jr., Donald L. Granger, James L. Cook, and *Andrew M. Lewis, Jr.

*Veterans Administration Medical Center and Department of Medicine, Division of Infectious Diseases, University of Utah Medical Center, Salt Lake City, Utah 84148; *National Institute of Allergy and Infectious Diseases, National Institutes of Health, Bethesda, Maryland 20205*

INTRODUCTION

Mouse peritoneal macrophages activated in vivo by chronic infection with Toxoplasma gondii or Bacillus Calmette-Guerin (BCG), or in vitro by lymphokines or endotoxin are capable of destroying target cells with abnormal growth properties by a nonphagocytic mechanism requiring direct contact (16,17,18,23,24). This cytotoxic reaction is based on a system of non-immunologic discrimination at the effector level; in this reaction activated macrophages have little or no cytolytic activity for target cells with normal growth characteristics and normal macrophages are not cytotoxic. In early studies, mouse embryo fibroblasts were used as target cells before and after spontaneous transformation in vitro. The phenomenon of spontaneous transformation in vitro is not well understood and suggests an inherent instability of the nontransformed cell phenotype. The ease of establishment of a spontaneously transformed cell line appears to be species dependent; establishment of a spontaneously transformed cell line from a human cell strain rarely if ever occurs (12); while, in practically all cases, murine cell strains develop spontaneously into transformed cell lines within three months of culture (30). The acquisition of unlimited capacity for in vitro proliferation distinguishes the spontaneous transformated cell lines from non-transformed cells. Spontaneously transformed cell lines, when cultured under conditions of extensive cell-to-cell contact, also acquire other abnormal growth properties that include loss of contact inhibition of cell proliferation as well as tumorigenic potential for syngeneic newborns and immunosuppressed

27

syngeneic adults (1).

Newly established transformed lines of mouse fibroblasts react differently than untransformed mouse fibroblasts when cocultivated with monolayers of cytotoxic activated macrophages (17). Activated macrophages did not destroy two allogeneic fibroblast cell strains differing from them at a strongly antigenic H-2 locus. In contrast, these macrophages were markedly cytolytic for the same allogeneic fibroblasts (and also for syngeneic fibroblasts) after the fibroblasts had spontaneously developed abnormal growth properties that included unlimited capacity to divide in vitro and loss of contact inhibition of cell division. Because H-2 antigens are more immunogenic than tumor-specific transplantation antigens or fetal antigens expressed on tumor cells, this study strongly suggested that changes associated with spontaneous in vitro transformation and the acquisition of abnormal growth properties by target cells, rather than a change in antigens, is responsible for their susceptibility to destruction by activated macrophages. These experiments showed that cells at incipient stages of neoplastic development were killed by contact with activated macrophages under conditions in which untransformed fibroblasts were not lysed.

These studies also showed that mouse or human fibroblasts transformed in vitro by simian virus 40 (SV40) or neoplastic cells that had developed spontaneously in vivo had the same marked susceptibility to the activated macrophage cytotoxic effect as fibroblasts that had spontaneously transformed during in vitro culture (13,14). As a result, we began to seriously consider the possibility that activated macrophages may have a homeostatic role in destroying cells that develop "abnormal growth" properties in vivo (14,17). Growth characteristics rather than the antigenic composition of the target cell seemed to determine whether or not the target cell was susceptible to cytotoxicity mediated by activated macrophages. Therefore, undefined factors related to normal and abnormal cell growth and the in vitro correlates of normal and abnormal cell growth, became important to further understanding of the activated macrophage cytotoxic reaction. These experiments elucidated a component of the transformed phenotype that had not been previously recognized. The key insight was that in addition to the abnormal growth properties that appear in parallel with in vivo or in vitro transformation (some of which are mentioned above), transformed cells also acquire a phenotypic susceptibility to activated macrophage induced cytotoxicity.

It subsequently became clear that not all transformed cells respond to activated macrophage induced cytotoxicity by undergoing cytolysis (6,9,19). This is the case, even though transformed cells appear to be uniformly susceptible to activated macrophage induced cytotoxic effect as measured by cytostasis. An example of the nonlytic phenotype is the murine L_{1210} leukemia. In addition, L_{1210} cells are highly tumorigenic. Grafts of less than 10 L_{1210} cells uniformly cause progressive tumor growth in syngeneic mice (28). L_{1210} cell growth in vivo is also relatively refractory to measures utilized to enhance host nonspecific resistance to tumor growth (15). This was shown in experiments that demonstrated that mice with chronic Toxoplasma gondii infection, and a persistent population of activated macrophages in the peritoneal cavity, have increased nonspecific resistance to some tumors but are nearly as susceptible to grafts of L1210 cells as are uninfected control mice that don't have a persistant population of activated macrophages in the peritoneal cavity or express increased nonspecific resistance to tumor growth. Since the cytotoxic response of L1210 cells to activated macrophages, cytostasis not progressing to cytolysis, represented a possible in vitro correlate for the high in vivo virulence of L1210 cells, it was of interest to examine biochemical changes that occur in transformed cell targets of activated macrophages.

CELLULAR ENERGY PRODUCTION IN THE ABSENCE AND PRESENCE OF OXYGEN

The results of these biochemical experiments demonstrate that activated macrophages cause a perturbation of energy metabolism in the transformed cells studied (9). The efficiency of cellular energy metabolism depends on whether or not oxygen is used as the terminal electron acceptor (20). Maximal energy yields from oxidizable organic substrates, including glucose, are realized only when oxygen is the terminal electron acceptor. When oxygen is not available as the terminal electron acceptor, all ATP required to maintain cellular metabolism must be produced by the relatively inefficient glycolytic pathway which anaerobically mobilizes the free energy intrinsic to the chemical bonds of glucose. Under anaerobic conditions, glucose or sugars that can be readily converted to glucose, must be present in the environment or glycolysis ceases and cell death ensues. Glycolysis can operate anaerobically because the pyruvate produced by the pathway can be reduced to lactate. The production of lactate is coupled to oxidation of the coenzyme nicotinamide adenine dinucleotide which allows the overall glycolytic process to continue in the absence of oxygen utilization.

However, when oxygen is present and can be utilized as an electron acceptor, the glycolytic breakdown of glucose, which occurs in the cytoplasm, is merely a preparatory step for further catabolism of pyruvate to CO_2 and H_2O. This occurs in the mitochondrial compartment by the combined activities of the tricarboxylic acid cycle and the electron transport chain. These two mitochondrial pathways couple the complete aerobic oxidation of glucose to the phosphorylation of ADP to ATP. The efficient utilization of the free energy intrinsic to the glucose molecule via aerobic glycolysis and mitochondrial oxidative phosphorylation (respiration) produces 36 moles ATP/mole glucose while the relatively inefficient production of ATP via anaerobic glycolysis yields only two moles ATP/mole glucose.

SUMMARY OF EXPERIMENTS THAT DEMONSTRATE PERTURBATION OF ENERGY HOMEOSTASIS IN L1210 LEUKEMIA CELLS AND OTHER TRANSFORMED CELLS INJURED BY CYTOTOXIC ACTIVATED MACROPHAGES

L1210 cells do not adhere to substrate when they are grown in vitro, and this property was exploited in studies designed to examine metabolic perturbations that occur in transformed cells after a period of contact with activated macrophages. Because L1210 cells are in contact with but not strongly adherent to macrophage monolayers, they can be removed from the macrophage monolayer after a period of cocultivation by gentle washing. They can then be washed, resuspended in fresh culture medium, and added to another tissue culture chamber for a second incubation. At this time, and free from the cytotoxic activated macrophage effector cells, biochemical changes that occur as a result of contact with activated macrophages can be measured.

Figure 1A shows that activated macrophage induced cytotoxicity causes prolonged stasis of L1210 cells that have been removed from activated macrophages and resuspended in fresh culture medium. The

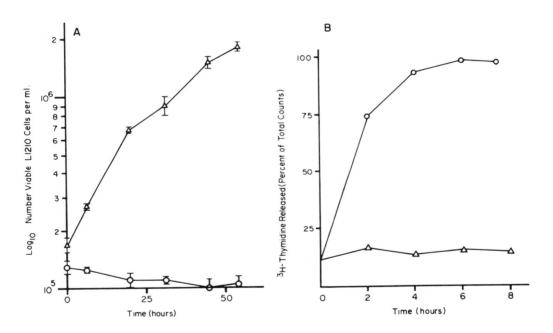

Figure 1A: Cytotoxic activated macrophage (CM) induced L1210 cell stasis is not reversed by removing target cells from macrophages and adding fresh culture medium. L1210 cells which had been incubated with CM for 40 h were removed, washed and reincubated for an additional 50 h (o). (Δ), uninjured L1210 cells. One-half the medium volume (0.5 ml) was replaced with fresh medium containing 10 mM glucose with 10% human serum each day. Each point is the mean ± SEM of triplicate cell counts. Figure 1B: CM injured L1210 cells require glucose to remain viable. Cytotoxic activated macrophage-injured L1210 cells incubated with culture medium minus glucose (o) or culture medium containing 10 mM glucose (Δ). See reference 9 for experimental details.

(Adapted from reference 9 with permission of the publisher.)

L1210 cells that had been cocultivated with cytotoxic activated macrophages failed to divide for an additional 50 hours despite removal from the cytotoxic activated macrophages and addition of fresh growth factors. Therefore, cytotoxic activated macrophage induced inhibition of L1210 cell proliferation persists for many hours beyond the time of removal from contact with cytotoxic activated macrophages. Although replication is suppressed, L1210 cells maintain almost complete viability for at least 90 hours as assessed by trypan blue exclusion (9).

When the cocultivation period of the cytotoxicity assay was extended and the culture medium was not supplemented with fresh nutrients, almost complete lysis of L1210 cells cultured with cytotoxic activated macrophages occurred between 72 and 96 hours. There was no detectable glucose in the medium on day four when L1210 cells died. Increasing the glucose concentration in the culture medium from 15.5 to 40 mM completely prevented L1210 cell death on day four. The interpretation was that L1210 cells and cytotoxic activated macrophages exhausted the supply of glucose during the four day culture period and this resulted in lysis of the L1210 cells. To examine these findings further, L1210 cells were incubated with cytotoxic activated macrophages for 24 hours with a nonlimiting glucose supply (20 mM under conditions of the assay). After the first incubation, L1210 cells were removed from cytotoxic activated macrophages and reincubated in the absence of macrophages (second incubation) in a culture medium lacking glucose but to which glucose or other substrate molecules could be added. Cytotoxic activated macrophage injured L1210 cells died within six hours when glucose was omitted from the culture medium of the second incubation (Figure 1B). As little as 0.25 mM glucose prevented lysis for six hours. Of numerous saccharides tested, only the sugars capable of supporting glycolysis, D-glucose (5 or 50 mM), D-mannose (5 or 50 mM), and fructose (50 mM) prevented lysis of cytotoxic activated macrophage injured L1210 cells during the second incubation period. If glycolysis was inhibited by 2-deoxy-D- glucose (20 mM inhibitor; 2 mM substrate), cytotoxic activated macrophage injured L1210 cells died in the presence of glucose or mannose (Table 1). Substrates for mitochondrial oxidative phosphorylation, pyruvate and glycerol (up to 50 mM each), did not prevent lysis of cytotoxic activated macrophage injured L1210 cells. Control L1210 cells maintain viability in culture medium without glucose or with 2-deoxy-D-glucose. Thus, cytotoxic activated macrophage injured L1210 cells require a sugar capable of maintaining glycolysis to remain viable.

Dependence on glycolysis for energy production could occur if cytotoxic activated macrophages interfered with mitochondrial oxidative phosphorylation. This was tested by measuring oxygen consumption of L1210 cells removed from cytotoxic activated macrophages after a 24-40 hour period of cocultivation (Table 2). Endogenous respiration of cytotoxic activated macrophage injured L1210 cells was consistently decreased six to seven-fold compared to control cells (9). This effect did not occur following cocultivation of L1210 cells with macrophages that had not differentiated to the cytotoxic activated stage. Decreased O_2 consumption of cytotoxic activated macrophage injured L1210 cells was not due to cell death because cell viability was >90%. Cytotoxic activated macrophage-induced inhibition of O_2 consumption reflects L_{1210} cell mitochondrial dysfunction because the bulk of O_2 consumed by uninjured L_{1210} cells was inhibited by either antimycin-A or oligomycin (Table 2). Antimycin-A inhibits mitochondrial electron transport at the level of cytochrome b (29) and oligomycin acts on the mitochondrial ATP synthetase complex (26). The degree of inhibition by cytotoxic activated macrophages (85%) was almost the same as maximal inhibition by oligomycin (87%).

If cytotoxic activated macrophages selectively inhibit mitochondrial respiration in L_{1210} target cells, the prediction would be that they would lose their Pasteur effect (depression of glycolysis upon exposure of anaerobically cultured cells to O_2) and exhibit an inappropriately high rate of glycolysis with O_2 present. Glycolytic rates of cytotoxic activated macrophage-injured L_{1210}

TABLE 1. Correlation between hexose requirement of cytotoxic activated macrophage injured L_{1210} cells and aerobic glycolysis of uninjured L_{1210} Cells

Additions to DEM-G*		Experiment 1£	Experiment 2∞
Substrate	Inhibitor	[^{3}H]Thymidine released	Lactate produced
		% total count	μ mol.h.10^5 cells
--	--	87	0
--	2DG	83	0
Glucose	--	17	24
Mannose	--	17	20
Glucose	2DG	78	0
Mannose	2DG	74	0

* Glucose and mannose concentrations were 2 mM; 2DG concentration was 20 mM.

£ First incubation, cocultivation with cytotoxic activated macrophages, lasted 24 h. Release during first incubation = 23%. Second incubation lasted 6 h.

∞ Log-phase L_{1210} cells were incubated in culture medium minus glucose with 2% dialyzed human serum plus substrates and/or inhibitor as shown. Glycolysis rates were calculated from triplicate samples taken at 0, 2, 4, and 6 h. The rates were linear for glucose and mannose during the 6 h incubation. Cell counts at the end of the 6 h incubation showed >95% viability in all experimental groups. See reference 9 for experimental details.

(Reprinted from reference 9 with permission of the publisher.)

cells conformed to this pattern (Figure 2). These findings provide an explanation for the death-preventing effect of glucose on cytotoxic activated macrophage-injured L_{1210} cells. Because cytotoxic activated macrophages induced almost complete inhibition of L_{1210} respiration, and hence mitochondrial ATP production, injured L_{1210} cells become dependent on glycolysis for chemical energy (ATP) production.

TABLE 2. <u>Endogenous</u> <u>respiration</u> <u>of</u> <u>cytotoxic</u> <u>activated</u> <u>macrophage</u> <u>injured L_{1210} cells</u>

No. of Experiments	L_{1210} cells cultured with:*	O_2 Consumption‡
		$\mu l \cdot h \cdot 10^6$ cells
6	Alone	7.4±0.3
4	Alone + ET (200 ng/ml)	7.2±0.4
2	Alone + MAF (10% vol/vol)	7.2±0.9
4	SM	6.9±0.7
6	CM	1.1±0.1
2	CM (MAF)	1.7±0.4
3	Alone (oligomycin inhibited)∞	0.9±0.1
3	Alone (antimycin A inhibited)∞	0.3±0.1

* For these experiments, L_{1210} cells were cultured alone or with macrophages for 24-40 h before respiration measurements. Cytotoxic activated macrophages (CM), peritoneal macrophages from mice infected intraperitoneally with 0.2 mg <u>Mycobacterium bovis</u>, strain BCG, 17-22 d before harvest and injected with 1 ml of 10% protease peptone 3 d before harvest. Final differentiation stimulus was provided by 20-200 ng ml^{-1} endotoxin. CM (MAF), same as CM except that the final differentiation stimulus was provided by a lymphokine preparation with macrophage activating factor activity. SM, peritoneal macrophages from normal mice injected intraperitoneally with 1 ml 10% protease peptone 3 d before harvest.

‡ Values are the mean ± SEM for the number of experiments shown.

∞ The effects of oligomycin and antimycin A were determined by injection into the respiration vessel to a final concentration of 0.1 and 0.01 μM, respectively. Previous experiments showed that these concentrations produced maximal inhibition of uninjured L_{1210} cell respiration at 2×10^6 cells/ml. See reference 9 for experimental details.

(Adapted from reference 9 with permission of the publisher.)

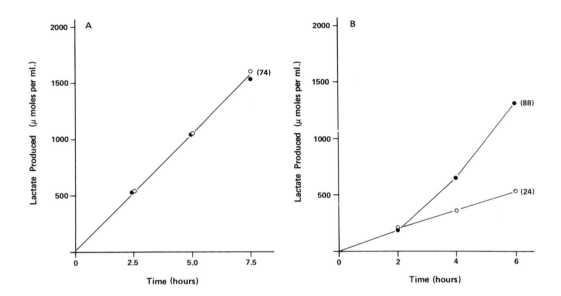

<u>Figure 2</u>. Aerobic (o) and anaerobic (●) glycolysis of cytotoxic activated macrophage-injured and uninjured L1210 cells. (A) L1210 cells which had been incubated for 20 h with cytotoxic activated macrophages before glycolysis measurements. (B) L1210 cells which had been incubated for 20 h without macrophages before glycolysis measurements. Numbers in parentheses are maximal rates of lactate production expressed as micromoles per hour per 10^5 cells. See reference 9 for experimental details.

(Reprinted from reference 9 with permission of the publisher.)

EVIDENCE THAT THERE ARE AT LEAST TWO TRANSFORMED CELL PHENOTYPIC RESPONSES TO CYTOTOXIC ACTIVATED MACROPHAGE INDUCED INHIBITION OF MITOCHONDRIAL RESPIRATION

There are at least two target cell responses to activated macrophage induced inhibition of mitochondrial respiration: stasis without progression to lysis (L1210 cell is an example of this phenotype), and stasis followed by lysis P815 cell is an example of the second phenotype). As described above, contact of L1210 cells with cytotoxic activated macrophages results in inhibition of proliferation and inhibition of mitochondrial respiration. Even when L1210 cells are removed from cytotoxic activated macrophages after a period of cocultivation, the inhibition of proliferation and the inhibition of mitochondrial respiration persists for a prolonged period (> 90 hours). As long as glycolytic substrate is available, this phenotype can survive cytotoxic activated macrophage-induced injury. When removed from cytotoxic activated macrophages, this phenotype eventually recovers both proliferative ability and mitochondrial respiration (10).

The prototype cell for the second phenotype is murine mastocytoma P815 which is also non-adherent when cultured in vitro. Identical perturbations of mitochondrial metabolism are measured in P815 cells

TABLE 3. Respiratory inhibition of neoplastic cells by cytotoxic macrophages.

Cell line*	Origin of cell line	Oncogenic agent	O_2 consumption $(\mu l \cdot h \cdot 10^6$ cells) of neoplastic cells after culture with:	
			Alone	CM
L1210	Mouse (DBA/2) lymphoblastic leukemia	Methyl-cholanthrene	7.2±0.4	1.1±0.1
P815	Mouse (DBA/2) mastocytoma	Methyl-cholanthrene	5.9±0.3	2.0±0.5
S180	Mouse (outbred) sarcoma	Unknown	14.2±0.9	1.3±0.4
TLX-9	Mouse (C57Bl) thymic lymphoma	X-ray	2.8	0.1
L10	Guinea pig (strain 2) hepatoma	Diethyl-nitrosamine	16.9±3.6	3.6±1.7
SV40 HE-1	Transformed hamster (LSH) embryo cell line	SV40 virus	10.0±2.1	1.2±0.2

* All maintained in vitro except for L10 cells which were harvested from strain 2 guinea pig ascites. Culture periods prior to endogenous respiration measurements were 24-40 hours except for P815 cell experiments (10 hours). SV40 HE-1 cells adhere to plastic and were removed by trypsin (0.25% in PBS, Difco Laboratories) treatment for five minutes. Values are the means±SEM for at least three experiments except for TLX-9 cells (one experiment). See reference 9 for experimental details.

(Reprinted from reference 9. with permission of the publisher.)

after cocultivation with cytotoxic activated macrophages as are detected in the L1210 phenotype (Table 3). However, this second phenotype responds to the stress of cytotoxic activated macrophage-induced changes, even in the presence of adequate glycolytic substrate, with stasis followed by lysis. The biochemical basis for a lytic or nonlytic response to cytotoxic activated macrophage-induced injury is unknown.

Table 3 also shows that cytotoxic activated macrophages cause inhibition of mitochondrial respiration in other transformed cells tested. Inhibition of oxygen consumption occurred regardless of species, tissue of origin, or whether the transformation event was spontaneous, induced by radiation, by a chemical carcinogen, or by an oncogenic virus.

EVIDENCE THAT THE NONLYTIC TRANSFORMED CELL PHENOTYPE MAY BE A MARKER FOR INCREASED TUMORIGENIC VIRULENCE

Good evidence exists that suggests expression of the nonlytic transformed cell phenotype confers increased resistance to host mediated antineoplastic surveillance. This correlation was possible because of the availability of a series of cells transformed by oncogenic DNA viruses (SV40 and adenovirus 2) whose in vivo biology was being studied by Lewis and Cook (5,22). At that point in time, these in vivo studies had defined three transformed cell phenotypes in terms of tumorigenicity: (i) nontumorigenic in adult syngeneic animals, (ii) tumorigenic in syngeneic adult but not in histoincompatible animals and, (iii) tumorigenic in syngeneic and histoincompatible adult animals (see Table 4). A brief summary of tumorigenic properties of SV40 transformed cells follows to provide background for interpretation of these in vivo studies as well as the in vitro experiments that were performed using the same series of cells.

Efforts to induce tumors in mice, rats, guinea pigs, rabbits, and primates by innoculating SV40 subcutaneously has been unsuccessful (8,21,27). Although not causing tumors when injected in vivo, SV40 does transform cells from these species growing in tissue culture (4,11,25,31). However, like the virus itself, SV40 transformed cells from these species are usually nontumorigenic when grafted into adult syngeneic immunocompetent animals. SV40 transformed cells from mice, and rats, resemble mouse embryo fibroblasts recently spontaneously transformed by prolonged in vitro culture (discussed in the first part of this review) with regard to their low tumorigenic potential. Like mouse embryo fibroblasts spontaneously transformed in in vitro culture, SV40 transformed mouse or rat cells may be a tissue culture approximation of an incipient stage of neoplastic transformation. Similar to spontaneously transformed mouse embryo fibroblasts, SV40 transformed mouse cells become tumorigenic in adult syngeneic mice only if the SV40 transformed cells have been maintained in tissue culture for a prolonged period of time or the immune response of the host has been suppressed (11).

The hamster is the exception to the rule that SV40 is nontumorigenic (4,8). SV40 innoculated subcutaneously into newborn hamsters induces tumors after a latent period of three to nine months. Likewise, hamster cells transformed in vitro by SV40 are highly tumorigenic when transplanted into adult syngeneic immunocompetent hosts. In fact, in sharp contrast to the other species mentioned above, the tumorigenic potential of SV40 transformed hamster cells is quite remarkable. Lewis and Cook (22) recently observed that SV40-transformed inbred LSH hamster cells grafted in histoincompatible adult CB hamsters induced tumors almost as efficiently as in syngeneic animals. It should be mentioned parenthetically that the immunocompetence of the hamster has been found to be equivalent to that of other species when carefully evaluated (2,3,7). Therefore, the evidence is now very strong that in the hamster, SV40 infection, either in vitro or in vivo, produces transformed cells with increased tumorigenic potential or "virulence" when compared to in vitro or in vivo SV40 induced transformation events in other species. The point for emphasis is that cells from species such as the mouse and rat possess in vitro abnormal growth characteristics of transformed cells after infection with SV40 and yet are not tumorigenic in syngeneic immunocompetent adult animals. SV40 transformed hamster cells have the same abnormal in vitro growth characteristics as SV40 transformed cells from other rodent species but in addition have high tumorigenic potential. The species dependency for tumorigenicity of SV40-transformed cells provides not only a model for examining factors that affect malignancy of transformed cells but also an experimental system for identification of factors responsible for ehanced tumorigenicity defined as the ability of transformed cells to grow in a histoincompatible host.

Recent experiments show that mouse and hamster peritoneal activated macrophages were cytolytic for nontumorigenic SV40 transformed mouse and rat cells (6). However, the highly tumorigenic SV40-transformed hamster fibroblasts, as defined by their ability to grow in allogeneic animals, were relatively resistant to the cytolytic effect of cytotoxic activated macrophages (6). These experiments demonstrate that SV40-transformed hamster fibroblasts have the same phenotypic response to the activated macrophage induced cytotoxic effect as another highly malignant cell, the L_{1210} mouse lymphoma which include (i) resistance to the lytic injury induced in neoplastic target cells by activated macrophages, (ii) susceptibility to a reversible cytostasis that persists for a variable period of time (48-120 hours) before cell proliferation resumes (iii) respiration is markedly reduced making them dependent on glycolysis for ATP generation (Table 3 shows the markedly decreased O_2 consumption of SV40-transformed hamster cells - SV40HE1 - that developed 24 hours after contact with activated macrophages). These experiments show that four different lines of SV40 transformed hamster cells (SV40HE1, SV40HE2, SV40HE3, and THK-1t) which have enhanced malignancy as demonstrated by the capability of growing progressively in allogeneic hosts, in addition, have the nonlytic response to cytotoxic activated macrophage induced injury.

It is important to emphasize that the nonlytic transformed phenotype appears to be a marker for enhanced tumorigenicity and not tumorigenicity per se. Transformed but nontumorigenic target cells or transformed cells of low tumorigenicity are highly sensitive to lysis induced by activated macrophages. Examples include TCMK, SV40RE1, SV40RE2, and Ad2HE7 cells (see Table 4), and mouse embryo fibroblasts recently transformed by in vitro culture (see above).

TABLE 4. Tumor-inducing capacity and response to cocultivation with cytotoxic activated macrophages of virus-transformed rodent cells.

Cell line	Species, strain of origin	Cells (log)/TPD50*: Host of origin	Cells (log)/TPD50*: Histoincompatible host (strain)†	Response to cocultivation with cytotoxic activated macrophages cytostasis	Response to cocultivation with cytotoxic activated macrophages cytolysis
TCMK-1	Mouse, C3H/Mai	> 8.5		+	+
SV40RE1	Rat, Sprague-Dawley	> 8.5		+	+
SV40RE2	Rat, Sprague-Dawley	> 8.5		+	+
SV40HE1	Hamster, LSH	4.2	5.0 (CB)	+	0
SV40HE2	Hamster, LSH	3.6	5.5 (CB)	+	0
SV40HE3	Hamster, LSH	3.5	3.5 (CB)	+	0
THK-1t	Hamster, LSH	< 2.5	< 2.5 (CB)	+	0
Ad2HE7	Hamster, LSH	> 8.5		+	+
Ad2HTL3-1	Hamster, LSH	4.1	> 7.5 (CB)	+	+

* Cells (log)/TPD50, logarithm of number of tissue culture cells required to produce subcutaneous tumors in 50% of the surviving adult animals. TPD, tumor producing dose. TPD50 > 8.5 = no tumors developed during a 3-mo observation period after subcutaneous challenge with 108 tissue culture cells. For tumor challenge procedure, see reference 5.

† The inbred CB strain of hamster differs from the LSH strain at a major histoincompatibility locus.

Adapted from reference 6.

However, other transformed cells that are clearly tumorigenic in adult syngeneic immunocompetent animals also have the lytic phenotype, i.e., respond to activated macrophage induced inhibition of proliferation and inhibition mitochondrial respiration by lysis in culture medium containing an adequate supply of glucose (6,9). Examples include a line of Ad2-transformed hamster cells (Ad2HTL3-1), a diethylnitrosamine induced guinea pig hepatoma (L10) and the mouse mastocytoma (P815). Ad2HTL3-1 cells, although tumorigenic in syngeneic adult hamsters, are nontumorigenic in allogeneic hamsters (Table 4). The guinea pig L10 hepatoma, a lytic transformed cell phenotype, is responsive to BCG stimulated nonspecific active immunotherapy. In fact, the guinea pig - L10 system is the classic immunotherapy model used by Zbar, Rapp, and their colleagues to define many of the basic principles of nonspecific active immunotherapy (32).

We need to examine many more transformed cells before any meaningful generalization can be made. However, it appears the subgroup of transformed cells that resist the cytolytic effect of activated macrophages may represent a phenotype inherently more resistant to host antineoplastic defense than transformed cells with the lytic phenotype which may be, as a group, more sensitive to host antineoplastic defense. Therefore, it is possible that tumorigenic cells with the lytic phenotype may be more responsive to agents administered to enhance host antineoplastic defense (BCG, C. parvum, etc.) while tumorigenic cells with the nonlytic phenotype may be inherently more refractory to measures designed to enhance the antineoplastic response of the host. Finally, since many malignant cells have the lytic phenotype, it is important to reiterate that factors determining tumorigenicity for immunocompetent syngeneic animals are not necessarily related to resistance to activated macrophage induced lysis as measured by the in vitro assay we employ.

Acknowledgements: These studies were supported by the American Cancer Society Grant (H-139) and Veterans Administration, Washington, D.C. . We thank Gwenevere South for typing the manuscript.

REFERENCES

1. Aaronson, S.A. and Todaro, G.J. (1968): Science, 162:1024-1026.

2. Billingham, R.E. and Hildemann, W.H. (1958): Ann. N. Y. Acad. Sci., 73:676-686.

3. Billingham, R.E., Sawchuck, G.H., and Silvers, W.K. (1960): Proc. Natl. Acad. Sci. U.S.A., 46:1079-1090.

4. Butel, J.S., Tevethia, S.S., and Melnick, J.L. (1972): Adv. Cancer. Res., 15:1-55.

5. Cook, J.L. and Lewis, A.M.,Jr. (1979): Cancer Res., 39:1455-1461.

6. Cook, J.L., Hibbs, J.B.,Jr., and Lewis, A.M.,Jr. (1980): Proc. Natl. Acad. Sci. U.S.A., 77:6773-6777.

7.   Duncan, W.R. and Streilein, J.W. (1978): <u>Transplantation</u>, 25:12-16.

8.   Eddy, B.E. (1964): <u>Prog. Exp. Tumor Res.</u>, 4:1-26.

9.   Granger, D.L., Taintor, R.R., Cook, J.L., and Hibbs, J.B.,Jr. (1980): <u>J. Clin. Invest.</u>, 65:357-370.

10.   Granger, D.L. and Hibbs, J.B.,Jr. (1981): <u>Federation Proceedings</u>, 40:761.

11.   Hargis, B.J. and Malkiel, S. (1979): <u>J. Natl. Cancer Inst.</u>, 63:965-967.

12.   Hayflick, L. and Moorhead, P.S. (1961): <u>Exp. Cell. Res.</u>, 25:585-621.

13.   Hibbs, J.B.,Jr. (1973): <u>Science</u>, 1890:868-870.

14.   Hibbs, J.B.,Jr. (1974): <u>J. Natl. Cancer Inst.</u>, 53:1487-1492.

15.   Hibbs, J.B.,Jr., Lambert, L.H.,Jr., and Remington, J.S. (1971): <u>J. Infec. Dis.</u>, 124:587-592.

16.   Hibbs, J.B.,Jr., Lambert, L.H.,Jr., and Remington, J.S. (1972): <u>Nature N. Biol.</u>, 235:48-50.

17.   Hibbs, J.B.,Jr., Lambert, L.H.,Jr., and Remington, J.S. (1972): <u>Science</u>, 117:998-1000.

18.   Kaplan, A.M., Morahan, P.S., and Regelson, W. (1974): <u>J. Natl. Cancer Inst.</u>, 52:1919-1921.

19.   Krahenbuhl, J.L., Lambert, L.H.,Jr., and Remington, J.S. (1976): <u>Cell Immunol.</u>, 25:279-293.

20.   Lehninger, A.L. (1975): <u>Biochemistry</u> Worth Publishers, Inc., New York.

21.   Lewis, A.M.,Jr. (1973): In: <u>Biohazards in Biological Research</u>, edited by A. Hellman, M.N. Oxman, and R. Pollack, (Cold Spring Harbor Laboratory) pp 96-113. Cold Spring Harbor, NY.

22.   Lewis, A.M.,Jr. and Cook, J.L. (1980): <u>Proc. Natl. Acad. Sci.</u> USA, 77:2886-2889.

23.   Meltzer, M.S., Tucker, R.W., and Breuer, A.C. (1975): <u>Cellular Immunol.</u>, 17:30-42.

24.   Piessens, W.F., Churchill, W.H., and David, J.R. (1975): <u>J. Immunol.</u>, 114:293-299.

25.   Rabson, A.S., O'Conner, G.T., Kirschstein, R.L., and Branigan, W.J. (1962): <u>J. Natl. Cancer Inst.</u>, 29:765-788.

26. Racker, E. (1976): Lecture 4: the coupling device. In: A New Look at Mechanisms in Bioenergetics. pp 67-87. Academic Press, Inc., New York.

27. Shah, K. and Nathanson, N. (1976): Am. J. Epidemiol. 103:1-12.

28. Skipper, H.E., Schabel, F.M.,Jr., and Wilcox, W.S. (1964): Cancer Chemother Rep., 35:1-111.

29. Slater, E.C. (1967): Methods Enzymol., 10:48-57.

30. Todaro, G.J. and Green, H. (1963): J. Cell Biol. 17:299-312.

31. Tooze, J. (1973): In: The Molecular Biology of Tumor Viruses, Cold Spring Harbor Laboratory, pp. 350-402. Cold Spring Harbor, New York.

32. Zbar, B., Wepsic, H.T., Borsos, T., and Rapp, H.J. (1970): J. Natl. Cancer Inst., 44:473-481.

*Mediation of Cellular Immunity in Cancer by
Immune Modifiers*, edited by M. A. Chirigos
et al., Raven Press, New York © 1981.

Variations in the Capacity for Prostaglandin Production by Resident and Elicited Macrophages

Robert J. Bonney, P. Davies, and J. L. Humes

*Departments of Immunology and Biochemistry, Merck Institute for Therapeutic Research,
Rahway, New Jersey 07065*

Macrophages elicited by TG broth showed a decreased response to zymosan for the release of PGE_2 and $6KF_{1\alpha}$ compared with resident populations (2,14,15). In these studies we show that populations of peritoneal macrophages obtained from mice pretreated with certain other eliciting stimuli also show marked decreases in their capacity to synthesize PG in response to zymosan compared to resident cells exposed to the same agent. The decreased production of PG was observed in populations of macrophages elicited by BCG and CP. These changes were accompanied by changes characteristic of elicited cells such as in the activities of 5′-nucleotidase and leucine aminopeptidase.

INTRODUCTION

Mononuclear phagocytes isolated from the peritoneal cavity of mice and maintained in culture secrete a variety of products (2,6) capable of influencing certain biological responses. One class of products that will be discussed here are the prostaglandins which have been implicated in the regulation of immune responses (10,17), in bone resorption (7) and tumor cell killing (13,20).

Mouse peritoneal macrophages from specific pathogen-free mice differ significantly in many biochemical functions from cells that have been elicited in similar mice by i.p. injection of a sterile inflammatory stimulus such as thioglycollate broth (TG). The elicited cells show faster adherence and spreading on surfaces (18), display increased pinocytic activity (18), and contain higher levels of lysosomal acid hydrolases (LAH) (4). In addition, certain membrane enzymes such as leucine aminopeptidase (23) and alkaline phosphodiesterase (9) are elevated whereas the activity of another membrane-associated enzyme, 5′-nucleotidase, is decreased (8) in elicited cells compared with resident cells. Elicited mononuclear phagocytes cultured from animals previously treated with an inflammatory stimuli secrete a number of products not released by resident populations. Examples of these products are neutral proteinases such as plasminogen activator (22), elastase (5,24), and collagenase (25).

We have recently shown that resident peritoneal macrophages synthesize and release large quantities of certain oxygenation products of arachidonic acid (AA), notably prostaglandin E_2 (PGE_2) and 6-keto prostaglandin $F_{1\alpha}$ ($6KF_{1\alpha}$) in response to inflammatory stimuli such as zymosan (14), antigen-antibody complexes (3), and phorbol myristate acetate (1). It is well established that such cells also release a large proportion of their lysosomal acid hydrolases (LAH) in a selective manner in response to inflammatory stimuli (19). In marked contrast, peritoneal macrophages from TG-treated mice show a diminished capacity for the synthesis of AA oxygenation products (14) and for the selective release of LAH (2). These observations show that the source and the environment from which mononuclear phagocytes are obtained will influence the nature of their biochemical responses to a given stimulus.

In this report we will discuss the regulation of PGI_2 and PGE_2 synthesis and secretion from resident, Bacillus-Calmette Guerin (BCG) and Corynebacterium parvum (C. parvum) - elicited macrophages.

MATERIALS

Animals.
Male Swiss Webster mice (HLA-SW/ICR SPF) were purchased from Hilltop Lab Animals, Inc., Scottdale, Pa. The mice, 15 to 25 g, were fed a standard pellet diet and water ad libitum.
Chemicals.
M199 medium and porcine serum were from Grand Island Biological Co., Grand Island, N.Y. Zymosan was from ICN, K&K Labs, Inc., Plainview, N.Y. The zymosan particles were suspended in phosphate-buffered saline (PBS), boiled, and centrifuged three times. The final pellet was suspended in PBS at a concentration of 20 mg/ml and stored frozen. Suspensions of zymosan were diluted in culture medium and sonicated immediately before addition to the cells. Bacillus Calmette-Guerin (BCG, Phipps-TMC-1069) was from the Trudeau Institute, Saranac Lake, N.Y. and Corynebacterium parvum (CP) from Wellcome Research Labs, Beckenham, England.

METHODS

Tissue culture.
Macrophages were collected by peritoneal lavage from untreated mice or from mice that had received an i.p. injection of BCG, 1×10^7 cells or CP, 1.4 mg dry weight. Cells were lavaged with 5 ml of M199 containing 100 units/ml of penicillin and streptomycin, 20 units/ml heparin, and 1% HIPS and cultured as described (2,3).
Labelling of cellular phospholipids with ^{3}H-AA.
One microcurie of ^{3}H-AA was added to cultures in 4 ml of M199 containing 1% HIPS. After 4 hr approximately 50 to 60% of the label was taken up by the cells.
Harvest of media and cells for PG and enzymatic assays.
At the termination of the experiments, media were collected and divided for subsequent analysis. Two milliliters of isotonic saline containing 0.1% Triton X-100 was then added to the plates and the lysed cells were removed with a rubber policeman.
Enzyme assays.
Lactate dehydrogenase (LDH) was assayed by determining the rate of oxidation of reduced nicotinamide adenine dinucleotide at 340 nm. Leucine aminopeptidase was assayed by the method of Wachsmuth (23) and 5′-nucleotidase by the method of Edelson and Cohn (8). Lysozyme was assayed by the method described by Gordon et al. (11).
DNA was determined by the method of Setaro and Morley (21) and protein by the method of Lowry et al. (16).

Extraction and chromatography of ^{3}H-PG.

Citric acid was added to the culture media to a final concentration of 0.03 M and 50 μg of PGE_2, 30 μg of $PGF_{2\alpha}$, and 30 μg of AA were added as chromatographic standards. The acidified media were then extracted and chromatographed as described (14,2). The areas corresponding to authentic PGE_2 and $6KF_{1\alpha}$ on the chromatograms were cut out and the radioactivity was determined by counting in 10 ml Aquasol with a Packard 3255 Liquid Scintillation Spectrometer.

RESULTS AND DISCUSSION

Mononuclear phagocytes elicited with CP were much less responsive to zymosan for the release of PG than resident cells (Table 1). The decreased capacity of CP-elicited cells to synthesize ^{3}H-AA oxygenation products was recently confirmed by radioimmunoassay for PGE (15). In a quantitatively similar manner the release of PG was also depressed in cells obtained from mice that had received an i.p. injection of BCG 21 days previously (Table 2). Particularly striking was the loss of ability of the stimulated cells to synthesize $6KF_{1\alpha}$ when stimulated with zymosan as illustrated by the change in the ratio of PGE_2 to $6KF_{1\alpha}$ synthesis.

In order to place the above findings in perspective with other criteria used to characterize resident and elicited macrophages, we assayed 5′-nucleotidase and leucine aminopeptidase activities in these cultures. Cells from BCG, and CP-treated mice all exhibited decreased specific activities of 5′-nucleotidase and increased specific activity of leucine aminopeptidase (Table 3).

There are several explanations that could account for the difference in the amount of PG produced by elicited and resident macrophages when challenged in culture with zymosan. These include a) differences in the amount of zymosan phagocytosed, b) altered rates of phospholipid deacylation for the production of AA, c) differences in the activity of fatty acid cyclooxygenase, and d) defective secretion of newly synthesized PG.

We have recently tested 3 of these possibilities using macrophages elicited by thioglycollate broth and stimulated with zymosan (15) or phorbol myristate acetate (1) and have concluded that there is a great difference in the rate of phospholipid deacylation between resident and TG-elicited macrophages. It is still possible that there is a difference in the PG-cyclooxygenase activity between the two cell populations. This difference could occur by an increased generation of a destructive oxygen moiety during the interaction of the newly recruited cells with the eliciting inflammatory agent. Such oxygen radicals have been shown to destroy the cyclooxygenase and, to a greater extent, PGI_2 synthetase in ram seminal vesicles (12). The greater sensitivity of the PGI_2 synthetase to be destroyed by oxygen radicals may explain the altered rate of PGE_2 and $6KF_{1\alpha}$ produced by elicited macrophages. However, it remains to be shown if either of these two mechanisms are operational in CP or BCG-elicited macrophages.

TABLE 1. Macrophages from Corynebacterium parvum-treated mice release less prostaglandins than resident macrophages[a]

	DNA Content	PG Secretion		
		^{3}H-PGE$_2$	^{3}H-6KF$_{1\alpha}$	
	(µg/plate)	(cpm/µg DNA)		
A. Resident 15.9 $\pm$ 2.4				Ratio PGE$_2$/6KF$_{1\alpha}$
Additions				
None		80 $\pm$ 3	28 $\pm$ 0	2.8
Zymosan, 50 µg/ml		1155 $\pm$ 59	374 $\pm$ 42	3.1
B. CP-Elicited 16.7 $\pm$ 0.6				
Additions				
None		5 $\pm$ 0.5	2.0 $\pm$ 0	2.5
Zymosan, 50 µg/ml		57 $\pm$ 8	12.0 $\pm$ 3	4.8
Zymosan, 200 µg/ml		82 $\pm$ 6	15.0 $\pm$ 1	5.5

[a]Cells were harvested from mice that had received an i.p. injection of 1.4 mg of CP 7 days previously or from untreated mice and cultured as described in Materials and Methods. Cells from untreated mice incorporated 0.6 µCi of ^{3}H-arachidonic acid in 4 hr whereas cells derived from CP-treated mice incorporated 0.64 µCi. Cells were harvested 4 hr after the addition of zymosan. The results are the mean $\pm$ S.D.; N = 3. Reproduced with the permission of the publishers from Humes et al. (15).

TABLE 2. <u>Macrophages from BCG-treated mice release less prostaglandins than resident macrophages</u>[a]

	DNA Content	PG Secretion		
		^{3}H-PGE$_2$	^{3}H-6KF$_{1\alpha}$	
	(µg/plate)	(cpm/µg DNA)		
A. Resident				
	9.9 ± 3.1			Ratio
Additions				PGE$_2$/6KF$_{1\alpha}$
None		44 ± 18	25 ± 11	1.8
Zymosan, 50 µg/ml		415 ± 72	176 ± 29	2.4
Zymosan, 200 µg/ml		793 ± 144	361 ± 69	2.2
B. BCG-Elicited				
	8.4 ± 0.8			
Additions				
None		29 ± 11	7 ± 2	4.1
Zymosan, 50 µg/ml		286 ± 37	32 ± 3	8.9
Zymosan, 200 µg/ml		422 ± 72	48 ± 9	8.8

[a]Cells were harvested from mice that had received an i.p. injection of BCG 3 weeks previously or from untreated mice and cultured as described in Materials and Methods. Resident cells incorporated 0.85 µCi of ^{3}H-AA and BCG cells incorporated 0.71 µCi ^{3}H-AA. The cultures were harvested 4 hr after the addition of zymosan. The results are the mean ± S.D.; N = 3. Reproduced with permission of the publishers from Humes <u>et al</u>. (15).

TABLE 3. <u>The activity of 5′-nucleotidase and leucine aminopeptidase in resident and elicited macrophages</u>[a]

In Vivo Treatment	Enzyme Specific Activities	
	5′-Nucleotidase	Leucine aminopeptidase
	units/mg protein	
None	42.0 ± 0.84	7.0 ± 0.11
CP	0.7 ± 0.04	16.3 ± 0.82
BCG	15.7 ± 2.90	21.5 ± 4.09

[a]Peritoneal macrophages were isolated from untreated mice and from mice receiving an i.p. injection of CP (7 days) or BCG (7 days) and cultured for 24 hr as described in Materials and Methods. The media were withdrawn and the cells washed three times with PBS and collected in PBS containing 0.1% Triton X-100. The two enzymes were assayed as described in Materials and Methods. The results are the mean ± S.D.; N = 3. Reproduced with permission of the publishers from Humes <u>et al</u>. (15).

REFERENCES

1. Bonney, R. J., Wightman, P. D., Dahlgren, M. E., Davies, P., Kuehl, F. A., Jr. and Humes, J. L. (1980): Biochim. Biophys. Acta, 633: 410-421.

2. Bonney, R. J., Wightman, P. D., Davies, P., Sadowski, S., Kuehl, F. A., Jr. and Humes, J. L. (1978): Biochem. J., 176: 433-442.

3. Bonney, R. J., Wightman, P. D., Naruns, P., Richardson, T. G., Davies, P., Galavage, M. and Humes, J. L. (1979): Prostaglandins, 18: 605-616.

4. Cohn, Z. A. and Benson, B. (1965): J. Exp. Med., 121: 153-164.

5. Dahlgren, M. E., Davies, P. and Bonney, R. J. (1980): Biochim. Biophys. Acta, 630: 338-351.

6. Davies, P. and Bonney, R. J. (1979): J. Reticulo. Society, 26: 37-47.

7. Dowsett, M., Eastman, A. R., Easty, D. M., Easty, G. C., Powles, T. J. and Nevine, A. M. (1976): Nature, 263: 72-74.

8. Edelson, P. J. and Cohn, Z. A. (1975): J. Exp. Med., 144: 1581-1595.

9. Edelson, P. J. and Erbs, C. (1978): J. Exp. Med., 147: 77-85.

10. Gery, I. and Davies, P. (1979) In: Biology of Lymphokines Edited by S. Cohen, E. Pick and J. J. Oppenheim, pp. 347-367. Academic Press, New York.

11. Gordon, S., Todd, I. and Cohn, Z. A. (1974): J. Exp. Med., 139: 1228-1248.

12. Ham, E. A., Egan, R. W., Soderman, D. D., Gale, P. H. and Kuehl, F. A., Jr. (1979): J. Biol. Chem., 243: 2191-2198.

13. Hibbs, J. B., Lambert, L. H. and Remington, J. S. (1972): Nature New Biol., 235: 48-50.

14. Humes, J. L., Bonney, R. J., Pelus, L., Dahlgren, M. E., Sadowski, S. J., Kuehl, F. A., Jr. and Davies, P. (1977): Nature, 269: 149-151.

15. Humes, J. L., Burger, S., Galavage, M., Kuehl, F. A., Jr., Wightman, P. D., Dahlgren, M. E., Davies, P. and Bonney, R. J. (1980): J. Immunol., 124: 2110-2116.

16. Lowry, O. H., Rosebrough, N. J., Farr, A. L. and Randall, R. J. (1951): J. Biol. Chem., 193: 265-275.

17. Pelus, L. and Strausser, H. (1977): Life Sciences, 20: 903-911.

18. Rabinovitch, M. and DeStefano, M. J. (1973): Exp. Cell Res., 77: 323-331.

19. Schorlemmer, H. V., Davies, P., Hylton, W., Gugig, M. and Allison, A. C. (1977): Br. J. Exp. Pathol., 58: 315-326.

20. Schultz, R. M., Pavlidis, N. A., Stylos, W. A. and Chirigos, M. A. (1978): Science, 202: 320-321.

21. Setaro, F. and Morley, C. (1976): Anal. Biochem., 71: 313-321.

22. Unkeless, J. C., Gordon, S. and Reich, E. (1974): J. Exp. Med., 136: 834-846.

23. Wachsmuth, E. D. (1975): Exp. Cell Res., 96: 409-416.

24. Werb, Z. and Gordon, S. (1975): J. Exp. Med., 142: 346-360.

25. Werb, Z. and Gordon, S. (1975): J. Exp. Med., 142: 361-377.

Mediation of Cellular Immunity in Cancer by Immune Modifiers, edited by M. A. Chirigos et al., Raven Press, New York © 1981.

The Roles of Lymphokine and Prostaglandin in the Regulation of Mouse Macrophage Activation for Tumor Cell Killing

Stephen W. Russell, *Steven M. Taffet, and Judith L. Pace

*Division of Comparative Pathology, Colleges of Veterinary Medicine and Medicine, University of Florida, Gainesville, Florida 32610; *Department of Bacteriology and Immunology, University of North Carolina School of Medicine, Chapel Hill, North Carolina 27514*

INTRODUCTION

Interest in the activation of macrophages for tumor cell killing, now that the phenomenon has been confirmed in many laboratories, is focusing on how activation is induced and regulated, and how killing is mediated. Basic understanding of these areas should help investigators harness the complex process of macrophage activation for possible therapeutic use, perhaps through biological response modifiers designed to augment and focus the process selectively.

Under a variety of conditions it appears that activation of mouse macrophages for tumor cell killing proceeds through one or more noncytotoxic, intermediate stages (3, 10, 13). Once developed, the expression of cytolytic activity is evanescent, disappearing in most cases within 24 hours (1, 2, 9, 10, 14). The following, brief overview summarizes results from our laboratory which pertain to the induction and negative regulation in vitro of mouse macrophage activation for tumor cell killing.

MATERIALS AND METHODS

Male, C3H/HeN mice, 6-8 weeks old, were obtained from ARS/Harland (Madison, WI). Modified Eagle's medium was supplemented with antibiotics, glutamine, sodium bicarbonate and HEPES (17). Assay medium was further supplemented to a final concentration of 10% with fetal bovine serum (Sterile Systems, Inc., Logan, UT). Purified bacterial lipopolysaccharide (LPS) from Escherichia coli 0111:B4 (6) was a gift from Dr. D. C. Morrison, Emory University, Atlanta, GA. Limulus amebocyte lysate (LAL), obtained from Cape Cod Associates, Woods Hole, MA was

49

used to assay reagents for endotoxin (5) at a sensitivity level of
0.13 ng/ml. Culture supernates from spleen cells stimulated with 2
μg/ml Con A for 72 hr in serum-free medium (7) served as a source of
lymphokine. Control supernates, to which Con A was added after the
cells were removed, were prepared from unstimulated spleen cells.
Both lymphokine-rich and control preparations were concentrated by
vacuum dialysis and fractionated using Sephadex G-100. Prostaglandin
E_2 (PGE) and indomethacin were obtained from Sigma Chemical Co., St.
Louis, MO. PGI_2 was obtained as a gift from Dr. John Pike, Upjohn
Co., Kalamazoo, MI. PGE produced by macrophages was assayed in
culture supernates by a modification (17) of the radioimmunoassay
described by Jaffe et al. (4). Macrophage monolayers were prepared
from either resident peritoneal macrophages (17) or peritoneal exudates induced by the intraperitoneal injection of 1 ng LPS in 1 ml
endotoxin-free phosphate buffered saline (7,8). Evidence of activation for tumor cell killing was obtained using a 16 hour ^{51}Cr release
assay wherein the targets were P815 mastocytoma cells (11, 17).

INDUCTION OF THE ACTIVATED STATE

Macrophage populations obtained directly from progressively growing
tumors (12, 13), macrophages derived from regressing Moloney sarcomas
and allowed to lose their cytolytic activity in vitro (13, 14), and
macrophages exposed in vitro to low doses of lymphokine (3, 10) are in
a noncytotoxic state which has been operationally referred to as
"primed" (10, 13). By primed it is meant that at least some cells in
these populations have been prepared to do something -- in this case
kill tumor cells -- but will not do so unless they are exposed to an
additional stimulus or combination of stimuli. Upon delivery of the
second signal, provided, for example, by low concentrations (pg-to-
ng/ml) of LPS, the primed cells respond by rapidly developing cytolytic activity. A key question, then, is whether lymphokine acting
alone, i.e., without the second signal, primes macrophages, activates
them for tumor cell killing, or has both capabilities. In our system
we have not been able to activate macrophages fully with lymphokine, a
finding which is concordant with results obtained previously by
Weinberg and Hibbs (19) using long term (60 hr) visual or radioisotope
release assays.
The inability of lymphokine to activate macrophages fully is illustrated in Figure 1. In this experiment a lymphokine-rich culture
supernate was concentrated 20-fold and applied to a Sephadex G-100
column prepared for use under conditions free of detectable endotoxin.
The eluted fractions were assayed for endotoxin using the LAL assay.
Each fraction was also assayed for evidence of lymphokine (cytotoxic)
activity, as previously described (7). Briefly, macrophages were
exposed to test material, both in the absence and presence of added
LPS (3 ng/ml). No fraction, at the dilution employed (1:10), induced
cytolytic activity in this experiment unless LPS was also present.
With LPS added a broad area of activity was revealed (Figure 1) between the approximate molecular weights of 25,000-70,000 daltons. It
has consistently been our finding that lymphokine does not activate
macrophages for tumor cell killing, even when concentrated up to
4-fold, providing that the system is free of detectable endotoxin.

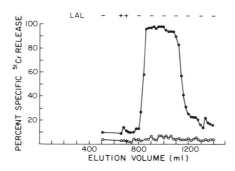

FIG. 1. Culture supernate from concanavalin A-stimulated
spleen cells was concentrated 20-fold (vacuum dialysis)
and fractionated using a Sephadex G-100 column (5x90 cm)
equilibrated with 0.01 M potassium phosphate buffer, pH
7.2, containing 0.15 M NaCl. Fractions (10 ml each) were
collected at a flow rate of 60 ml/hr. While the uncon-
centrated supernate was free of detectable endotoxin by
the Limulus amebocyte lysate (LAL) assay (sensitivity
level 0.13 ng/ml), the concentrated material was slightly
positive. All LAL positive material eluted from the
Sephadex column in the void volume, however. Fractions
also were assayed for lymphokine (cytolytic) activity
with (●) or without (o) 3 ng/ml added LPS. Most of the
lymphokine activity, which was detected only in the presence of LPS, was found between the column markers
bovine serum albumin (M.W. 67,000) and chymotrypsinogen A
(M.W. 25,000).

Synergistic interaction between LPS and lymphokine in the activation of macrophages for tumor cell killing has been described (3, 10);
however, the full extent of such synergism is only now becoming apparent. For example, the relation between LPS and lymphokine is such
that cytolytic activity will be induced in macrophages when either of
the two is present in low concentration, providing that the other is
present in high concentration (7). The observation that large amounts
of lymphokine will synergize with minute quantities of LPS to effect
activation may be key to explaining at least some of the claims that
lymphokine activates when used in high enough concentration.

LOSS OF CYTOLYTIC ACTIVITY

Schultz and his colleagues (16) have postulated that PGE negatively feeds back on the process of macrophage activation to inhibit tumor cell killing. As described below, our recent findings (17) confirm this hypothesis and indicate generally how interference is mediated.

The first indication that PGE was involved in the negative regulation of activation stemmed from observations that indomethacin (10^{-6}M) prevented the loss of cytolytic activity after mouse resident peritoneal macrophages had been activated by exposure to 100 ng/ml LPS. Further, the levels of killing reached in the presence of indomethacin were significantly increased over levels attained in the absence of the cyclooxygenase inhibitor. Radioimmunoassay for PGE in macrophage culture supernates revealed that the hormone accumulated rapidly following stimulation with LPS -- approximately 3×10^{-9}M within 1 hour and a maximum of 10^{-8}M after 4 hours. To determine if these concentrations were sufficient to suppress cytolytic activity, monolayers were first treated with 100 ng/ml LPS and 10^{-6}M indomethacin. The latter drug prevented the macrophages from synthesizing any of their own PGE. When various doses of PGE were added to the culture, 10^{-8}M shut off killing, while 10^{-9}M had a variable effect, ranging from 20% reduction to complete suppression of cytolytic activity, depending on the experiment. $PGF_{2\alpha}$ had no effect in the same system, and PGI_2 was much less efficient at inhibiting cytotoxicity, despite the fact the PGI_2 induced a whole cell cyclic AMP response comparable to that obtained with PGE_2 (S. Taffet and S. Russell, manuscript in preparation). The latter result suggests that more than activation of adenylate cyclase and induction of a generalized cyclic AMP response is needed to effect shut off. This hypothesis is supported by other experiments we have performed. For example, PGE did not negatively regulate cytolytic activity unless it was added to macrophages in conjunction with activator (17). This has been a consistent finding in spite of the fact that exposure of macrophages to PGE in the absence of LPS stimulates significant increases in intracellular levels of cyclic AMP within minutes (S. Taffet and S. Russell, unpublished observations).

It is emphasized that many more studies will be needed before the relations PGE has to macrophage activation are fully understood. However, from the information accumulated to date it can be concluded that: (i) PGE negatively regulates nonspecific tumor cell killing mediated in vitro by LPS-stimulated resident peritoneal macrophages; (ii) PGE acts in this system by shutting off cytolytic activity rather than by preventing its development; (iii) LPS-stimulated macrophages produce PGE in quantities sufficient to limit the expression of cytolytic activity; and (iv) the negative regulatory effect of PGE is dependent on more than increased intracellular levels of cyclic AMP, at least as measured on a whole cell basis.

MAINTENANCE OF CYTOLYTIC ACTIVITY BY LYMPHOKINE

We had noted that macrophages cultured in the presence of lymphokine tended not to lose their cytolytic activity as rapidly as those cultured in medium alone or in dilutions of fractionated, control supernate. This impression was confirmed in prospective studies wherein macrophages retained increasingly greater amounts of cytolytic

activity after 24 hours of preincubation with LPS when increasing
amounts of lymphokine were included in the culture medium (18). Since
to a certain extent this finding mimiced the effect of indomethacin,
the ability of macrophages to produce PGE in response to LPS stimulation was examined.   No difference was found between cultures which
contained either medium, fractionated control supernate, or lymphokine.   Subsequent studies showed that the maintenance effect was,
instead, caused by lymphokine inducing in macrophages a state of
decreased sensitivity to PGE.   In the presence of lymphokine 1,000
times more of the hormone (10^{-5}M, rather than 10^{-8}M) was required to
shut off cytotoxicity, compared to medium alone or control material.
Lymphokine was shown not to produce this effect by interfering with
the cyclic nucleotide response of macrophages to PGE.

DISCUSSION

Based on the results reviewed here, the roles that lymphokine and
prostaglandin have in regulating macrophage activation for tumor cell
killing are summarized in Figure 2.

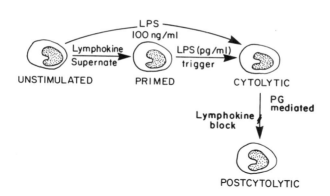

FIG.2. Acquisition and loss of tumoricidal
activity by mouse peritoneal macrophages.

Lymphokine-rich supernates of Con A-stimulated mouse spleen cell
cultures potentially contain at least two activities which are
relevant to the activation of mouse peritoneal macrophages for tumor
cell killing. One of these prepares macrophages -- primes them -- to
respond to a second signal, provided in examples given here by LPS,
which then triggers the onset of cytolytic activity. The second
activity that has been associated with lymphokine is maintenance of
macrophage-mediated, nonspecific tumoricidal activity. Accumulating
evidence suggests that lymphokine maintains tumoricidal activity by
interfering with the negative-regulatory effects of PGE. Whether or
not these two lymphokine activities are due to the same or different
molecule(s) remains to be determined.

Understanding the roles of lymphokine and PGE in the process of macrophage activation may prove to be of particular importance in the design and use of biological response modifiers for therapeutic purposes. For example, macrophages in at least some progressively growing tumors are primed (12, 13). It may be possible, therefore, to activate these cells fully if the required second signal can be delivered in an appropriate manner. We emphasize that the use of LPS as a second signal should be viewed as a model for what are probably more "physiologic" molecules that can have the same triggering effect. There is suggestive evidence, for example, that such molecules are present in preparations of Gram positive bacteria which are free of detectable endotoxin (15). Other approaches might include the use of modifiers that would interdict PGE production by intratumoral macrophages and/or tumor cells or, on the other hand, reduce the responsiveness of activated macrophages to the negative regulatory effects of PGE. All of these would appear to be areas wherein biological response modifiers might be helpful in harnessing activated macrophages for tumor cell killing in vivo.

ACKNOWLEDGEMENTS

The authors thank Ms. Judith McCallister for typing the manuscript. The work was supported, in part, by U.S.P.H.S. research grants CA 31199 and CA 31202. Steve M. Taffet was supported by training grant CA 09057 and Stephen W. Russell was the recipient of Research Career Development Award CA 00497.

REFERENCES

1. Fidler, I. J., Darnell, J. H., and Budmen, M. B. (1976): J. Immunol., 117:666-673.
2. Hibbs, J. B., Jr. (1975): Transplantation, 19:81-87.
3. Hibbs, J. B., Jr., Taintor, R. R., Chapman, H. A., Jr., and Weinberg, J. B. (1977): Science, 197:279-282.
4. Jaffe, B. M., Behrman, H. A., and Parker, C. W. (1973): J. Clin. Invest., 52:398-405.
5. Levine, J., Tomasulo, P. A., and Oser, R. S. (1970): J. Lab. Clin. Med., 75:903-911.
6. Morrison, D. C. and Leive, L. (1975): J. Biol. Chem., 250:2911-2919
7. Pace, J. L. and Russell, S. W. (1981): J. Immunol., (In press).
8. Pace, J. L., Taffet, S. M. and Russell, S. W. (1981): J. Reticuloendothel. Soc., (In press).
9. Poste, G. and Kirsh, R. (1979): Cancer Res., 39:2582-2590.
10. Ruco, L. P. and Meltzer, M. S. (1978): J. Immunol., 121:2035-2042.
11. Russell, S. W. (1981): In: Methods for Studying Mononuclear Phagocytes, edited by D. O. Adams, P. Edelson, and H. Koren, (In press).
12. Russell, S. W. and McIntosh, A. T. (1977): Nature (Lond.), 268:69-
13. 71, Russell, S. W., Doe, W. F., and McIntosh, A. T. (1977): J. Exp. Med.146:1511-1520.
14. Russell, S. W., Gillespie, G. Y., and McIntosh, A. T. (1977): J. Immunol., 118:1574-1579.
15. Schreiber, R. D., Ziegler, H. K., Calamai, E. G., and Unanue, E. R.(1981): Fed. Proc. 40:1002.
16. Schultz, R. M., Pavlidis, N. A., Stylos, W. A., and Chirigos, M. A. (1978): Science, 202:320-321.

17. Taffet, S. M. and Russell, S. W. (1981): J. Immunol., 126:424-427.
18. Taffet, S. M., Pace, J. L., and Russell, S. W. (1981): J. Immunol., (In press).
19. Weinberg, J. B. and Hibbs, J. B., Jr. (1979): J. Reticuloendothel. Soc., 26:283-293.

Mediation of Cellular Immunity in Cancer by Immune Modifiers, edited by M. A. Chirigos et al., Raven Press, New York © 1981.

Activating Pathways of Macrophage Interleukin 1 Production, Ia and FcR Expression

Joost J. Oppenheim, Stefanie N. Vogel, Patricia S. Steeg, and Robert N. Moore

Cellular Immunology Section, Laboratory of Microbiology and Immunology, National Institute of Dental Research, National Institutes of Health, Bethesda, Maryland 20205

INTRODUCTION

There is considerable evidence that macrophages play an important role as effector cells in tumor immunity. However, macrophages must be activated to attain their tumoricidal capabilities, and this frequently involves the participation of lymphocytes. Conversely, macrophages play an essential role in inducing lymphocyte mediated immunological responses. Thus, multiple interactions occur between macrophages and lymphocytes during the induction phase of immunity with both positive and negative consequences which can either amplify or suppress immunity. Therefore understanding the mechanisms of immune induction will provide many unique opportunities for mod ification of the biological response to tumors.

In this report we will consider the exogenous and endogenous signals involved in activating macrophages and lymphocytes to participate in the immune response. We will use the term "activation" in the general sense of denoting any increase in the activity of these cells that serves to amplify host defense mechanisms. The macrophage-lymphocyte interactions are bidirectional since exogenous stimulants induce both cell types to produce endogenous "hormone-like" signals or "cytokines" that amplify each others functional capabilities. Macrophages are activated by exogenous stimulants to increase their production of a wide variety of enzymes, complement and clotting components, as well as cytokines such as colony stimulating factors (CSF), interferon (IF), and an immuno-enhancing activity called lymphocyte-activating factor (LAF) which was recently renamed interleukin 1 (IL 1). IL 1 is a 12,000-15,000 MW polypeptide that in conjunction with exogenous stimulants activates T lymphocyte proliferation, lymphokine (IL 2) production (17) and differentiation. IL 1 also augments immunoglobulin production by B lymphocytes (12). Activated lymphocytes in turn produce lymphokines such as macrophage activating factor(s) (MAF), CSF and IF which can induce macrophage activation, proliferation and differentiation.

Macrophages can be activated by one of two major pathways. Stimulants that can activate cultures of purified macrophages or cell line macrophages presumably activate them directly. Other agents activate other cell types such as fibroblasts or lymphocytes to activate macrophages either through the production of soluble factors (cytokines) or by cell contact dependent mechanisms. In this paper we will document these pathways of macrophage activation and the consequent production of IL 1 and the enhanced expression of phenotypic markers such as Ia and receptors for the Fc portion of the immunoglobulin molecule (FcR) by macrophages. This lymphokine induced macrophage differentiation may promote Ia dependent tumor immunity and FcR mediated "antibody dependent cellular cytotoxicity" (ADCC).

DIRECT ACTIVATION OF MACROPHAGES

We have used IL 1 production as an indicator of macrophage activation since the degree of IL 1 production has been correlated with the degree of macrophage stimulation (7). A wide variety of stimulants can act directly on macrophages to produce IL 1 (11). These include particulate materials such as latex and bentonite, adjuvants such as lipopolysaccharide endotoxin (LPS) and mycobacterial peptidoglycolipids, and agents that affect membrane functions such as dimethylsulfoxide (DMSO), colchicine, mycostatin and phorbol myristic acetate (PMA).

We will consider PMA in greater detail because it has many fascinating biological effects. PMA is a well known tumor promotor (2), is a comitogen which is manifested by its enhancement of the lymphostimulatory effect of lectins (6), induces T cell growth factor (TCGF or IL 2) production by lymphocytes (4), can substitute for macrophages in T cell induction (14), enhances thymocyte mitogenic factor production by epidermal cells (15), and is directly mitogenic for human T lymphocytes (20). PMA is also a most potent activator of macrophages. PMA activates murine macrophages directly to secrete many products including oxygen intermediates (5), plasminogen activator (22) and IL 1 (9). We therefore tested the capacity of human mononuclear cells (MNC) incubated for 48 hrs with PMA and various analogues to produce mitogenic IL 1 activity for murine (C3H/HeJ) thymocytes (Table 1). While several of these compounds induced the production of a thymocyte mitogenic activity by the MNC, neither the parent phorbol compounds nor any of the phorbol derivatives tested were directly mitogenic for thymocytes. The interpretation of these results are complicated by the fact that PMA is mitogenic for human T lymphocytes and can potentially induce them to produce IL 2, which is also mitogenic for murine thymocytes. However, supernatants of PMA stimulated MNC did not support the growth of an IL 2 dependent T cell line and therefore contained predominantly IL 1 uncontaminated by IL 2.

The parent phorbol molecule stimulated only low levels of IL 1 production by MNC. Phorbol dibenzoate (PDB) was moderately active, phorbol dibenzoate (PDD) more so and PMA was the most active in inducing MNC to produce thymocyte mitogenic activity. The capacity of the various congeners of PMA to induce IL 1 production correlates with their capacity to induce inflammatory reactions and promote tumor growth since PMA > PDD > PDB is the order of activity in all these assays and phorbol is inactive. This suggests that the capacity of PMA to activate macrophages, as indicated by the production of growth factors, correlates with its tumor promoting capacity, despite its immunostimulating effects.

TABLE 1. Effect of Phorbol Derivatives on Il 1
Production by Human MNC

Stimulant of cultured MNC[*]	Dose µg/ml	^{3}H TdR Incorporation by C3H/HeJ thymocytes	
		118 dil. of MNC sup	Stimulant only
None	–	242 ± 42[**]	122 ± 6
Phorbol	1.0	760 ± 335	150 ± 4
"	0.1	3,000 ± 921	N.D.
"	0.01	3,400 ± 1,142	N.D.
Phorbol myristic acetate (PMA)	1.0	63,033 ± 8,253	272 ± 32
	0.1	34,202 ± 1,400	N.D.
	0.01	3,478 ± 507	N.D.
Phorbol dide-canoate (PDD)	1.0	69,159 ± 9,538	127 ± 5
	0.1	9,147 ± 1,125	N.D.
	0.01	2,044 ± 415	N.D.
Phorbol dibenzoate (PDB)	1.0	51,599 ± 1,998	108 ± 14
	0.1	793 ± 269	N.D.
	0.01	1,153 ± 269	N.D.

[*] 4×10^6 MNC/ml cultured for 48 hrs.

[**] Mean ± S.E.M of ^{3}H TdR incorporated in cpm.

INDIRECT MACROPHAGE ACTIVATION

Phytohemagglutinin (PHA), a classical T lymphocyte mitogen which
induces lymphocyte-derived IL 2 production, to our surprise, also
induced the production of IL 1 (8). Direct stimulation of the P388D$_1$
macrophage cell line with PHA results in little or no IL 1 production
nor does the addition of unstimulated lymphocytes to the cell line
cells. However, when either syngeneic DBA/2 mouse or xenogeneic
guinea pig lymphocytes were pulsed with PHA and added to the P388D$_1$
macrophages, considerable thymocyte mitogenic factor production
ensued. This activity was macrophage-derived IL 1 rather than lymphocyte derived IL 2 since in this study the guinea pig lymphocyte
derived mitogenic factor did not induce mouse thymocyte proliferation.
Therefore, this induction of IL 1 production was not genetically
restricted and was based on an indirect lymphocyte-mediated process.
The explanation for these findings remains unclear, but other studies,
as will be discussed, suggest that lymphokines and or cell contact
mediated mechanisms may account for the PHA induced IL 1 production.

Cytokine Mediated Macrophage Activation

The supernatants of antigen stimulated spleen cell cultures contain a factor that activates adherent mouse peritoneal cells and P388D$_1$ macrophages to produce IL 1 activity (7). Since these supernatants also activated macrophages to become tumoricidal, this lymphokine was hypothesized to be a macrophage activating factor (7). However, it has also been observed that L-cell line as well as lymphocyte-derived mediators can activate macrophages to produce IL 1. Chromatographic analysis of supernatants of the L-cell as well as concanavalin A (Con A) stimulated murine spleen cells revealed that these mediators have the characteristics of colony stimulating factor (CSF) and that these IL 1 inducing activities could be inhibited by antibody to CSF (10). In addition, purified L-cell CSF (provided by R. K. Shadduck) induced macrophage IL 1 production. Thus, genetically unrestricted immunologically nonspecific cytokines can induce macrophages to produce IL 1.

Cell-Contact Dependent Macrophage Activation

Lymphocytes activated by antigens can also activate macrophage IL 1 production in a cell-contact dependent, genetically restricted manner (1). Unanue and coworkers (21) have reported that murine T lymphocytes sensitized to Listeria monocytogenes can, in conjunction with the bacterial antigen, activate macrophages to produce a factor that is mitogenic for thymocytes. Neither the bacterial antigen nor the lymphocytes by themselves had an effect. The induction process exhibited antigen specificity since neither unsensitized lymphocytes nor unrelated antigen activated the macrophages. The effect is apparently not due to a mediator since separation of the sensitized lymphocytes and Listeria from the macrophages by a cell-impermeable membrane blocks the effect. The most intriguing observation is that only syngeneic lymphocytes which share the Ia subregion of the H-2 complex with the macrophages were effective in activating macrophages. This requirement for Ia region homology in cell contact dependent, lymphocyte-macrophage interactions is the mirror image of the genetic restriction of macrophage-lymphocyte interaction that is seen in antigen presentation. This suggests the possibility that such interactions may occur simultaneously and be bidirectional.

Thus, stimulation of lymphocytes can indirectly result in the activation of macrophages by either Ia restricted cell-contact or mediator-dependent pathways. Such activated macrophages exhibit more active secretory and metabolic processes which presumably can enhance their anti-tumor effects.

Cytokine Induced Differentiation of Macrophages

Stimulants that enhance macrophage differentiation presumably also have the capacity to enhance their anti-tumor activity. In this regard it has been observed that lymphokine-rich culture supernatants of Con A stimulated mouse spleen cells induce the appearance of membrane receptors for Fc (FcR) on macrophages from LPS resistant C3H/HeJ mice, thus normalizing their capacity to bind and phagocytose IgG antibody coated sheep erythrocytes (23). (Table 2). This activity of the lymphokine rich supernatant can be mimicked by highly purified β

TABLE 2. FcR Dependent Phagocytosis of Opsonized
Sheep Erythrocytes by C3H/HeJ Macrophages

Culture stimulant[1]	Phagocytosis (Mean $\pm$ S.E.M. cpm ^{51}Cr)
None	6,672 $\pm$ 545
Con A supernatant (1:10 dil)	17,677 $\pm$ 416
β interferon (10 u/ml)	21,568 $\pm$ 583
None	7,623 $\pm$ 554
Con A supernatant (CS) 1:20 dil)	12,433 $\pm$ 320
CS + anti γ interferon	3,177 $\pm$ 480
None	9,619 $\pm$ 944
Dibutyryl cAMP (10^{-4}M)	17,692 $\pm$ 330

1. Cultures performed in duplicate and incubated for 48 hrs prior to
   phagocytosis assay (23).

interferon (kindly provided by Dr. William Stewart), has the chromatographic properties of γ interferon (24) and is inhibitable by rabbit
antisera against partially purified γ interferon (kindly provided by
Dr. Howard Johnson via Dr. William Farrar). In contrast, purified CSF
(provided by Dr. R. Stanley) did not induce macrophage FcR expression,
The induction of C3H/HeJ macrophage FcR expression can be mimicked by
dibutyryl cAMP and cAMP agonist (25). The lymphokine rich supernatants also elevate the macrophage levels of intracellular cAMP, which
suggests that the lymphokine induced expression of FcR is mediated by
cAMP. Since interferon has also been shown to induce FcR on normal
murine macrophages (13) IF may thus enhance phagocytic functions and
potentially promote ADCC reactions (16).
     We also investigated whether macrophages could be induced to express
Ia antigen (Ia$^+$). This is an important phenotypic marker since Ia$^+$
but not Ia$^-$ macrophages are able to participate in cell contact
dependent lymphocyte activation (3). We observed that potent
macrophage stimulants such as LPS and CSF did not affect macrophage Ia
antigen expression, but that Con A induced spleen cell supernatants
induced a significant proportion (30-80%) of murine thioglycollate
elicited peritoneal macrophages to become Ia$^+$ (19). Furthermore, up
to 90% of P388D$_1$ Ia$^-$ cell line macrophages incubated for two to four
days with the lymphokine rich supernatants also become Ia$^+$ (Table 3).
In addition to exhibiting this phenotypic change, the Ia$^+$ P388D$_1$
macrophages developed the functional capability of serving as active
stimulator cells in an MLR. Thus, in contrast with the non-stimulatory
capacity of untreated P388D$_1$ cells, the Ia$^+$ became able to induce
lymphoproliferative reactions to alloantigens. As was observed for FcR,
the induction of Ia expression by macrophages may also be mediated by
IF (Table 4). Induction of Ia expression by lymphokine-rich supernatants was blocked by the anti γ interferon antiserum (18) and
could be mimicked by murine fibroblast supernatants containing β
interferon. CSF failed to induce this conversion.

TABLE 3. INCUBATION OF P388D[1] MACROPHAGES WITH CON A SUPERNATANT
INCREASES THEIR Ia ANTIGEN EXPRESSION

Diluttion of Con A sup	Con A sup[3] A.TH anti-A.TL serum[5]	Mean cytotoxicity index $\pm$ S.E.M[2]	
		Con A sup Balb/c anti-CKB serum[6]	Control sup[4] A.TH anti-A.TL serum[5]
1:20	89.5 + 3.6	0	2.1 + 2.1
1:80	90.6 + 2.8	0	7.0 + 2.7
1:320	45.9 + 4.8	0	3.5 + 3.5
1:1280	31.8 + 1.8	0	6.9 + 3.5

1. 5×10^3 P388D[1] (Ia^d) cells were incubated in 200 µl supernatants in
enriched McCoy's 5-a medium for five days and the percentage of Ia
cells determined by antiserum and complement mediated cytotoxicity.
2. Cultures performed in quadruplicate.
3. Concanavalin A stimulated spleen cell supernatant, prepared with
C3H/HeN (Ia^k) spleen cells.
4. Control spleen cell supernatant supplemented with Con A, prepared
from CeH/HeN Ia^k) spleen cells.
5. Detects both k and d haplotypes.
6. Detects k, but not d haplotypes.

TABLE 4. P388D[1] Macrophage Ia Antigen Expression[1] Induced by
β Interferon Containing L Cell Supernatant

L cell supernatant added (Units β interferon/ml[2])	Mean cytotoxicity index $\pm$ S.E.M[3] (A.TH anti-A.TL + complement)
2.0	31.0 + 1.9
0.5	26.4 + 2.4
0.125	11.8 + 1.8
0.031	0
None	0

1. 5×10^3 P388D[1] macrophages were incubated for three days in 200 µl
IF (in enriched McCoy's 5-A medium) and the percentage of Ia$^+$ cells
determined.
2. Supernatant of L[929] cells induced with Poly I: Poly C (25 µg/ml) in
medium containing 100 µg/ml DEAE-dextran.
3. Cultures performed in triplicate.

Since Ia$^+$ but not Ia$^-$ macrophages can act as accessory cells in
the antigenic activation of lymphocytes, these observations suggest that
interferon produced by activated lymphocytes may by promoting macrophage Ia antigen expression, enhance antigen induced lymphocyte
activation, thus resulting in a positive feedback loop that may
facilitate specific tumor immunity (16).

CONCLUSION

Either immunoenhancing stimulants or the tumor antigens themselves, can by activating macrophages, augment the host response to tumors through mediator or cell-contact dependent bidirectional macrophage-lymphocyte interactions. We have described the means by which such macrophage-lymphocytes interacions lead to the generation of cytokines such as IL 1, CSF and IF. These endogenous signals by activating lymphocytes and promoting macrophage Ia and FcR expression enhance the capacity of these cells to maintain host integrity. The afferent limb of the immune response thus offers a multiplicity of opportunities for modifying the biological response.

REFERENCES

1. Beller,D.I.,Farr,A.G.,and Unanue,E.R.(1978): Fed.Proc.37:91-96.

2. Berenblum, I.(1969): Prog.Exp.Res.,11:21-30.

3. Cowing,C.,Pincus,S.H.,Sachs,D.H.,and Dickler,H.B.(1978): J.Immunol., 121:1680-1686.

4. Farrar,J.J.,Fuller-Farrar,J,Simmon,P.L.,Hilfiker,M.L.,Stadler,B.M., and Farrar,W.L.(1980). J.Immunol.,125:2555-2558.

5. Greenberger,J.S.,Newburger,P.E.,Karpas,A.,and Moloney,W.C.(1978.: Cancer Res.,38;3340-3348.

6. Mastro,A.M.,and Mueller,G.C.(1974): Exp.Cell.Res.,88:40-46.

7. Meltzer,M.S.,and Oppenheim,J.J.(1977). J.Immunol.,118:77-83.

8. Mizel,S,B.,Oppenheim,J.J.,and Rosenstreich,D.L.(1978): J.Immunol., 120:1497-1503.

9. Mizel,S.B.,Rosenstreich,D.L.,and Oppenheim,J.J.(1978): Cell.Immunol., 40:230-235.

10. Moore,R.N.,Oppenheim,J.J.,Farrar,J.J.,Carter,C.S.,Waheed,A.,and Shadduck,R.K.(1980): J.Immunol.,125:1302-1305.

11. Oppenheim,J.J.,Mizel,S.B.,and Meltzer,M.S.(1979): In: The Biology of Lymphokines, edited by S.Cohen,E.Pick,and J.J.Oppenheim,pp.7-11. Academic Press, New York.

12. Oppenheim,J.J.,Moore,R.,Melig-Meyling,G.,Togawa,A.,Wahl,S., Mathieson,B.,Dougherty,S.,and Carter,C.(1980: In Regulatory Role of Macrophages in Immunity,edited by E.R.Unanue,and A.S.Rosenthal, pp.379-398. Academic Press,New York.

13. Rabinowitch,M.,and Manejias,R.E.(1978): Cell.Immunol., 39:402-406..

14. Rosenstreich,D.L.,and Mizel,S.B.(1979): J. Immunol.,123:1749-1754.

15. Sauter,D.N.,Carter,C.,Katz,S.A.,and Oppenheim,J.J.(1981): Clin. Res."(in press)".

16. Schultz,R.M.(1980): In Lymphokine Reports 1:63-97.

17. Smith,K.A.,Lachman,L.B.,Oppenheim,J.J.,and Favata,M.D.(1980): J. Exp. Med.,151:1551-1556.

18. Steeg,P.,Moore,R.N.,and Oppenheim,J.J.(1981): Fed.Proc."(in press)".

19. Steeg,P.,Moore,R.N.,and Oppenheim,J.J.(1980): J.Exp.Med."(in press)".

20. Touraine,J.L.,Hadden,J.W.,Touraine,F.,Hadden,E.M.,Estensen R.,and Good,R.A.(1977): J.Exp.Med.,145:460-465.

21. Unanue,E.R.(1980): N.Eng.J.Med.,303:977-985.

22. Vassali,J.D.,Hamilton,J.,and Reich,E.(1971): Cell,11:695.

23. Vogel,S.N.,and Rosenstreich,D.L.(1979): J.Immunol.,123:2842-2850.

24. Vogel,S.N.,and Rosenstreich,D.L.(1981): Fed.Proc."(in press)".

25. Vogel,S.N.,Weedon,L.L.,Oppenheim,J.J.,and Rosenstreich,D.L.(1980): J.Immunol."(in press)".

ACKNOWLEDGEMENTS

We are grateful to Dr. Harvey Klein of the NIH Blood Bank for a plentiful supply of white blood cell buffy coats and to Dr. Monte Meltzer for his constructive critique of this manuscript.

Mediation of Cellular Immunity in Cancer by Immune Modifiers, edited by M. A. Chirigos et al., Raven Press, New York © 1981.

Macrophage Activation for Tumor Cytotoxicity: Characterization of Noncytotoxic Intermediates During Lymphokine Activation

Monte S. Meltzer, Luigi P. Ruco, Janis K. Lazdins, and Edward J. Leonard

Immunopathology Section, Laboratory of Immunobiology, Division of Cancer Biology and Diagnosis, National Cancer Institute, National Institutes of Health, Bethesda, Maryland 20205

Recent reports from several laboratories suggest that macrophage activation for nonspecific tumoricidal activity during an immune response occurs only after completion of a series of reactions (1,12,13). Development of macrophage tumoricidal activity may be analogous to blood coagulation or complement-mediated hemolysis in that the final event requires multiple reactions, each in a defined sequence. Initial reaction(s) are independent of the immune response per se and depend only upon inflammation. T-cells best able to release macrophage-active lymphokines(LK) nonspecifically but preferentially accumulate at inflammatory sites (7). Blood monocytes are also recruited or accumulate at inflammatory sites and there differentiate into competent mononuclear phagocytes. These immature, blood-derived inflammatory macrophages are 10-20 fold more responsive to lymphocyte-derived activation stimuli than cells in the resident tissue macrophage population (10). Activation of these inflammatory precursors to the fully cytotoxic macrophage effector cell requires completion of two additional reaction stages: macrophages must first be exposed to one stimulus to enter into a receptive or primed state in which they are not yet cytotoxic but can then respond or be triggered by certain other stimuli to develop full functional activity (11,12). The ultimate stimulus in this reaction sequence may in fact be contact between activated cytotoxic macrophages and tumor target cells (6).

It should be noted at the outset that completion of each of these intermediary reactions within the activation sequence (differentiation of monocyte precursors into inflammatory macrophages, exposure of inflammatory cells to priming stimuli, interaction of primed, noncytotoxic macrophages with trigger signals and contact between activated tumoricidal macrophages and sensitive target cells) must occur within a relatively short time interval (8-16 hr). Each stage of macrophage activation is completely dependent upon the simultaneous presence of localized activation signals and responsive cellular intermediates. The nature of the activation signal and the responsive cell differs from stage to stage. However, ability of these intermediary cells to

65

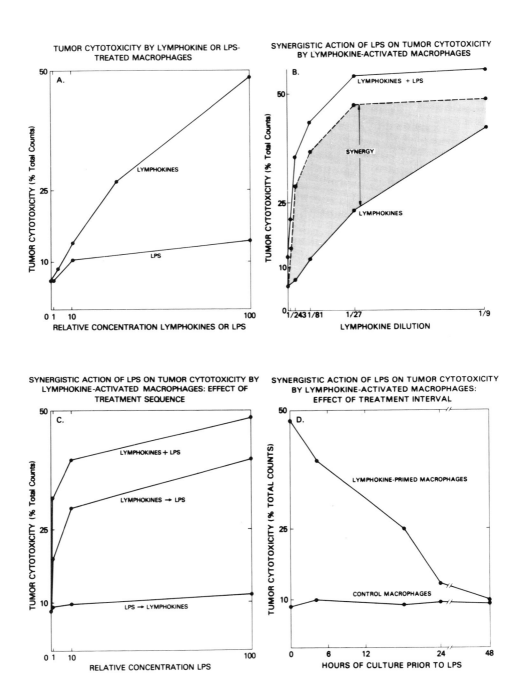

FIG.1. Synergistic action of LPS on tumor cytotoxicity by LK-activated macrophages.

respond to activation signals is short-lived and decays with time. Current evidence suggests that this loss of macrophage responsiveness occurs both in vivo and in vitro and is irreversible (8,9).

The interaction of LK and endotoxic lipopolysaccharides (LPS) from Gram-negative bacteria for development of macrophage tumoricidal activity provides a model regulatory system for control of macrophage effector function and illustrates many of the preceding points (1,12,13). Peritoneal exudate macrophages treated with as little as 1/30 dilution of LK for 4-8 hr prior to addition of tumor target cells were strongly cytotoxic (Figure-1A) (9). LPS, however, was much less effective than LK as an in vitro activation stimulus. In fact, tumor cytotoxicity by macrophages treated with up to 1 ug/ml LPS alone was minimal. Although macrophages treated with LPS alone had little or no cytotoxic activity, 1 ng/ml LPS (1000-fold less) significantly increased tumoricidal activity of LK-activated macrophages (Figure-1B) (4,12). The interaction of LPS and LK for development of macrophage cytotoxic activity was synergistic: if the slight direct effect of LPS is subtracted from the combined activity of LPS and LK throughout the LK dose-response, significant increases in cytotoxic activity persist (shaded area). This synergistic interaction was critically dependent upon treatment sequence (Figure-1C). Macrophages treated with suboptimal concentrations of LPS (1 ng/ml) or LK (1/300 dilution) alone had little or no tumoricidal activity. However, cells treated simultaneously with LK and LPS for 6 hr were strongly cytotoxic; macrophages treated first with LK for 5 hr and then with LPS for 1 hr were also tumoricidal. In contrast, cells treated with LPS for 1 hr and then exposed to LK for 5 hr showed little or no cytotoxic activity. Thus, macrophages exposed to low concentrations of LK are not cytotoxic but undergo changes to become receptive or primed to an LPS signal (trigger) and develop strong cytotoxic activity. The reverse treatment is ineffective (3,12). Furthermore, the synergistic effect of LPS on development of cytotoxic activity by LK-activated macrophages was also dependent upon treatment interval (Figure-1D). Macrophages primed by exposure to low concentrations of LK remained receptive to the LPS trigger for only a short time. LK-primed cells progressively lost ability to develop cytotoxic activity after LPS treatment with time in culture.

Activity in LK supernatants that activates inflammatory macrophages for nonspecific tumor cytotoxicity elutes from Sephadex G-100 as a single peak in the 50,000 mw region (Figure-2A). This activity is heat-labile (80% loss at 56°C/30 min), inactivated at pH $\leq$ 4 or $\geq$ 10 and sensitive to proteolytic enzymes (Pronase)(Figure-2B) (2,5). Macrophages cultured in low concentrations of LK fractions eluted from Sephadex G-100 failed to develop tumoricidal activity without an LPS trigger signal. The activity in LK supernatants that primes macrophages for the LPS trigger also elutes as a single peak in the 50,000 mw region.

That macrophages can be activated by LK alone at high concentrations (1/50) suggests an LPS-like signal may be present in these LK supernatants. (Figure-3). Macrophages cultured for 4 hr in low concentrations of LK (1/300) developed strong tumoricidal activity after exposure to 10 ng/ml LPS for 1 hr; LK or LPS treatment alone was inef-

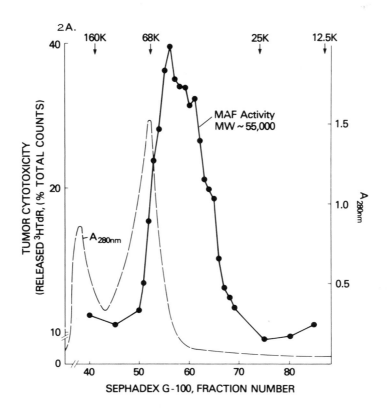

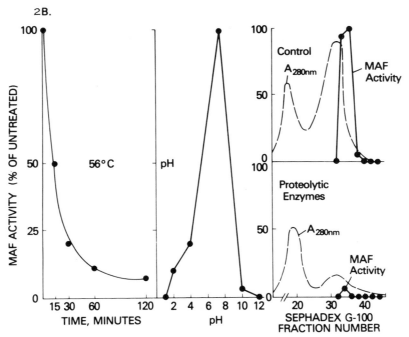

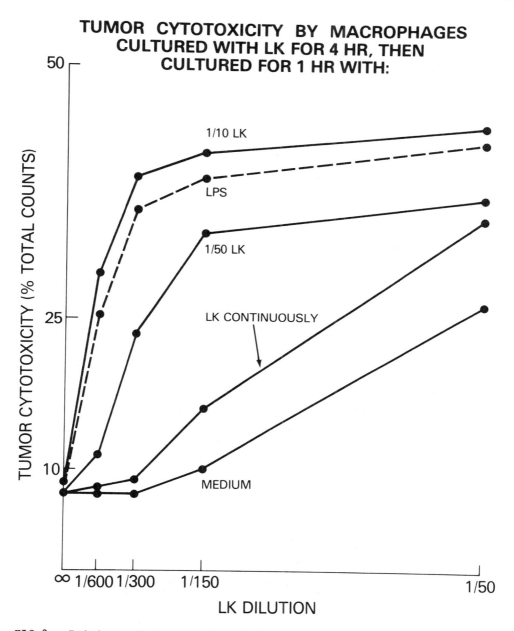

TUMOR CYTOTOXICITY BY MACROPHAGES CULTURED WITH LK FOR 4 HR, THEN CULTURED FOR 1 HR WITH:

TUMOR CYTOTOXICITY (% TOTAL COUNTS)

1/10 LK

LPS

1/50 LK

LK CONTINUOUSLY

MEDIUM

∞ 1/600 1/300 1/150 1/50

LK DILUTION

FIG.3. Priming and trigger signals in LK supernatants.

fective. Macrophages exposed to low concentrations of LK for 4 hr also developed strong tumoricidal activity after a 1 hr culture in high concentrations of LK (1/10 or 1/50). Again, either treatment alone was ineffective.

Culture manipulations associated with washing adherent macrophages had little or no effect on development of cytotoxic activity: tumor

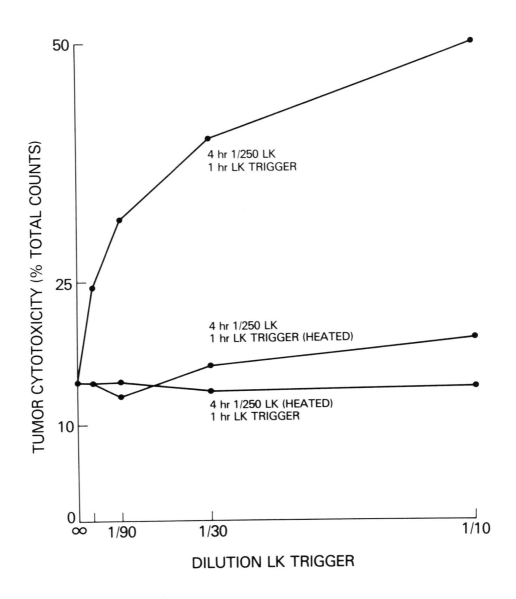

FIG. 4. Heat sensitivity of LK priming and trigger signals.

cytotoxicity by macrophages cultured continuously in 1/50 LK for 5 hr was comparable to that by macrophages cultured in 1/50 LK for 4 hr, washed in medium then cultured in 1/50 LK for an additional hr. It should be noted, however, that cytotoxic activity of macrophages cultured continuously in LK for 5 hr was slightly but reproducibly greater than that of cells incubated in LK for 4 hr and then in medium for 1 hr. This increased cytotoxic activity may reflect increased activation of

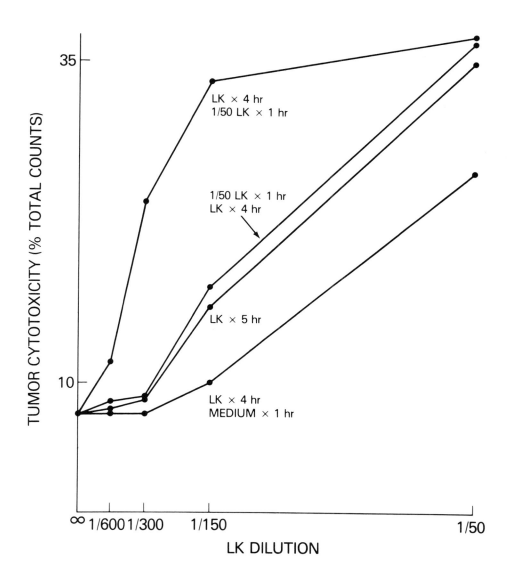

FIG.5. Priming and trigger signals in LK supernatants: effect of treatment sequence.

macrophages by LK during the additional hr (note that the length of time for optimal LK activation is about 8 to 12 hr) or loss of cytotoxic activity over the hr by LK-activated cells incubated in medium.

Thus, the preceding results show that with LK alone or with LK and LPS, macrophage activation can be divided into two stages: cells ex-

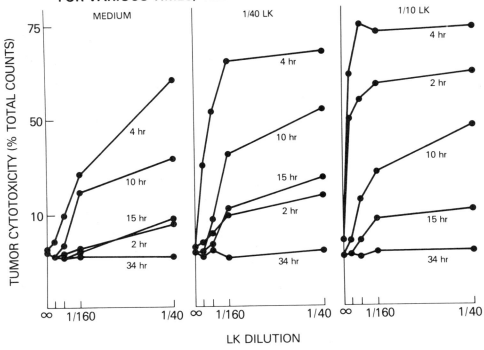

TUMOR CYTOTOXICITY BY MACROPHAGES CULTURED WITH LK FOR VARIOUS TIMES, THEN CULTURED FOR 1 HR WITH:

FIG.6. Time required for LK-primed macrophages to become receptive to LK trigger signals.

posed to one signal, such as low concentrations of LK, enter into a receptive or primed state in which they are not yet active but can then be triggered by another signal (LPS, high concentrations of LK) to develop full cytotoxic activity. LK with both priming and triggering activities have been characterized in supernatants of spleen cell preparations after either specific antigen- or mitogen-stimulation.

That the second LK signal (trigger) in this two stage regulatory system is not contaminating LPS can be demonstrated by two approaches. First, LPS activity in this system is heat stable. LPS trigger signals remain unaffected by temperatures as high as 80° to 100°C for 30 min (12,14). In contrast, both LK priming and triggering signals were completely destroyed by 60°C for 30 min (Figure-4). Second, we have previously shown that 5 to 25 ug/ml polymyxin B will inhibit the activity of up to 20 ug/ml LPS, but not that of LK (4,8). Similar effects of polymyxin B have been shown in other systems (14). In contrast, this antibiotic had little or no effect on either the priming or trigger signals in LK supernatants.

We have described an obligate treatment sequence for development of tumor cytotoxicity by macrophages treated with LK and LPS: strong

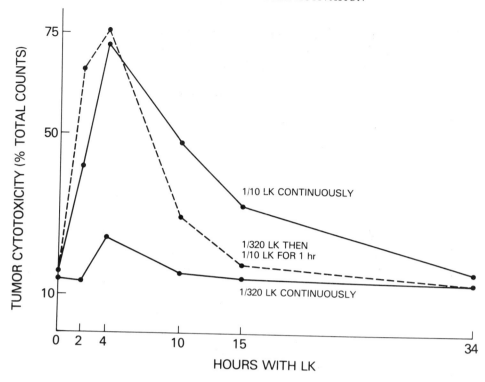

FIG.7. Tumor cytotoxicity by LK-activated macrophages.

tumoricidal activity was evident with cells treated simultaneously with LPS and LK or with cells treated first with LK and then with LPS; macrophages treated with LPS before LK treatment, however, had little or no cytotoxic activity. Similar effects of treatment sequence were shown with macrophages treated with LK alone (Figure-5). Optimal development of tumoricidal activity occurred with macrophages treated (primed) with low concentrations of LK and then treated (triggered) with high concentrations. For example, tumor cytotoxicity by macrophages treated with 1/150 LK for 4 hr and then 1/50 LK for 1 hr was equivalent to that by cells treated with 1/50 LK for the full 5 hr. In contrast, cells treated with 1/50 LK for 1 hr and then with 1/150 LK for 4 hr were much less cytotoxic. The effect of treatment sequence was evident throughout the LK dose-response.

Macrophages cultured in low concentrations of LK require an optimal time to develop receptiveness to LK trigger signals (Figure-6). Cells were cultured in dilutions of LK for 2 to 3 hr, washed and exposed to 1/10 or 1/40 LK for an additional hr. The optimal response by these primed macrophages to the LK trigger signal was observed after 4 hr of LK treatment. Ability of LK-primed macrophages to respond to LK trigger signals and develop cytotoxic activity decreased with time in culture so that by 15 to 34 hr these cells were unresponsive.

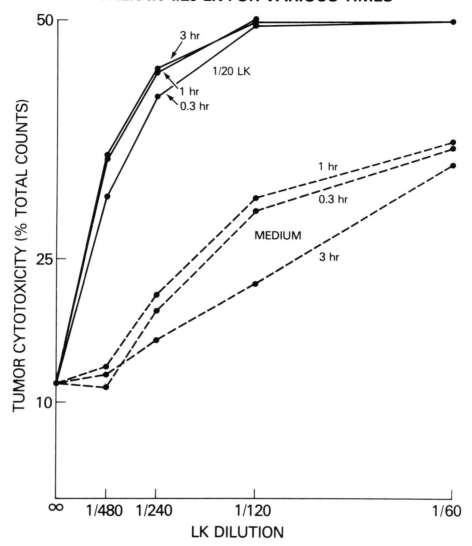

**TUMOR CYTOTOXICITY BY MACROPHAGES
CULTURED WITH LK DILUTIONS FOR 4 HR,
THEN IN 1/20 LK FOR VARIOUS TIMES**

FIG.8. Time required for LK-primed macrophages to respond to LK trigger
signals.

It should also be noted that macrophages continuously incubated in
low concentrations of LK do not develop significant levels of cytotoxic
activity at any time through 34 hr (Figure-7). For example, macrophages cultured continuously in 1/320 LK show only weak cytotoxic
activity throughout 34 hr. Yet macrophages cultured in 1/320 LK for
various times and then exposed to 1/10 LK for only 1 hr behave compara-

**TUMOR CYTOTOXICITY BY MACROPHAGES CULTURED IN
LK FOR 4HR, THEN IN LK FOR 1 HR: EFFECT OF TEMPERATURE**

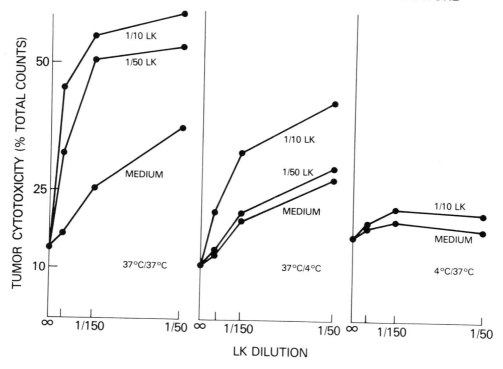

FIG. 9. Tumor cytotoxicity by LK-primed macrophages exposed to LK trigger signals: effect of temperature.

bly, in terms of both time course and levels of cytotoxic activity, to cells continuously incubated in 1/10 LK.

The optimal time required for LK-primed macrophages to be exposed to LK trigger signals was less than 20 min (Figure-8). Macrophages cultured in LK dilutions for 4 hr and then incubated in the LK trigger for various times responded maximally by 20 min. This maximal response to the LK trigger persists through 3 hr. Even though the response of LK-primed macrophages to LK trigger signals was relatively rapid compared to the 4 hr priming interval, both macrophage responses to LK were temperature dependent (Figure-9). Tumor cytotoxicity by macrophages primed at 37°C and then exposed to the LK trigger at 4°C was much less than that by cells treated with both signals at 37°C. Macrophages primed at 4°C and then exposed to the LK trigger at 37°C showed little or no cytotoxic activity. The effects of temperature were not due to loss of macrophage viability: no differences in LK dose-response were detected between cells treated for 5 hr with LK at 37°C and cells held at 4°C for 5 hr and then treated with LK for 5 hr at 37°C.

Operationally, LK supernatants contain priming signals effective at low concentrations and trigger signals effective only at high concentrations. To date, however, we have been unable to separate priming and trigger signals in LK supernatants by physicochemical characteristics: both activities are heat-labile; both elute from Sephadex G-100 in the 50,000 mw region. Priming and trigger signals in LK supernatants, while functionally different, could result from interactions of macrophages with a single molecular species: inflammatory mononuclear phagocytes would bind or respond to this molecule and undergo a series of changes (alterations in number or affinity of surface receptors, development of new intracellular effector compartments or of coupling systems to transduce receptor signals to effector compartments) that transform the cell into a competent intermediate; this intermediate receives signals from the same molecule to become an activated tumoricidal macrophage. By any of these mechanisms, the LK priming and trigger signals described here form the basis of regulatory system that sets the threshold and determines the onset of macrophage effector function.

REFERENCES

1. Hibbs, J.B.,Jr., Taintor, R.R., Chapman, H.A.,Jr. and Weinberg,J.B. (1977): <u>Science</u> 197:279-282.
2. Leonard, E.J., Ruco, L.P. and Meltzer, M.S. (1978): <u>Cell.Immunol.</u> 41:347-357.
3. Meltzer, M.S., Ruco, L.P., Boraschi, D. and Nacy, C.A. (1979): <u>J.Reticuloendothel.Soc.</u> 26:403-415.
4. Meltzer, M.S., Ruco, L.P. and Leonard, E.J. (1980): <u>Adv.Exp.Med. Biol.</u> 121:381-398.
5. Meltzer, M.S., Wahl, L.M., Leonard, E.J. and Nacy, C.A. (1980): In: <u>Proceedings of the Second International Lymphokine Workshop</u>, edited by A.L. de Weck, pp. 161-168. Academic Press, New York.
6. Marino, P.A. and Adams, D.O. (1980): <u>Cell.Immunol.</u> 54:26-37.
7. Rosenstreich, D.L., Blake, J.T. and Rosenthal, A.S. (1971): <u>J.Exp. Med.</u> 134:1170-1178.
8. Ruco, L.P. and Meltzer, M.S. (1977): <u>Cell.Immunol.</u> 32:203-215.
9. Ruco, L.P. and Meltzer, M.S. (1977): <u>J.Immunol.</u> 119:889-896.
10. Ruco, L.P. and Meltzer, M.S. (1978): <u>J.Immunol.</u> 120:1054-1062.
11. Ruco, L.P. and Meltzer, M.S. (1978): <u>Cell.Immunol.</u> 41:35-51.
12. Ruco, L.P. and Meltzer, M.S. (1978): <u>J.Immunol.</u> 121:2035-2042.
13. Russel, S.W., Doe, W.F. and McIntosh, A.T. (1977): <u>J.Exp.Med.</u> 146:1511-1546.
14. Weinberg, J.B., Chapman, H.A.,Jr. and Hibbs, J.B.,Jr. (1978): <u>J.Immunol.</u> 121:72-80.

*Mediation of Cellular Immunity in Cancer by
Immune Modifiers*, edited by M. A. Chirigos
et al., Raven Press, New York © 1981.

In Vivo Correlation of Macrophage Tumoricidal Activity, Natural Killer Cell Augmentation, and Delayed Type Hypersensitivity by Immune Modifiers

Michael A. Chirigos, Anna Bartocci, and Elizabeth Read

Viruses and Disease Modification Section, Division of Cancer Treatment, National Cancer Institute, National Institutes of Health, Bethesda, Maryland 20205

INTRODUCTION

The vital role of the cellular elements of the immune system in host defense against neoplasia, as well as infectious organisms, has been amply demonstrated. Immune modifiers have the potential to benefit man in the treatment of, not only cancer, but also in immuno deficiency, chronic infections, and autoimmunity. There appears to be a close relationship between the ability of biologic and synthetic agents to enhance host antitumor resistance and their capacity to stimulate or enhance specific cellular components of the immune system, e.g., macrophage, natural killer cells (NKC), T-cells and B-cells. Increasing evidence suggests that the activated macrophage and enhanced natural killer cell are major effectors of tumor surveillance. It then becomes important to better understand the mechanism by which the biologic and chemical immune modifying agents are involved in the pharmacological control of the cellular components of the immune system. By judiciously controlling macrophage or natural killer cell activity to express a tumoricidal or tumorstatic effect, through agents capable of enhancing this effect, it is possible to combine a tumor cytoreductive therapy with a macrophage activating or NK cell enhancing agent leading to a more marked decrease in primary tumor or metastatic disease.

This chapter describes the immunological and tumor responses achieved with several immune modifiers employing two tumor systems. An attempt was made to correlate the beneficial effect achieved when the immune modifying agent was combined with cytoreductive therapy.

MATERIALS AND METHODS

Tumor Cell Lines

Tumor cell lines were maintained <u>in vitro</u> in RPMI-1640 supplemented with 10% fetal calf serum and 50 µg/ml gentamycin (M109 alveolar carcinoma, which arose spontaneously in a BALB/c mouse; YAC-1, a Moloney virus induced lymphoma of A/sn origin; and MBL-2, a Moloney virus inducer leukemia of C57 Bl/6 origin. For *in vivo* studies the *in vivo* passaged tumor cell lines were used (M109 and MBL-2).

Mouse Strains Used

BALB/c males were used for M109 studies; C57 Bl/6 males were used for MBL-2 tumor studies; and CD_2F_1 male mice were used for interferon induction studies, DTH response and macrophage and NK cell *in vivo* studies. All mice were obtained from the Mammalian Genetics and Animal Production Section, DCT, National Cancer Institute, NIH, Bethesda, MD. All animals weighed at least 23 gm and were 6-8 weeks old before they were used for experimentation.

Assay Procedures

Natural Killer (NK) Cytotoxicity Assay

A conventional ^{51}Cr release assay was employed as previously described (8). In brief, $2.0x10^4$ radiolabeled tumor cells (100μCi of ^{51}Cr, SA 250-800 mCi/mg, per $1.0x10^7$ tumor cells at 37°C for 45 minutes) in 0.1 ml volume were added to graded numbers of splenic effector cells in round bottom 96-well microliter plates. Triplicate cultures were maintained in a humidified CO_2-in air incubator at 37° for 4 hours. At the end of the incubation period the plates were centrifuged for 10 minutes at 800xg and a volume of 0.1 ml of supernatant was removed and measured in a γ-counter. The percent cytotoxicity was calculated from the formula:

$$\% \text{ specific lysis} = \frac{\text{Experimental CPM} - \text{SR CPM}}{\text{MR CPM} - \text{SR CPM}} \times 100$$

SR: Spontaneous Release was determined by incubation of $2.0x10^4$ tumor cells in 0.2 ml of RPMI-1640. MR: Maximum release of radioactivity was determined by freezing and thawing of $2.0x10^4$ tumor cells, four times in an acetone-dry ice bath.

Macrophage Activation Assay

Our previously described technique (10) was used to measure the ability of the test agents to produce growth inhibitory macrophages. Briefly, for the *in vivo* macrophage activation the agents were administered i.p. on day 0. Peritoneal Exudate cells (PEC) were harvested on D1, D3 and D6. Approximately $8x10^5$ activated macrophages were seeded onto 16 mm wells and incubated at 37°C in an atmosphere of 5% CO_2 in air for two hours. The monolayers were then washed three times with RPMI-1640 to eliminate nonadherent cells. The remaining adherent monolayers were overlaid with approximately $8x10^4$ viable MBL-2 cells. The ratio of macrophages to tumor cells was 10:1 at the beginning of each experiment. All cultures were again incubated for 48 hours and viable MBL-2 cells were determined by trypan blue dye exclusion. The percent inhibition of MBL-2 cells due to macrophage interaction was calculated by:

$$\% \text{ inhibition} = 1 - \frac{\text{Mean of MBL-2 cells from drug treated macrophages}}{\text{Mean of MBL-2 cells from nontreated macrophages}} \times 100$$

Delayed Hypersensitivity Reaction

The DTH reaction was studied in 8-10 week old CD_2F_1 male mice. Sheep red blood cells (SRBC) were washed 3 times with sterile PBS and brought to a concentration of 1×10^9 cells per ml. Experimental groups received test agent intraperitoneally in a 0.25 ml volume. On day 0, mice were injected s.c. with 1×10^8 SRBCs into the left hind footpad. Test agent was given either on day 0 or prior to day 0 intraperitoneally. On day 4, 1×10^8 SRBC were injected s.c. into the right hind footpad; 24 hours later the thickness of both footpads was measured with a gravity-sensitive calibrated measuring device and the thickness of both footpads recorded. The time intervals selected between the sensitizing and challenging doses as well as the concentration of SRBC used were those that were found to be optimal.

Interferon Assay

CD_2F_1 male mice were injected intraperitoneally with test agent and bled at various time intervals. Serum was collected for assay of interferon by a modification of the micro CPE inhibition method previously described (1) employing L929 mouse cells and vesicular stomatitis virus.

RESULTS

Six agents which have been reported to possess the capacity to exert an immune modulating effect were examined for their capacity to: (1) exert an antitumor effect; (2) activate macrophage tumoricidal activity; (3) induce host interferon; (4) augment NK cell cytotoxicity; and (5) enhance delayed type hypersensitivity (DTH) to sheep red blood cells.

Results in Table 1 show that interferon, MVE$_2$, Poly ICLC and Cytoxan treatment resulted in significant increases in median survival time of MBL-2 tumor inoculated mice. This increase in survival time correlated with the capacity of interferon, MVE2 and Poly ICLC to enhance macrophage tumoricidal activity.

TABLE 1

Correlation of Antitumor Activity, Enhanced Macrophage Tumoricidal

Activity and Interferon Induction by Various Immune Modifiers

Treatment[a]	Increase in MST 0/0[b]	Macrophage Cytotoxicity 0/0[c]	Maximum IF Titer at Indicated Time and Drug Dosed
Cytoxan, 50 mg/kg	140	Not Tested	Not Tested
Interferon, 10^5 U/mouse	270	94	–
MVE2, 25 mg/kg	270	90	500U (48 hrs) 100 mg/kg
Poly ICLC, 4, mg/kg	220	72	2,500U (24 hrs) 4 mg/kg
Levan, 10 mg/kg	120	50	300U (48 hrs) 100 mg/kg
Mannozym, 1 mg/kg	120	16	400U (72 hrs) 100 mg/kg
Lentinan, 5 mg/kg	130	0	300U (48 hrs) 100 mg/kg

[a] 10^6 MBL-2 leukemia cells inoculated i.p. into C57 B1/6 mice and treated daily i.p. with agent for 5 consecutive days.

[b] Percent increase in median survival time calculated with the formula $\frac{\text{MST treated}}{\text{MST non-treated}}$ X 100 = % increase

[c] Macrophage tumoricidal activity: % inhibition of MBL-2 leukemia cell replication above tumor bearing control values. Mice sacrificed on day 6.

[d] CD_2F_1 mice inoculated i.p. with drug and exsanguinated at different time periods (up to 72 hrs) for serum.

All the test agents were found to induce interferon detectable in serum at various time intervals. MVE2 and Poly ICLC induced the highest titers of interferon which correlated with their capacity to exert an antitumor effect and enhance macrophage tumoricidal activity.

The six agents were again tested for their capacity to enhance macrophage tumoricidal activity and augment NK cytotoxicity (Table 2). Animals were sacrificed at different time intervals after treatment for testing peritoneal macrophage and splenic NK cell activity. Mannozym, MVE2 and Poly ICLC significantly enhanced both macrophage tumoricidal activity and NK cell cytotoxicity. Levan treatment resulted in only macrophage enhancement. The peak activity varied with each agent. Mannozym and MVE2 effects peaked at 72 hours and Poly ICLC at 24 hours. It is of interest that these peak times of activity correlate with the peak time of interferon levels but for the exception of Levan. Macrophage tumoricidal activity enhanced by Levan, however, was relatively high over the 6 day observation.

TABLE 2

Response of Macrophages and Natural Killer Cell Activity after

In Vivo Treatment with Immune Modifiers

Test Agent	Dose mg/kg	Day 1		Day 3		Day 6	
		$M\phi$ [a]	NK [b]	$M\phi$	NK	$M\phi$	NK
Levan	50	63	8	68	12	81[c]	7
Lentinan	100	37	9	17	11	65	9
Mannozym	4	16	8	95[d]	25[c]	20	7
MVE2	25	15	2	93[d]	15[c]	91[c]	5
Poly ICLC	4	75[d]	50[d]	50	20	30	3

[a]Macrophage tumoricidal activity: % inhibition of MBL-2 leukemic cell replication above normal control values.

[b]Natural Killer Cell augmentation: % cytotoxicity above controls inoculated with PBS. Target cells (YAC). Effector: Target cell ratio of 100:1.

[c]$p<0.002$.

[d]$p<0.001$.

The delayed type hypersensitivity response (DTHR) is considered a good model for measuring the cellular immune response (Table 3). All six agents were found to enhance the DTHR significantly.

TABLE 3

Augmentation of Delayed Type Hypersensitivity

by Immune Modifiers

SRBC	Treatment[a] Test Agent	Dose mg/kg	Day[b]	Footpad Swelling (mm)	P values
D0	Saline	–	0	0.24	
D0	Interferon	$1 \times 10^5 U^c$	0	0.41	<0.01
D0	Levan	50	–6	0.48	<0.001
D0	Lentinan	100	–6	0.54	<0.001
D0	Mannozym	4	–3	0.42	<0.01
D0	MVE2	25	–3	0.55	<0.001
D0	Poly ICLC	4	–1	0.50	<0.001

[a]Treatment with test agent was by the i.p. route.

[b]Day of treatment which gave maximum response for each agent. Minus sign (–) denotes treatment prior to first challenge with SRBC.

[c]Units of interferon injected per mouse.

MVEs of various molecular weights were examined for their macrophage activating capacity (Fig. 1).

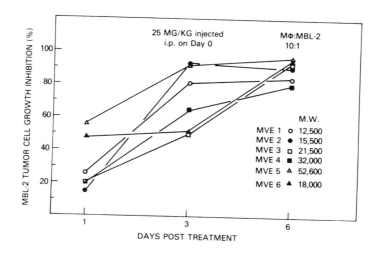

Fig. 1. Activation of tumoricidal macrophages _in vivo_ by treatment with MVEs.

Significant increases in macrophage tumoricidal activity was observed with the 6 MVEs. Maximum effect was achieved by the sixth day after treatment. These results confirm that the MVEs activate macrophage _in vivo_, and when tested for their tumoricidal activity on MBL-2 leukemia cells _in vitro_, an 80 to 95% tumoricidal effect is achieved. At the peak time of macrophage activity (day 6 post treatment), no preferential effect on activity based on molecular weight was apparent.

The alveolar carcinoma M109 cell line was employed to assess whether the tumor retarding effect associated with MVE treatment could be related to macrophage activated tumoricidal activity. BALB/c mice were inoculated s.c. with the M109 tumor and distributed to MVE2 treated and placebo treated groups. Mice were continuously monitored for survival and growth of local tumor. In addition, treated and control mice were sacrificed for peritoneal macrophages which were tested _in vitro_ for their tumoricidal activity on MBL-2 tumor cells.

Results in Fig. 2 (Panel D) show that all 6 MVEs were effective in increasing survival time over placebo treated controls and macrophage tumoricidal activity was markedly increased after only one treatment. In the corollary study (Panels A, B and C), tumor growth was markedly repressed till after the third treatment (A). The rate of death resulting from tumor correlated with the rate of tumor growth (C). Of particular interest was the host macrophage response (Panel B). Macrophage tumoricidal activity of tumor bearing controls increased slowly and represent an "armed" macrophage response. In contrast, macrophage

activity was markedly enhanced in the treated tumor bearing mice. A 64
to 78 tumoricidal activity was expressed by macrophages harvested at
days 10, 17 and 24, but markedly decreased by day 31 after the fourth
treatment. The three parameters appeared to coincide, i.e., increase
in rate of tumor growth, rate of death and decrease in macrophage
tumoricidal activity. Whether macrophages become hyporesponsive to MVE
treatment and lose their tumoricidal capacity is presently under investigation.

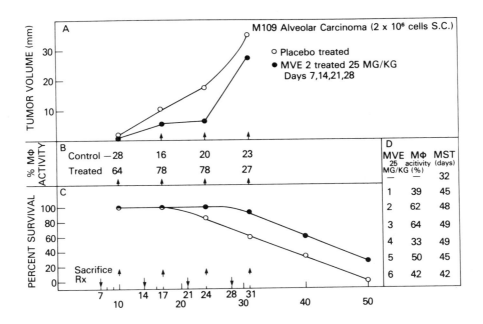

Fig. 2. Effect of MVE treatment on M109 tumor growth, survival time,
and macrophage activity.

A highly beneficial antitumor effect was achieved when MVE2 and MVE6
were combined with Cytoxan cytoreductive therapy. Treatment with increasing concentrations of Cytoxan resulted in persistent increases
in survival time of mice inoculated with MBL-2 leukemia (Fig. 3). One
treatment with MVE2 or 6 was ineffective. In contrast, remarkable
synergism was achieved when Cytoxan was combined with MVE treatment.
In every case where Cytoxan was combined with single or multiple
treatment with MVE, the combined treatment led to significant increases
in survival time and in most cases, a large percentage of animals surviving greater than the 50 day observation period.

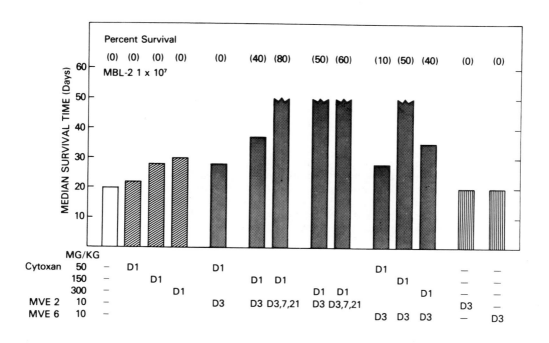

Fig. 3. Combination of marginally effective Cytoxan chemotherapy and immune modifier resulting in a strong synergistic effect against MBL-2 leukemia.

DISCUSSION

It is of interest to note that of the six immune modifiers tested, those which exerted a significant antitumor effect were also potent macrophage activators. Since direct exposure of MBL-2 tumor cells to the 3 most active agents (i.e., interferon, MVE2, Poly ICLC) in vitro does not result in appreciable cell death, the cytoreductive effect achieved in vivo appears to be due to activated macrophages exerting a nonspecific, but selective, tumor cell cytotoxicity. Results of previous studies show that interferon or MVE6 treatment in MBL-2 inoculated mice results in a significant increase in the number of dead tumor cells in peritoneal exudates as well as the recovery of markedly activated tumoricidal macrophages from the same peritoneal exudates (3). It is tempting to speculate that the response achieved with MVE2 and Poly ICLC, and to some degree Levan, may be due to their capacity to induce interferon. From previous studies it was established that the capacity of interferon inducers to activate macrophages was selectively neutralized by anti-interferon antibody (11). These results established the important role that endogenously generated interferon plays in in macrophage function. The lower antitumor and macrophage activation effects achieved by Levan, Mannozym and Lentinan may be due to the lower doses used in the treatment regimen compared to the higher doses used in testing the capacity of these agents to induce interferon.

Mannozym, MVE2, and Poly ICLC were effective in both enhancing macrophage activity and augmenting NK cell cytotoxicity. Augmentation of mouse NK cell cytotoxicity was reported to occur with pyran Poly IC and interferon (2,6,7,9,12). Results in the present study show that Mannozym, Poly ICLC (a polyinosinic:polycytidylic acid stabilized with poly-L-lysine) and MVE2 (a low molecular weight pyran) also augment NK cell cytotoxicity. This augmented effect on both NK cells and macrophages could be due to the ability of these agents to induce endogenous interferon.

The DTH response can be used as an *in vivo* model to moniter the cellular immune response of an animal. All six agents significantly stimulated the DTH response indicating them to be effective *in vivo* stimulators of T-cells. MVE6 has been reported to reconstitute the depressed T-cell population of tumor bearing mice (15) and mice exposed to whole body irradiation (16). Poly ICLC has also been shown capable of enhancing the mitogenic response of splenic lymphocytes to PHA (5).

Based on enhanced macrophage tumoricidal activity, the degree of activity attained by the 6th day after treatment by each of the MVEs, did not appear to distinguish one from the other. All six were found to be equally effective in macrophage enhancement as well as augmenting NK cell cytotoxicity (2), stimulating the DTH response or serving as adjuvants to tumor cell vaccines (4).

Of particular interest was the correlation noted between the tumor growth retarding effect of MVE2 treatment resulting in longer survival time to enhanced macrophage tumoricidal activity. Since these results were achieved with MVE2 monotherapy, it would appear that macrophage activation was instrumental in retarding the growth of the tumor. Snodgrass *et al.* (14) studied the histopathology of C57 B1/6 mice bearing the Lewis lung carcinoma and treated with pyran (MVE6). The mice treated with pyran, in contrast to controls, were characterized by a shift from a predominance of neutrophils to a predominance of histiocytes and lymphocytes in the connective tissue of the subcutaneous tumor. Similarly, marked infiltration of macrophages and lymphocytes were found surrounding the M109 tumor in mice treated with pyran (13). The rate of growth of the 16/C mammary adinocarcinoma was also shown to be markedly depressed by the intralisional treatment with MVE2 and MVE6 (3).

The remarkable synergistic antitumor effect achieved against the MBL-2 tumor could be due to Cytoxan's cytoreductive effect decreasing the number of tumor cells significantly, and the residual tumor cells, escaping Cytoxan cytotoxicity, were subsequently killed by the combined MVE activated tumoricidal macrophages and augmented NK cell cytotoxicity.

The bulk of evidence to date indicates that when immune modifying agents, particularly macrophage activators, T-cell restorative agents and NK cell augmenting agents, are combined with cytoreductive therapy (chemotherapy, surgery or irradiation) a more beneficial response is achieved. The future successful use of immunoregulating agents in augmenting the tumor debulking procedures rests with our understanding the cellular elements being regulated by these agents and the most judicial time, route, and dose that each agent should be employed.

ACKNOWLEDGMENTS

The skillful technical assistance of Roy Welker and Melanie Mitchell is gratefully acknowledged. We wish to thank Vicki Sutton and Julie Ewers for proofing and typing this manuscript.

REFERENCES

1. Armstrong, J.A. (1971): Appl. Microbiol. 21:723-725.

2. Bartocci, A., Papademetriou, V., and Chirigos, M.A. (1980): J. Immunopharmacol. 2(11):149-158.

3. Chirigos, M.A. (in press): In Pestka, S. (Ed.): Interferons: Methods of Enzymology. New York, Academic Press, 1981.

4. Chirigos, M.A., and Stylos, W.A. (1980): Cancer Res. 40:1967-1972.

5. Chirigos, M.A., Papademetriou, V., Bartocci, A., Read, E., and Levy, H.B. (1981): Int. J. Immunopharmacol. (in press).

6. Djeu, J.Y., Heinbaugh, J.A., Holden, H.T., and Herberman, R.B. (1979): J. Immunol. 122:175-181.

7. Gidlund, M., Orn, A., Wigzell, H., Senik, A., and Gresser, I. (1978): Nature 273:259-262.

8. Kiessling, R., Hochaman, P.S., Haller, O., Shearer, G.M., Wigzell, H., and Cudkowicz, G. (1977): Eur. J. Immunol. 7:655-662.

9. Santoni, A., Pucceti, A., Riccardi, C., Herberman, R.B., and Bonmasser, E. (1979): Int. J. Cancer 24:656-663.

10. Schultz, R.M., and Chirigos, M.A. (1978): Cancer Res. 38:1003-1007.

11. Schultz, R.M., and Chirigos, M.A. (1979): Cell Immunol. 48:52-58.

12. Senik, A., Gresser, I., Maury, C., Gidlund, M., Orn, A., and Wigzell, H. (1979): Cell Immunol. 44:186-200.

13. Schultz, R.M., Papamathiakis, J.D., Luetzler, J., Ruiz, P., and Chirigos, M.A. (1977): Cancer Res. 37:358-364.

14. Snodgrass, M.J., Morahan, P.S., and Kaplan, A.M. (1975): J. Natl. Cancer Inst. 55:455-462.

15. Stylos, W.A., Chirigos, M.A., Lengel, C.R., and Lyng, P.J. (1978): Cancer Immunol. Immunother. 5:165-172.

16. Stylos, W.A., Chirigos, M.A., Lengel, C.R., and Weiss, J.F. (1978): Cancer Treat. Rep. 62:1831-1836.

Mediation of Cellular Immunity in Cancer by
Immune Modifiers, edited by M. A. Chirigos
et al., Raven Press, New York © 1981.

Effects of Inhibitors and Products of Arachidonic Acid Metabolism on Macrophage-Mediated Cytotoxicity Induced by Interferon and Lipopolysaccharide

Richard M. Schultz and William T. Jackson

Lilly Research Laboratories, Eli Lilly and Company, Indianapolis, Indiana 46285

Activated macrophages have been implicated as important, if not crucial, participants in natural surveillance against neoplasia by differentiating normal from transformed cells and selectively killing transformed cells by a nonimmunologic contact—mediated mechanism (for review, see Ref. 26). Numerous agents, including bacterial lipopoly-saccharide (LPS) (1, 31), muramyl dipeptide from bacterial cell walls (38), fibroblast interferon (IFN) (28), pyran copolymer (29), double-stranded RNA (1), and lymphokine preparations (25) induce resting macrophages to become nonspecifically tumoricidal in vitro. Despite our considerable knowledge about agents that induce macrophage activation, little is known about biochemical mechanisms that regulate this process.

Macrophages contain considerable amounts of arachidonic acid in their phospholipids, and they are capable of synthesizing various oxygenation products via the cyclooxygenase and lipoxygenase pathways (22,35). Macrophages activated by some stimuli, including LPS, have been shown to synthesize and release large amounts of prostaglandin E_2 (PGE_2) (6, 15, 34). Macrophage—derived PGE_2 has been shown to be an important regulator of lymphocyte reactivity (6, 10, 37) and natural killer (NK) activity (39).

We recently showed that PGE_1 and PGE_2, administered in vitro or in vivo, suppressed the cytotoxic activity of IFN—treated macro-phages in a dose—dependent manner (33, 34). PGE_2 apparently inhi-bits macrophage cytotoxicity by increasing intracellular levels of cyclic AMP (32). Although the macrophage functions of tumor cytotox-icity and PGE_2 production completely dissociate (17, 34), we have proposed that PGE_2 production by activated macrophages could allow for negative feedback inhibition to limit cell activities. In this chapter, we attempt to characterize the role of endogenous and exoge-nous prostaglandins on modulating macrophage cytotoxic activity induced by LPS and fibroblast IFN.

MATERIALS AND METHODS

Mice

Male BALB/c mice, 6 to 8 weeks old, were purchased from Charles Rivers Breeding Laboratories, Portage, MI. All animals weighed at least 20 g before they were used as a source of resident peritoneal macrophages.

Reagents

Partially-purified mouse fibroblast interferon (specific activity $>10^7$ ref. units/mg protein) was purchased from Calbiochem-Behring Corp., San Diego, CA. Lipopolysaccharide B (E. coli 055:B5) was obtained from Difco Laboratories, Detroit, MI. Prostaglandins E_2 and $F_{2\alpha}$ (PGE$_2$ and PGF$_{2\alpha}$), indomethacin, and phorbol 12-myristate 13-acetate (PMA) were purchased from Sigma Chemical Co., Saint Louis, MO. Eicosa-5,8,11,14-tetraynoic acid (ETYA) was kindly donated by Dr. W. E. Scott of Hoffman-LaRoche, Inc., Nutley, NJ.

Indomethacin (10^{-3}M) was prepared in Dulbecco's phosphate-buffered saline (PBS), pH 7.2 and sonicated immediately before use. Concentrated solutions of PMA and ETYA were initially prepared in dimethyl sulfoxide (DMSO) and further diluted in PBS before testing. DMSO at the concentrations used had no effect on macrophage cytotoxic activity.

Cell Cultures

Tumor cell cultures. P815 mastocytoma cells were maintained as suspension cultures in RPMI-1640 medium supplemented with 20 percent heat-inactivated (56°C for 30 min) fetal calf serum, 50 μg/ml gentamicin solution, and 25 mM HEPES buffer (RPMI-FCS). Viability of the cells was determined by the trypan blue exclusion test.

Peritoneal macrophages. Noninduced peritoneal macrophages were harvested from BALB/c mice as previously described (30), washed in RPMI-1640 medium, and approximately 4×10^5 macrophages were seeded into 16-mm wells on tissue culture cluster[24] plates (Costar, Cambridge, MA) in 1.0 ml RPMI-FCS. The cultures were incubated for 90 min, and macrophage monolayers were washed thoroughly with jets of medium before use in experiments; by this means it was estimated that >95% of the cells had morphological and phagocytic properties of macrophages.

Macrophage Activation Assay

Our technique for measuring the ability of IFN or LPS to produce cytotoxic macrophages _in vitro_ has previously been described (25).

Monolayers of macrophages in 16-mm wells were treated with IFN or LPS at a final concentration of 1000 units/ml or 10 µg/ml respectively. Agents tested for inhibitory activity on macrophage function were added in 100-µl aliquots simultaneously with the activating agents. The macrophages were then overlaid with 4×10^4 P815 mastocytoma cells contained in 1 ml of RPMI-FCS. All cultures were incubated at $37°C$ in an atmosphere of 5 percent CO_2 in air, and viable tumor cells were counted after 48 hr with a hemacytometer. The ratio of macrophages to target cells was approximately 10:1 at the beginning of each experiment. The percentage growth inhibition of P815 cells due to macrophage-drug interaction was calculated by comparison to P815 cells grown in the presence of normal resting macrophages alone.

Prostaglandin Assay

Five $\times 10^5$ normal resting macrophages, previously purified by adherence, were seeded into 16-mm wells on tissue culture cluster[24] plates in 2.0 ml RPMI-FCS. The resultant macrophage monolayers were treated with either partially-purified IFN at 1000 units/ml, LPS at 10 µg/ml, or PMA at 10 ng/ml culture medium. The cultures were allowed to incubate at $37°C$ in 5% CO_2 in air. The prostaglandin synthetase inhibitor, indomethacin, was added to some of the cultures at $10^{-7}M$ as a control. Cell-free supernatants were collected at various times and analyzed for PGE_2 using a commercially available radioimmunoassay kit.

RESULTS

Effects of LPS and IFN on Macrophage Cytotoxic Activity and PGE$_2$ Production

When resting macrophages are incubated with various amounts of either LPS or mouse fibroblast IFN *in vitro* and challenged with P815 mastocytoma targets, the dose response curves for induction of macrophage cytotoxicity are quite different (Fig. 1). At optimal activating concentrations, LPS (10 µg/ml) provides a much weaker stimulus (46% cytotoxicity) than IFN (97% at 10,000 U/ml).

We also tested the ability of LPS and IFN to induce macrophage secretion of PGE_2. Treatment of macrophages with LPS (10 µg/ml), but not fibroblast IFN (1000 U/ml), stimulated optimal PGE_2 release by 24 hr of incubation (Ref. 34 and Table 1). Indomethacin ($1 \times 10^{-7}M$) completely inhibited PGE_2 secretion by treated macrophages.

Effects of Exogenously-Added Prostaglandins on Macrophage Cytotoxic Activity

Normal mouse macrophages were treated with either IFN (1000 U/ml) or LPS (10 µg/ml) in the presence or absence of exogenous prostaglan-

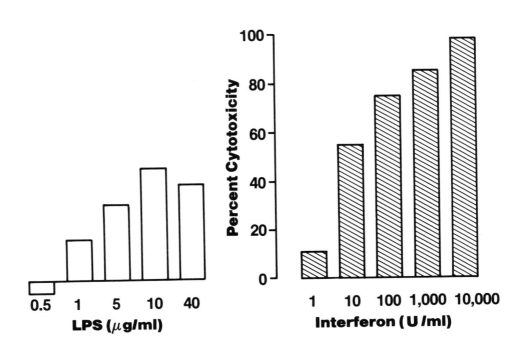

FIG. 1. Concentration response for macrophage activation by LPS and
IFN <u>in vitro</u>

TABLE 1. Influence of LPS and IFN on macrophage PGE$_2$ secretion

	PGE$_2$ (ng/ml)	
Activator	w/o indomethacin	w/indomethacin
None	10	0
LPS	44	0
IFN	9	0

dins, and the amount of macrophage cytotoxicity induced by 48 hrs was
measured. The cytotoxicity of IFN-activated macrophages was strongly
inhibited by exogenous PGE$_2$ (Figure 2). In contrast, the cytotoxicity
of LPS-activated macrophages which secrete large amounts of PGE$_2$ was
very mildly inhibited by exogenous PGE$_2$. Prostaglandin F$_{2\alpha}$ was
without effect on the cytotoxic activity of LPS- and IFN-treated macrophages.

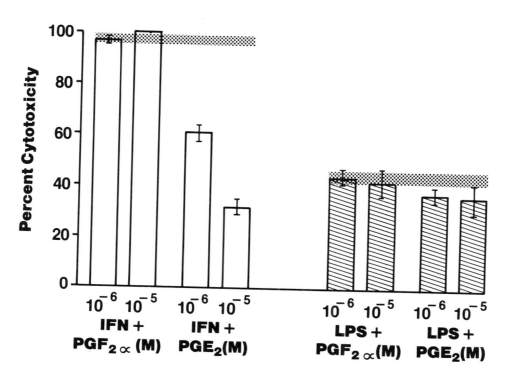

FIG. 2. Effect of in vitro prostaglandin treatment on cytotoxic activity of activated macrophages. Macrophages were simultaneously treated with either IFN or LPS and various molar concentrations of $PGF_{2\alpha}$ and PGE_2. The horizontal bars represent the cytotoxic activity of IFN- or LPS-treated macrophages respectively in the absence of prostaglandins ± SEM.

Effect of Prostaglandin Synthesis Inhibitors on Macrophage Activation by LPS

Since LPS is a potent trigger for PGE_2 release by macrophages and provides a weaker stimulus for macrophage activation than IFN, we tested whether endogenous PGE production may limit the cytotoxic activity induced by LPS. Macrophages were treated with LPS at 10 µg/ml in the presence of the cyclo-oxygenase inhibitor, indomethacin and ETYA, an acetylene analogue of arachidonic acid that blocks both the cyclo-oxygenase and lipooxygenase pathways. These inhibitors of arachidonic acid metabolism had no effect on the amount of macrophage cytotoxicity induced by LPS (Table 2).

TABLE 2. Effect of Indomethacin and ETYA on Induction
of Macrophage Cytotoxicity by LPS

Compound	Molar Concentration	Percent Cytotoxicity
Buffer		41
Indomethacin	1×10^{-6}	37
	1×10^{-7}	40
ETYA	1×10^{-5}	40
	1×10^{-6}	46

Effect of PMA on Macrophage Cytotoxicity

The potency of tumor promoters in experimental carcinogenesis has been reported to correlate with PGE_2 secretion by macrophages exposed to promoter in vitro (3). In this regard, PMA has been shown to be a potent trigger for PGE_2 release from mouse peritoneal macrophages, occurring within 2 hr after exposure in vitro (2, 5, 27). We tested whether PMA would interfere with activated macrophage function. PMA, even in concentrations as low as 10 ng/ml, markedly reduced macrophage-mediated cytotoxicity of P815 targets (Table 3). The addition of indomethacin (1×10^{-7}M) to the reaction mixture partially reversed this suppression, indicating the possible involvement of endogenous prostaglandins.

TABLE 3. Combined Effects of PMA and Indomethacin
on Macrophage Activation

Activator	PMA (10 ng/ml)	Indomethacin (1×10^{-7}M)	Percent Cytotoxicity
LPS	−	−	37
	+	−	9
	+	+	29
	−	+	36
IFN	−	−	85
	+	−	24
	+	+	58
	−	+	94

DISCUSSION

Although prostaglandins are frequently described as ubiquitous products of cellular metabolism, quantitative comparisons of macrophages with other lymphoid cells in terms of PGE synthesis suggest that the former is likely to be the major source of PGE in lymphoid cell mixtures and inflammatory exudates (10, 37). Studies from several labaoratories, including our own, have shown that resident peritoneal macrophages from specific pathogen-free mice synthesize and release large quantities of

PGE_2 in response to diverse stimuli including endotoxic LPS (6, 15, 34), zymosan (11), antigen–antibody complexes (23), neutral protease (5), and PMA (2, 3, 5, 27).

The time course for PGE_2 release from macrophages varies with the inducer. For example, significant increases in synthesis and release of PGE_2 are observed within 3 hours after the addition of LPS, and levels continue to increase for 24 hours (34). In contrast, PMA triggers significant PGE_2 release from macrophages as early as 15 min, and levels continue to rise, reaching a maximum by 2 hours (5, 27). The synthesis of PGE_2 in both cases was completely inhibited by indomethacin.

There is abundant evidence that exogenous PGE are potent inhibitors of several macrophage activities, including random locomotion (8) collagenase and plasminogen activator secretion (41, 42), release of lysosomal hydrolases (43), cell spreading and adhesion (4), and response to migration inhibitory factor (MIF) (14). In addition, we demonstrated that exogenous PGE_1 and PGE_2 suppress the cytotoxicity of IFN–activated macrophages, even when applied after the macrophages reached full morphologic activation (34). However, PGE exerted their strongest inhibitory effect when presented simultaneously with IFN. PGE required concentrations of $> 10^{-8}M$ to suppress tumor killing by IFN–treated macrophages in vitro (32). However, Gemsa and co–workers demonstrated that the process of phagocytosis enhances the sensitivity of the macrophage to PGE, along with a subsequent release of PGE, providing a sensitive control mechanism that may regulate macrophage function under physiologic conditions (9).

Macrophage functions of tumor cytotoxicity and PGE_2 release completely dissociate, since certain potent activation stimuli including antigen–induced lymphokine and fibroblast–derived IFN do not make macrophages release more PGE_2 than buffer–treated controls (17, 34). Moreover, macrophage–mediated tumor cell killing appears to be completely independent of the cyclo–oxygenase pathway of prostaglandin synthesis (17, 36). However, Meltzer and Wahl showed that antigen–induced lymphokine and LPS acted synergistically in increasing both PGE_2 secretion and in vitro tumor cytotoxicity (17).

The contribution of macrophage–borne PGE_2 to the self–regulation of macrophage function remains to be fully elucidated. Since certain activation stimuli such as LPS induce macrophages to release PGE_2, we have proposed that PGE_2 may act as a local feedback inhibitor of the activated tumoricidal state (24). In this regard, Kennedy and Stobo demonstrated that LPS–treated macrophages are capable of responding to self–synthesized prostaglandin by elevating cAMP levels and also down–regulating their receptors for prostaglandins (13). In the present study, PGE_2 was able to potently inhibit IFN–induced macrophage–mediated cytotoxicity, but had minor effect on that induced by LPS. Our failure to modulate macrophage activation by LPS with exogenous PGE_2 treatment may be related to the observation that macrophages become desensitized to the inhibitory effects of PGE_2 after prolonged exposure to PGE_2 (21).

Several reports have indicated that cyclo–oxygenase inhibitors can enhance the tumoricidal activity of activated macrophages in vitro. Prosser and associates demonstrated that indomethacin $(10^{-6}M)$ inhibited PGE_2 production and enhanced the tumor cytotoxicity of macrophages activated by BCG cell wall material (20). Resident peritoneal macrophages from tumor–bearing mice have been reported to release significantly more PGE_2 spontaneously in culture (19). In this regard, it is interesting that Farram and Nelson demonstrated that indomethacin was capable of enhancing the tumoricidal activity of macrophages harvested from the peritoneal cavities of mice bearing the C-4 tumor (7). Studies by Keller (12) and our own laboratory show that the tumor promoter, PMA inhibits the acquisition of tumoricidal function by macrophages in vitro. In the present study, indomethacin enhanced the cytotoxic activity of macrophages simultaneously exposed to PMA and either IFN or LPS. In contrast, indomethacin did not enhance the responsiveness of macrophages treated with LPS alone.

The studies described in this chapter show that endogenous and exogenous PGE_2 may modulate the tumoricidal activity of macrophages in vitro. The inhibitory effect of PGE_2 on macrophage function appears to be complex, being dependent on the nature of the activation stimulus, the concentration of PGE_2 added to the macrophage cultures, and the time of addition of PGE_2 relative to exposure to activation stimulus. Since many tumors produce high concentrations of PGE_2 (18, 40), the possibility exists that macrophage surveillance of neoplasia might be compromised by elevated PGE_2 in the microenvironment of the tumor. Lynch and Salomon reported that the cyclo-oxygenase inhibitor, indomethacin, inhibits tumor growth and potentiates nonspecific immunotherapy by bacterial agents in mice (16). Further studies are clearly needed to determine whether cyclo-oxygenase inhibitors enhance the therapeutic efficacy of macrophage activating agents in experimental animal tumor models.

SUMMARY

Fibroblast interferon (IFN) and bacterial lipopolysaccharide (LPS) can both independently induce noncytotoxic macrophages to kill tumor cells in vitro. However, the concentration curves for their induction are quite different. Bacterial LPS at an optimal inducing concentration (10 µg/ml) provides a much weaker stimulus (46 percent cytotoxicity) for macrophage activation than fibroblast IFN (85 percent cytotoxicity at 1000 U/ml). Studies were carried out to see if variations in arachidonic acid metabolism may account for this difference. Treatment of macrophages with LPS, but not fibroblast IFN, stimulated macrophages to release prostaglandin E_2 (PGE_2). Exogenously-added PGE_2 at $> 1 \times 10^{-6}M$ markedly inhibited the tumor cytotoxicity of IFN-treated macrophages, but had minor effect on cytotoxicity induced by LPS. These results suggest that PGE_2-producing macrophages become desensitized to PGE_2. Indomethacin ($1 \times 10^{-7}M$) inhibited PGE_2 secretion by LPS-treated macrophages in vitro. However, indomethacin and an inhibitor of both cyclo-oxygenase and lipooxygenase, eicosa-5,8,11,14-tetraynoic acid, did not markedly enhance induction of cytotoxicity by LPS. Since suboptimal levels of IFN can augment LPS activation of macrophages, the limiting factor in in vitro LPS activation appears to be the strength of the activating signal, rather than the level of endogenous PGE_2 production. The tumor-promoting phorbol 12-myristate 13-acetate (PMA) is a potent trigger of PGE_2 release from mouse peritoneal macrophage. Macrophages treated with PMA become refractory to activation by IFN or LPS unless PGE_2 production is blocked with indomethacin. The results suggest that both exogenously-applied and endogenously-produced PGE_2 can modulate the cytotoxic activity of macrophages in vitro.

REFERENCES

1. Alexander, P., and Evans, R. (1971): <u>Nature (London) New Biol.</u>, 232: 76–78

2. Brune, K., Glatt, M., Kalin, H., and Peskac, B.A. (1978): <u>Nature,</u> 274: 261–263.

3. Brune, K., Kalin, H., Schmidt, R., and Hecker, E. (1978): <u>Cancer Letters,</u> 4: 333–342.

4. Cantarow, W.D., Cheung, H.T., and Sundharadas, G. (1978): <u>Prostaglandins,</u> 16: 39–46.

5. Chang, J., Wigley, F., and Newcombe, D. (1980): <u>Proc. Natl. Acad. Sci., USA,</u> 77: 4736–4740.

6. Ellner, J.J., and Spagnuolo, P.J. (1979): <u>J. Immunol.,</u> 123: 2689–2695.

7. Farram, E., and Nelson, D.S. (1980): <u>Cell. Immunol.,</u> 55: 283–293.

8. Gallin, J.I., Sandler, J.A., Clyman, R.I., Manganiello, V.C., and Vaughan, M. (1978): <u>J. Immunol.,</u> 120: 492–496.

9. Gemsa, D., Seitz, M., Kramer, W., Till, G., and Resch, K. (1978): <u>J. Immunol.,</u> 120: 1187–1194.

10. Goldyne, M.E., and Stobo, J.D. (1980): <u>J. Invest. Dermatol.,</u> 74: 297–300.

11. Humes, J.L., Bonney, R.J., Pelus, L., Dahlgren, M.E., Sadowski, S.J., Kuehl, F.A., anbd Davies, P. (1977): <u>Nature,</u> 269: 149–151.

12. Keller, R. (1979): <u>Nature,</u> 282: 729–731.

13. Kennedy, M.S., and Stobo, J.D. (1980): <u>Clin. Res.,</u> 28: 351A.

14. Koopman, W.J., Gillis, M.H., and David, J.R. (1973): <u>J. Immunol.,</u> 110: 1609–1614.

15. Kurland, J.I., and Bockman, R. (1978): <u>J. Exp. Med.,</u> 147: 952–957.

16. Lynch, N.R., and Salomon, J.-C. (1979): <u>J. Natl. Cancer Inst.,</u> 62: 117–121.

17. Meltzer, M.S., and Wahl, L.M. (1979): <u>Fed. Proc. II,</u> 38: 933.

18. Owen, K., Gomolka, D., and Droller, M.J. (1980): <u>Cancer Res.,</u> 40: 3167–3171.

19. Pelus, L.M., and Bockman, R.S. (1979): <u>J. Immunol.,</u> 123: 2118–2125.

20. Prosser, F.H., Nichols, S.V. and Nichols, W.K. (1979): Fed. Proc. II, 38: 962.

21. Remold-O'Donnell, E. (1974): J. Biol. Chem., 249: 3615-3622.

22. Rigaud, M., Durand, J. and Breton, J.C. (1979): Biochim. Biophys. Acta, 573: 408-412.

23. Rouzer, C.A., Scott, W.A., Kempe, J., and Cohn, Z.A. (1980): Proc. Natl. Acad. Sci., USA, 77: 4279-4282.

24. Schultz, R.M. (1980): Medical Hypotheses, 6: 831-843.

25. Schultz, R.M., and Chirigos, M.A. (1978): Cancer Res., 38: 1003-1007.

26. Schultz, R.M., and Chirigos, M.A. (1980): In: Advances in Pharmacology and Chemotherapy, Vol. 17, edited by R.J. Schnitzer, pp. 157-193, Academic Press, New York.

27. Schultz, R.M., Chirigos, M.A., and Olkowski, Z.L. (1980): Cell. Immunol., 54: 98-106.

28. Schultz, R.M., Papamatheakis, J.D., and Chirigos, M.A. (1977): Science, 197: 674-676.

29. Schultz, R.M., Papamatheakis, J.D., and Chirigos, M.A. (1977): Cell. Immunol., 29: 403-409.

30. Schultz, R.M., Papamatheakis, J.D., Luetzeler, J., Ruiz, P., and Chirigos, M.A. (1977): Cancer Res., 37: 358-364.

31. Schultz, R.M., Pavlidis, N.A., and Chirigos, M.A. (1978): Cancer Res., 38: 3427-3431.

32. Schultz, R.M., Pavlidis, N.A., Stoychkov, J.N., and Chirigos, M.A. (1979): Cell. Immunol., 42: 71-78.

33. Schultz, R.M., Pavlidis, N.A., Stylos, W.A., and Chirigos, M.A. (1978): Science, 202: 320-321.

34. Schultz, R.M., Stoychkov, J.N., Pavlidis, N., Chirigos, M.A., and Olkowski, Z.L. (1979): J. Reticuloendothel. Soc., 26: 93-102.

35. Scott, W.A., Zrike, J.M., Hamill, A.L., Kempe, J., and Cohn, Z.A. (1980): J. Exp. Med., 152: 324-335.

36. Shaw, J.O., Russell, S.W., Printz, M.P., and Skidgel, R.A. (1979): J. Immunol., 123: 50-54.

37. Stenson, W.F., and Parker, C. W. (1980): J. Immunol., 125: 1-5.

38. Taniyama, T., and Holden, H.T. (1979): Cell. Immunol., 48: 369-374.

39. Tracey, D.E., and Adkinson, N.F. (1980): <u>J. Immunol.</u>, 125: 136–141.

40. Trevisani, A., Ferretti, E., Capuzzo, A., and Tomasi, J. (1980): <u>Br. J. Cancer,</u> 41: 341–347.

41. Vassalli, J., Hamilton, J., and Reich, E. (1976): <u>Cell,</u> 8: 271–281.

42. Wahl, L.M., Olsen, C.E., Sandberg, A.L., and Mergenhager, S.E. (1977): <u>Proc. Natl. Acad. Sci., USA,</u> 74: 4955–4958.

43. Zurier, R.B., Dukor, P., and Weissman, G. (1971): <u>Clin. Res.,</u> 19: 453–457.

Mediation of Cellular Immunity in Cancer by Immune Modifiers, edited by M. A. Chirigos et al., Raven Press, New York © 1981.

Activation of Spontaneous Monocyte-Mediated Cytotoxicity in Humans by X-Irradiation and Cis-Diamnedichloroplatinum

Andrew V. Muchmore, and Eugenie S. Kleinerman

Cellular Immunology Section, Metabolism Branch, Division of Cancer Biology and Diagnosis, National Cancer Institute, National Institutes of Health, Bethesda, Maryland 20205

One of the inescapable conclusions of this conference is that mammalian immune systems possess a highly developed and easily demonstrated form of antigen independent cell mediated cytolysis. A multiplicity of investigators have demonstrated the existence of mononuclear lymphoid cells capable of directly lysing target cells in the absence of pre-existing immunity. A host of in vitro models have been developed to assay such spontaneously cytotoxic cells and this type of in vitro and in vivo killing has been termed natural cytotoxicity (NC), spontaneous cytotoxicity, or natural killing (NK) (1-3). Common to all these models is the demonstration of target cell lysis which appears in the absence of pre-existing immunity, and is independent of the addition of exogenous antibody or lectin. Cellular characterization of these assays have shown that monocytes, T-cells, T-cells with some of the characteristics of monocytes, and non-T non-B small lymphocytes are all capable of killing target cells under the appropriate circumstances. One important variable in all of such assays is the type of target cell employed. Thus such simple manipulations as whether a target cell is carried in tissue culture or passed in vivo profoundly affects observed lysis. Some of the confusion surrounding this phenomena appears to be the result of generalizations which tend to lump all spontaneous cell mediated cytotoxicity under a single heading; it appears reasonable to propose that existing data is consistent with the hypothesis that a whole range of non-immune spontaneously cytotoxic cells exist which are capable of killing cell lines, tumor cells, and red blood cells.

We have extensively characterized one assay which we have termed spontaneous monocyte mediated cytotoxicity (SMMC). This assay measures the spontaneous lysis of xenogeneic red blood cell targets after a period of in vitro culture. The origin of the assay was based on the observation that freshly obtained human mononuclear cells failed to lyse chicken red blood cell targets but that human mononuclear cells cultured for seven days in low (2%) levels of serum were markedly cytotoxic (4). Further characterization of this phenomena revealed that more than 80% of the cytotoxicity found in these cultured cells was mediated by adherent phagocytic non-T cells with a receptor for the Fc portion of IgG (5). Perhaps the most interesting aspect of this assay is that the appearance of cytotoxicity coincides with the loss of a preformed suppressor cell (5). We have shown that a variety of in vitro maneuvers can stimulate suppressor cell activity and result in suppression of cytotoxic function (6). For example pokeweed mitogen markedly suppresses the appearance of cytotoxic cells and under appro-

priate circumstances can inhibit cytotoxicity even after cytotoxic
monocytes have been generated. The cell responsible for suppression
of monocyte mediated cytotoxicity in the presence of pokeweed mitogen
appears to be a radiosensitive lymphocyte. Thus this particular assay
of monocyte mediated cytotoxicity is somewhat unique in that it is
clearly under the influence of suppressor lymphocytes. We have utilized this assay to assess the in vitro and in vivo effects of various
chemotherapeutic agents on spontaneous monocyte mediated cytotoxicity.
The original rational of the experiments was to screen for agents
capable of inhibiting monocyte function. However as will be seen, we
discovered that a variety of exceedingly useful chemotherapeutic drugs
act to enhance spontaneous monocyte mediated cytotoxicity. Interestingly several mechanisms for enhancement of monocyte function appear
operative since enhancement can be the result of inhibition of suppression or may result from direct monocyte activation. Finally early
results suggest that in vitro effects are mirrored in vivo, since a
group of patients with ovarian carcinoma and profoundly depressed spontaneous monocyte mediated cytotoxicty had restoration of monocyte function during chemotherapy.

     All of the methods have been previously described (4-6). Basically
7×10^6 human mononuclear cells are cultured in medium NCTC 109 in a
volume of 2ml with 2% FCS, penicillin, streptomycin, and L-glutamine for
5-7 days. The cells are vigorously aspirated, counted for viability and
assayed at various target to effector cell ratios usually against ^{51}Cr
labeled chicken red blood cell targets. The effectors and targets are
mixed in round bottomed microtiter dishes for 18 hours and assayed for
^{51}Cr release as previously described (7). All cultures are routinely
assayed for viability using tryan blue exclusion. None of the measures
employed resulted in a greater than 40% reduction in viability. This is
even more striking since the effect of these agents was actual enhancement of function. Cells treated with irradiation were irradiated in a
cesium irradiator prior to culture. Cells treated with cis-diammedi
chloroplatinum (II) (cis-DDP) were pulsed for fifteen minutes at 37
degrees centigrade at various concentrations of drug (10^0 to 10^{-6}
micromolar) and then excess drug was washed out prior to culture. In
all cases control cells were run in parallel with no drug.

     Previous work from our laboratory had suggested that PWM was
capable of stimulating a radio-sensitive suppressor lymphocyte. These
studies all employed irradiation of a putative suppressor population
with addition to an indicator culture. We wondered what would happen to
fresh mononuclear cells which had been irradiated prior to culture. To
asess this question we irradiated whole mononuclear cell preparations
with various doses of irradiation and then allowed them to sit in culture for seven days. On the fourth day these cells were harvested and
assayed for cytotoxicity against ^{51}Cr labelled CRBC's in the usual
manner. As can be seen in Table I very low doses of irradiation led to
marked enhancement of spontaneous cytotoxicity towards RBC targets.

     Since we knew from our studies with PWM that irradiation could
affect the suppressor lymphocyte which regulates expression of spontaneous monocyte cytotoxicity we suspected that this was the mechanism
of the observed enhancement. If this were the case then one would

expect to see earlier and enhanced killing with irradiated cells since suppressor influences would be at least partially negated. As seen in Table II this was exactly what was seen and we saw much earlier and enhanced killing with irradiation.

Table I

Effect of increasing doses of X-irradiation on Spontaneous Monocyte Cytotoxicity assayed on day 4

Dose of X-irradiation	5^{51}Cr Release
0 R	8+1
50 R	24+4
150 R	57+10
200 R	74+2
400 R	84+14

[1]Human mononuclear cells were irradiated at time 0 and allowed to incubate for 4 days. These cells were then harvested, counted for viability and assayed for ^{51}Cr release against chicken red blood cell targets in the standard fashion. Results are + 2 S.D. of quadruplicate determinations

Table II

X-irradiation induced enhancement of monocyte mediated cytotoxicity also induces earlier killing

Day of Harvest	no irradiation[1]	100R irradiation
Day 2	3+ 1	2+2
Day 4	8+1	57+10
Day 5	9+3	64+2
Day 7	50+10	72+3

[1] Results expressed as %^{51}Cr release + 1 S.E.. In this experiment human mononuclear cells were irradiated with 100 R and harvested at the times noted.

Thus our data suggested the presence of a radiosensitive suppressor cell and experiments were designed to characterize the cell being affected by irradiation. Using Percoll gradients to separate cells into monocyte enriched and lymphocyte enriched populations we irradiated each subpopulation and recombined the cells. As seen in Table III irradiation appeared to act exclusively on the lymphocyte population.

However not all DNA toxic agents effect lymphocyte suppression. For example, in a series of related studies we examined the effect of Cis-DDP on spontaneous monocyte mediated cytotoxicity. We have previously shown that in contradistinction to irradiation, cis DDP seems to exert all of it's stimulatory effects by directly activating monocyte function leading to enhanced and earlier killing by human monocytes (8). Table IV compares enhancement of spontaneous monocyte mediated killing after treatment at the initiation of culture with either low doses of

X-irradiation or cis-DDP.

Table III

The effect of irradiation is on the lymphocyte suppressor cell

Cells[1]	%[51]Cr Release
L	2
M+L	11
M+L*	42
M*+L	12

[1]Human mononuclear cells were separated on Percoll gradients into monocyte enriched (M) and lymphocyte enriched populations (L) Some of these populations were irradiated (*) with 250R prior to re-mixing and culture for 5 days. These cultured cells were then assayed for cytotoxicity as usual

Table IV

Comparison of X-irradiation and cis-DDP for their ability to stimulate monocyte mediated cytotoxicity

Effect	X-irradiation enhancement	cis-DDP enhancement
Dose	low (50R)	low (1 nanomolar)
Present thoughout assay?	no	no
Earlier killing?	yes	yes
Cell affected	suppressor lymphocyte	monocyte

We are now expanding these studies to examine other compounds capable of activating spontaneous monocyte mediated cytotoxicity *in vitro* using human mononuclear cells.

In addition we have demonstrated that the peripheral blood mononuclear leucocytes taken from patients with a variety of malignancies exhibited defective monocyte killing *in vitro*. Furthermore in a study of a group of these patients with Stage III or IV ovarian carcinoma receiving chemotherapy, we found that monocyte mediated cytotoxicity was enhanced by 100% to 1200% (average 500%) compared to their individual baseline values (9).

Thus we have presented data to suggest that X-irradiation and cis-DDP result in marked *in vitro* activation of monocyte mediated cytotoxicity. It appears that x-irradiation and cis-platinum clearly act via different mechanisms. Thus irradiation has a primary effect on a lymphocyte suppressor cell population whereas cis-platinum appears to act directly on the monocyte. In this respect it is interesting to note that in unpublished observations we have also noted stimulation of spontaneous monocyte mediated cytotoxicity by gold compounds and by old fashioned arsenicals. It is intriguing to speculate that many of the heavy metals used for chemotherapy prior the the advent of antibiotics might have acted by activating monocyte mediated cytolysis presumably of

both the fixed reticuloendothelial system as well as circulating monocytes and macrophages.

A central question addressed generally at this meeting is what role
spontaneous killer cells and NK cells play in host immune defense. A
variety of lines of evidence exist which suggest that these forms of
cytotoxicity may play a central role in immune defense against malignancies. Thus resistance to direct tumor innoculation or the occurence
of spontaneous tumors correlates well with some measures of NK activity.
We feel that NK, NC, and spontaneous monocyte mediated cytotoxicity
represent a spectrum of host defence all characterized by their appearance and activity in the absence of intentional immunization.

Our patient data suggests that defective spontaneous monocyte
mediated cytotoxicity is a general finding in patients with a variety
of solid malignancies, and at least in the small group of ovarian carcinoma patients studied, restoration of monocyte function was observed
during chemotherapy (9).

Perhaps the biggest outstanding question regarding this data is
whether restoration of spontaneous monocyte mediated cytotoxicity during
chemotherapy is a function of monocyte activation by the agents employed
or is a secondary phenomena related to removal of tumor burden. We are
unable to distingiush these two possibilities now but our in vitro data
strongly suggest that direct activation may play a very important role.

Taken in aggregate it is tempting to speculate that many cancer
chemotherapeutic agents owe their efficacy not only to their ability to
directly inhibit tumor cells but also to an ability to activate the
reticuloendothelial system leading to enhanced spontaneous cytotoxicity.

REFERENCES

1. Kiessling, R. Klein E., Wigzell H. 1975. Eur. J. Immunol. 5: 112-
   118.

2. Herberman, R.B., Nunn M.E., and Lavrin D.H. 1975. Int. J. Cancer
   15: 216-229.

3. Stutman, O., Dien P., Wison, R., and Lattime E.C., 1980. Proc.
   Natl. Acad. Sci. 77: 2895-2898.

4. Muchmore, A.V., Decker, J.M., and Blaese, R.M. 1977. J. Immunol.
   119: 1680-1685.

5. Muchmore, A.V., Decker, J.M., and Blaese, R.M. 1977. J. Immunol.
   119: 1686-1689.

6. Muchmore, A.V., Decker, J.M., and Blaese, R.M. 1979. J. Immunol.
   122: 65-70.

7. Muchmore, A.V., Decker, J.M., and Blaese, R.M. 1979. J. Immunol.
   122: 1152-1155.

8. Kleinerman, E.S., Zwelling, L.A., Muchmore, A.V. 1980. Cancer
    Research 40: 3099-3102.

9. Kleinerman, E.S., Zwelling, L.A., Howser, D., Barlock, A.,
    Young, R.C., Decker, J.M., Bull, J., and Muchmore, A.V. 1980.
    Lancet 2:1102-1105.

*Mediation of Cellular Immunity in Cancer by
Immune Modifiers*, edited by M. A. Chirigos
et al., Raven Press, New York © 1981.

Human Monocyte Direct Cytotoxicity to Tumor Cells

Albert F. LoBuglio, Perry Robinson, M. A. Chirigos, and Maxine Solvay

*Simpson Memorial Research Institute, University of Michigan Medical Center,
Ann Arbor, Michigan 48109*

Blood monocytes are a circulating component of the reticuloendothelial system and represent the cell population which responds to
chemotactic stimuli to provide a monocyte/macrophage infiltrate at
sites of inflammation or tumors. Our laboratory has been exploring the
potential interaction of these cells with tumor cells. We have shown
that blood monocytes have cytotoxic capacity in antibody dependent
cellular cytotoxicity to a variety of human malignant target cells
coated with either human (3) or rabbit antibody (4). We also reported
that coincubation of human monocytes with tumor cell targets resulted
in monocyte attachment to the target cell surface and inhibition of
tritiated thymidine incorporation into DNA by the tumor cells (1). The
studies reviewed in this report have characterized the direct cytolysis
of tumor cells by monocytes from normal donors, examined some potential
mechanisms of cytolysis and explored both in vivo and in vitro modulation of monocyte cytotoxicity.

METHODS

Monocyte Isolation

Monocytes were isolated from the peripheral blood of human donors
as previously described (4). This involved surface adherence of monocytes from mononuclear cell preparations obtained by Ficoll-Hypaque
separation. The unbound lymphocytes were rigorously washed out of the
tissue culture plates and the adherent monocytes obtained by gentle
brushing with a rubber policeman after a brief incubation in cold (4°C)
buffer containing EDTA and albumin. The monocyte preparations were
> 95% nonspecific esterase positive and > 95% viable by trypan blue
exclusion.

Tumor Cell Targets

Human tumor cell lines were grown in RPMI 1640 containing 10%
fetal calf sera (FCS) or pooled human serum. The cells were labeled by
the addition of 50 uC of tritiated thymidine 24 hours prior to cell
harvest. Cell suspensions were obtained by using brief incubation with

trypsin. The target cells were then washed, counted and resuspended to the appropriate cell concentration in RPMI 1640.

Direct Monocyte Cytotoxicity Assay

This assay is carried out by incubating 2×10^4 tritiated thymidine labeled HeLa cells (or other tumor cell lines) either alone or with varying numbers of isolated monocytes to produce effector:target (E/T) ratios from 10:1 to 1:1 in triplicate. The assay media is RPMI 1640 containing 5% FCS, penicillin and streptomycin (complete media) and can be carried out in microwell tissue culture trays (300 ul volume) or tissue culture tubes (2 ml volume) with identical results. At 48, 72 and 96 hours the supernate is sampled to determine the number of cpm released from the tumor cells incubated alone (spontaneous release) or in the presence of monocytes. The amount of supernate removed is replaced with fresh complete media at the 48 and 72 hour sampling times. At each time point, triplicate values for per cent cytotoxicity are calculated using the formula:

$$\% \text{ cytotoxicity} = \frac{A - B}{C - B} \times 100$$

A = Total cpm released to that point in time in the tumor-cell/monocyte culture.

B = Total cpm released to that point in time in the tumor cell alone culture (spontaneous release).

C = Total cpm in the 2×10^4 tumor cells.

These calculations are carried out with a computer program which provides the mean $\pm$ 1 SD of cytotoxicity at each time point and each E/T ratio examined. Spontaneous release over 96 hours generally ranged from 10-20% of total cpm.

Preincubation of Monocytes (Activation)

In order to examine the effects of preincubation of monocytes with interferon, a modification of the method of Van der Meer (6) for in vitro culture of monocytes without cell adherence was developed. Sheets of teflon were used to form teflon sleeves in tissue culture tubes and the tubes then sterilized. For in vitro activation, 1×10^6 monocytes were incubated in 1 ml complete media containing various doses of fibroblast interferon in these teflon sleeves for 18 hours at 37°. Two-thirds of the supernate was then discarded and the monocytes resuspended in the remaining media, counted and appropriate aliquots distributed to assay tubes containing target cells for the cytotoxic assay. Monocyte yield was 75-80% and viability > 95%.

Materials and Reagents

Partially purified fibroblast interferon was provided by NIH (M.A. Chirigos) 434,000 units per vial (Lot #45-13-12). Purified human lysozyme was provided by Elliot Osserman (Columbia University, New York). Tissue culture media and FCS was provided by GIBCO. Chemicals were obtained from Sigma. Indomethacin was obtained from Merck, Sharpe & Dohme Research Laboratory (West Point, PA) and PGE1 was obtained from the Upjohn Co. (Kalamazoo, MI). The endotoxin used was lipopolysaccharide E. coli 0111B4 (Difco).

RESULTS

Characteristics of Monocyte Direct Cytotoxicity

The coincubation of blood monocytes with tritiated thymidine labeled HeLa cells resulted in a progressive increase in radioactive cpm in the supernate above that seen with HeLa cells alone. A typical experiment is illustrated in Table 1.

Table 1. Direct Monocyte Cytotoxicity to Tumor Cells

E/T Ratio[b]	Per Cent Cytotoxicity[a]		
	48 hr	72 hr	96 hr
1:1	1.1 + 0.7	2.7 + 0.6	7.1 + 0.5
3:1	4.8 + 0.8	9.9 + 0.8	18.9 + 0.9
10:1	10.3 + 0.6	27.8 + 1.2	47.9 + 0.9

[a] Expressed as mean + 1 SD of triplicate values.
[b] Varying numbers of monocytes were added to 2×10^4 tritiated thymidine labeled HeLa cells to give appropriate E/T ratio.

As can be seen, the variation in cytotoxicity with the triplicate values is modest (small S.D.). The amount of cytotoxicity is clearly related to the number of monocytes in the assay (E/T ratio) as well as the duration of coincubation. The degree of cytotoxicity noted with 5 normal donors is illustrated in Table 2.

Table 2. Effect of E/T Ratio on Monocyte Cytotoxicity

E/T Ratio[b]	Per Cent Cytotoxicity[a]		
	48 hr	72 hr	96 hr
1:1	1.5 + 0.8	5.4 + 3.0	11.7 + 7.1
3:1	4.7 + 1.9	14.1 + 2.8	24.9 + 7.4
10:1	11.2 + 3.2	28.4 + 4.9	42.9 + 5.8

[a] Mean + 1 S.D. of per cent cytotoxicity from assays of 5 different monocyte donors.
[b] 2×10^4 H^3 labeled HeLa cells incubated with appropriate number of monocytes to achieve E/T ratios.

To be sure that the enhanced radioactive release in fact reflected a decrement in tumor cell numbers at 96 hours, we counted the tumor cells using a Coulter Channelyzer II to identify tumor cells which had two to three times the volume of blood monocytes. In 3 experiments at an E/T ratio of 10/1, the number of tumor cells in the monocyte cultures was decreased by 56, 52 and 53% compared to tumor cells cultured alone. To determine the requirement for viable monocytes, the effector cells were freeze thawed x 5 prior to addition of tumor cells or pretreated with 10^{-4}M N-ethyl maleimide. Both of these manipulations resulted in complete inhibition of cytotoxicity.

In order to examine the cytotoxic potential of normal monocytes to other malignant cell lines, we carried out cytotoxic assays (Table 3) against a variety of tritiated thymidine labeled human tumor cell lines including K-562 (myeloid leukemia), HCT-9 (adenocarcinoma of the colon), CEM (T-lymphoblast line), SK-Mel-28 and 23 (two melanomas).

Table 3. Monocyte Cytotoxicity to Tumor Cell Targets

	% Cytotoxicity (E/T = 10/1)		
Target Cells	48 hr	72 hr	96 hr
HeLa	10.3	27.8	47.9
K-562	10.0	15.3	22.0
HCT-9	12.2	17.4	21.8
CEM	17.6	41.1	55.6
SK-Mel-28	24.6	38.3	49.0
SK-Mel-23	2.1	3.9	5.6

All target cells were lysed to varying degrees by the normal monocytes although the SK-Mel-23 was quite resistant as compared to the other targets. This did not seem to be a characteristic of melanoma cells since the SK-Mel-28 was lysed as well as the HeLa target cell. We also examined the monocyte cytotoxic potential toward a human fibroblast cell line (P-10) as outlined in Table 4.

Table 4. Monocyte Cytotoxicity to Tumor and Fibroblast Cell Lines

		Per Cent Cytotoxicity[a]	
		HeLa	Fibroblast (P-10)
Donor 1	48 hr	29.0	− 3.9
	72 hr	52.5	− 5.2
	96 hr	63.0	− 3.6
Donor 2	48 hr	12.8	0
	72 hr	38.9	0
	96 hr	39.8	0

[a] Expressed as mean cytotoxicity of triplicate cultures carried out at an E/T ratio of 10:1.

No cytotoxicity was seen with the fibroblast targets while the same monocyte populations were quite cytotoxic to HeLa cells set up in the same experiments.

Thus, monocytes isolated from normal donors appear capable of cytotoxic activity toward a variety of human tumor targets and not to a fibroblast line. The cytotoxicity requires viable monocytes and is directly related to the number of effector cells and duration of coincubation.

In Vivo Modulation of Monocyte Cytotoxicity

We have examined the ability of monocytes isolated from patients with malignant lymphoma (5 non-Hodgkin's lymphoma and 2 Hodgkin's disease) and metastatic solid tumors (lung, breast and sarcoma) to carry out direct cytotoxicity (Table 5). For these studies, a normal donor and patient were examined concurrently on the same day.

Table 5. Monocyte Cytotoxicity in Malignant Disease

E/T Ratio	Per Cent Cytotoxicity[a]		
	48 hr	72 hr	96 hr
Normal (n=13)			
1:1	1.2 + 1.4	2.9 + 2.4	6.1 + 3.5
3:1	6.6 + 6.4	13.8 + 10.9	20.6 + 12.6
10:1	19.6 + 10.5	37.0 + 14.8	48.8 + 14.4
Lymphoma (n=7)			
1:1	1.7 + 1.5	2.7 + 1.8	5.4 + 2.9
3:1	4.0 + 2.8	8.4 + 4.4	14.7 + 5.6
10:1	14.6 + 7.1	31.9 + 10.4	48.0 + 12.4
Solid Tumor (n=6)			
1:1	1.9 + 1.6	3.3 + 2.0	6.1 + 2.8
3:1	5.3 + 2.9	12.0 + 7.6	17.6 + 10.4
10:1	18.5 + 6.7	33.3 + 12.1	43.7 + 12.7

[a]Expressed as mean ± 1 SD of 13 normal, 7 lymphoma and
6 patients with metastatic solid tumors.

These groups of patients did not have significant alteration of monocyte cytotoxicity. Further, when individual patients were examined, they all fell within the normal range. Thus, the presence of malignant disease does not appear to produce a striking alteration in monocyte cytotoxic potential.

Mechanism of Direct Monocyte Cytotoxicity

Since several in vitro animal macrophage cytotoxic systems are dependent on the presence of endotoxin (LPS), we have examined the role of this material in monocyte cytotoxicity. First, we compared monocyte cytotoxicity carried out in the presence of 5% FCS (Limulus assay positive) with cytotoxicity carried out in 5% fresh sterile and Limulus assay negative human serum (Table 6).

Table 6. Effect of FCS or Human Serum on Monocyte Cytotoxicity

Serum[b]	Per Cent Cytotoxicity[a]		
	48 hr	72 hr	96 hr
FCS	20.3 + 1.4	30.1 + 0.8	42.4 + 1.6
Human	28.8 + 1.2	43.2 + 2.6	53.7 + 0.3

[a]Expressed as mean ± 1 SD of triplicate values at a 10:1 E/T ratio.
[b]Assay carried out in 5% fetal calf serum or 5% human serum.

In multiple experiments of this type, cytotoxicity by monocytes in human serum was either greater than or comparable to monocyte cytotoxicity in the presence of FCS. Further, the addition of endotoxin (LPS) to our in vitro assay over a wide dose range had no effect at low doses and actually inhibited monocyte cytotoxicity at high doses.

A second mechanism examined involved the potential cytotoxic effect of thymidine released from monocytes. The addition of large doses of thymidine ($10^{-4}M$) to the tritiated thymidine labeled HeLa cells failed to enhance radioactive release beyond levels for spontaneous release. Further, deoxycytine which should reverse thymidine induced toxicity failed to inhibit monocyte cytotoxicity (Table 7).

Table 7. Deoxycytidine Effect on Monocyte Cytotoxicity

| | | Per Cent Cytotoxicity[a] | | |
		48 hr	72 hr	96 hr
Exp. 1	Monocytes	15 + 1	25 + 3	30 + 5
	Monocytes + DC[b]	15 + 1	25 + 1	30 + 2
Exp. 2	Monocytes	17 + 3	25 + 3	34 + 4
	Monocytes + DC	17 + 1	24 + 2	32 + 1

[a] Expressed as mean + 1 SD of triplicate values at a 10:1 E/T ratio.
[b] Deoxycytidine at a concentration of $10^{-5}M$.

The role of prostaglandins in monocyte cytotoxicity was explored by examining the effects of indomethacin and PGE_1 on the cytotoxic system. As seen in Table 8, indomethacin inhibition of cyclooxygenase did not reduce and, in fact, produced a modest increment in cytotoxicity.

Table 8. Indomethacin Effect on Monocyte Cytotoxicity

| | Per Cent Cytotoxicity[a] | |
Indomethacin	72 hr	96 hr
Control A[b]	28.2	37.4
Control B[b]	27.9	37.1
$10^{-4}M$	32.6	53.2
$10^{-5}M$	32.8	45.3
$10^{-6}M$	33.3	45.5
$10^{-7}M$	30.8	43.5

[a] Expressed as mean of triplicate values at an E/T of 10:1 at 72 and 96 hr.
[b] Control A was usual assay media. Control B included 100 λ of buffer used to add the indomethacin.

Consistent with a modest enhancement seen in cytotoxicity with indomethacin, the addition of PGE_1 produced a modest inhibition of cytotoxicity (Table 9).

Table 9. PGE₁ Effect on Monocyte Cytotoxicity

	Per Cent Cytotoxicity[a]	
PGE₁	72 hr	96 hr
Control A[b]	34.0	43.7
Control B[b]	31.9	42.6
10^{-5}M	26.9	32.3
10^{-6}M	26.7	33.3
10^{-7}M	27.4	34.7
10^{-8}M	.29.5	38.7

[a]Expressed as the mean of triplicate values at an E/T ratio of 10/1.
[b]Control A was usual assay media. Control B included 100 λ of buffer used to add PGE₁.

Thus, we were unable to find evidence that monocyte damage to tumor cells was related to endotoxin, thymidine or prostaglandins.

In Vitro Modulation of Monocyte Cytotoxicity

Le Marbre et al. (2) have reported that human lysozyme was able to produce in vitro enhancement of monocyte cytotoxicity using a different assay system. In collaboration with Elliot Osserman, we have examined the effect of a highly pure lysozyme preparation on monocyte cytotoxicity (Table 10).

Table 10. Lysozyme Effect on Monocyte Cytotoxicity

		Per Cent Cytotoxicity[a]			
Lysozyme	Donors:	A	B	C	D
None		46.0 ± 1.3	48.9 ± 3.6	34.6 ± 2.7	20.2 ± 0.6
25 ug		40.7 ± 2.2	45.9 ± 0.8	34.8 ± 3.0	18.4 ± 0.5
100 ug		35.6 ± 2.0	44.3 ± 3.3	30.6 ± 0.7	15.5 ± 1.1
500 ug		23.5 ± 2.5	36.1 ± 1.0	24.7 ± 1.4	5.6 ± 0.4

[a]Expressed as mean ± 1 SD of triplicate values at 96 hrs at a 10:1 E/T ratio by 4 normal donors (A-D).

We found no enhancement but rather a depression of monocyte cytotoxicity at high doses of human lysozyme. Egg white lysozyme produced no alteration of monocyte cytotoxicity at doses from 25-500 ug/ml.

Schultze et al. (5) have reported that fibroblast interferon is capable of enhancing murine macrophage cytotoxicity to tumor cells. We have examined the effects of fibroblast interferon on direct monocyte cytotoxicity. The simple addition of interferon to the co-culture of monocytes and tumor cells failed to alter monocyte cytotoxicity at doses of 100-2000 u/ml. In contrast, if monocyte cell suspensions were incubated with various doses of interferon for 18 hrs and then placed in co-culture with tumor cells, a consistent enhancement of cytotoxicity was seen (Table 11).

Table 11. Effect of Interferon on Monocyte Direct Tumor
Cell Cytotoxicity[a]

| | Interferon | Per Cent Cytotoxicity[b] | | |
		48 hr	72 hr	96 hr
Exp 1	0	13.8 + 3.5	26.4 + 3.3	38.6 + 3.2
	300 u	15.3 + 2.2	30.9 + 2.5	54.2 + 5.7
	1000 u	16.6 + 2.7	33.8 + 5.5	56.7 + 4.9
	2000 u	19.1 + 2.0	37.6 + 1.1	60.2 + 1.7
Exp 2	0	9.9 + 1.9	24.2 + 5.0	31.7 + 5.9
	300 u	27.9 + 2.7	48.1 + 2.0	59.5 + 0.7
	1000 u	26.4 + 7.7	47.9 + 6.6	64.6 + 2.9
	2000 u	19.7 + 5.3	44.4 + 6.8	61.5 + 5.5

[a]Monocytes (1×10^6/ml) were incubated in RPMI 1640 with 5%
FCS with varying doses of interferon (0-2000 u/ml) for 18
hrs and then used in the cytotoxicity assay at an E/T of
10:1.
[b]Expressed as mean + 1 SD of triplicate values.

In these studies, monocytes were incubated in teflon sleeves in a
1 ml volume of complete media containing varying doses of interferon.
At the end of the incubation, approximately 2/3 of the supernate was
discarded and the monocytes resuspended in the remaining media, counted
and appropriate volumes (to provide 2×10^5 monocytes) transferred to
assay tubes containing 2×10^4 HeLa cells and the volume brought up to
2 ml with fresh complete media. The cytotoxicity assay was then
carried out over 96 hours as previously described. The transfer of
monocytes to the assay tubes included 40-80 ul of media containing
0-200 u of interferon which was then diluted to 2 ml to result in
final concentrations of 0-100 u/ml interferon in the cytotoxic assay.
It was thus important to determine the effects of similar concentrations
of interferon (preincubated with monocytes) on HeLa cell proliferation,
viability and tritiated thymidine release. This was accomplished by
incubating interferon with monocytes in an identical fashion and then
transferring the cell free supernate to assay tubes to determine the
effect of such preincubated interferon on the HeLa cells in the absence
of monocytes (Table 12).
    The HeLa cells in experiment 1 underwent 3-4 cell doublings and in
experiment 2 between 2-3 cell doublings in the 96 hour study. At concentrations of interferon present in the interferon activated monocyte
study outlined in Table 11 (< 100 u/ml) little or no effect on cell
proliferation or thymidine release was noted due to interferon alone.
Interferon concentrations of 250 u/ml did produce moderate inhibition
of cell proliferation with minimal effects on spontaneous release of
tritiated thymidine. The cell viability of all HeLa cell cultures in
this experiment was > 98% by trypan blue exclusion. Thus, interferon
preincubation of monocytes appears capable of enhancing monocyte direct
cytotoxicity independent of direct interferon damage of tumor cell
targets.

Table 12. <u>Preincubated Interferon Effects on HeLa</u>
<u>Cells (96 hr culture)</u>

Interferon[a]		HeLa Cell Number x 10^4[b]	S.R.[c]
Exp. 1	None	25.6	15.7 ± 1.7
	50 u	27.0	14.5 ± 1.1
	125 u	18.3	15.2 ± 2.4
	250 u	14.0	16.1 ± 0.8
Exp. 2	None	9.5	21.1 ± 0.2
	50 u	11.8	22.0 ± 1.3
	125 u	9.5	22.4 ± 1.8
	250 u	7.3	26.2 ± 4.2

[a]Concentration of interferon/ml in the assay tube.
Interferon obtained from the supernate of monocytes
cultured in teflon sleeves as in Table 11.
[b]Mean of triplicate values for the number of HeLa cells
96 hrs after addition of 2 x 10^4 HeLa cells.
[c]Expressed as mean $\pm$ 1 SD spontaneous release of triplicate values at 96 hrs.

REFERENCES

1. King, G.W., File, J., and LoBuglio, A.F. (1978): <u>J. Allergy Clin.</u>
   <u>Immunol.</u> 62:283-288.
2. LeMarbre, P., Rinehart, J., Kay, N., Osserman, E., and Jacob, H.
   (1979): <u>Blood</u> 54, Suppl. 1, pg. 103A.
3. Shaw, G.M., Levy, P.C., and LoBuglio, A.F. (1978): <u>J. Immunol.</u>
   121:573-578.
4. Shaw, G.M., Levy, P.C., and LoBuglio, A.F. (1978):
   <u>J. Clin. Invest.</u> 62:1172-1180
5. Schultze, R., Papanatheakis, J., and Chirigos, M. (1977):
   <u>Science</u> 197:674-676.
6. Van der Meer, J., Bulterman, D., van Zwet, T., and van Furth, R.
   (1978): <u>J. Exp. Med.</u> 147:271.

This work was supported by the National Cancer Institute Grant
CA 25641-03.

Mediation of Cellular Immunity in Cancer by
Immune Modifiers, edited by M. A. Chirigos
et al., Raven Press, New York © 1981.

Immunoregulatory Effect of Human Chorionic Gonadotropin on Murine Peritoneal Macrophages

V. Papademetriou, A. Bartocci, *L. K. Steel, E. Read,
and M. A. Chirigos

*Virus and Disease Modification Section, Laboratory of Chemical Pharmacology, National Cancer Institute, and *Laboratory of Clinical Investigation, National Institute of Allergy and Infectious Diseases, National Institutes of Health, Bethesda, Maryland 20205*

Human Chorionic Gonadotropin (HCG) was suggested to possess important immunosuppressive properties. Several investigators reported that HCG suppresses the immune response against allografts and inhibits lymphocyte blastogenic response to mitogens. In this study, the effect of crude HCG on peritoneal macrophages has been examined. In vitro concentrations higher than 100 IU/ml were found to render macrophages cytotoxic against MBL-2 leukemia cells. Intraperitoneal, daily injections of 500 IU/mouse for a total of six or more treatments also rendered peritoneal macrophages cytotoxic. The in vivo HCG-activated macrophages were found to be suppressive for normal splenic lymphocytes at lymphocyte:macrophage ratios of 10:1 to 2.5:1. In vitro treatment of macrophages with HCG from 100 to 2500 IU/ml resulted in elaboration and release of high concentrations of prostaglandins, notably of the E series. The data presented in this study strongly suggest that some of the previously reported immunosuppressive activities of crude HCG may be mediated by macrophages through prostaglandin production.

KEYWORDS

Human Chorionic Gonadotropin, Macrophage, Prostaglandin, Blastogenesis

INTRODUCTION

Human Chorionic Gonadotropin (HCG), a normally produced hormone during pregnancy, has been shown to be secreted (besides choriocarcinoma) by a wide variety of non-trophoblast containing neoplasms (19,3). Horne et al.' (10) using an enzyme-bridge immunoperoxide technique examined 50 cases of breast cancer for tumor markers. They reported that, among other pregnancy specific tumor markers, HCG was found in 60% of the cases. Other investigators reported that pancreatic islet cell and breast carcinomas, which synthesize HCG, appear to behave in a more aggressive manner, as indicated by the presence of metastases, than do similar neoplasms which lack this secretory capacity (12,25). In the Framingham study (26) it was shown retrospectively, that abnormal HCG levels were present up to 26 months before the diagnosis of cancer was made. However in the same study a 20% borderline false positive HCG elevation in postmenopausal women was found, which diminishes the value of this hormone as a tumor marker.

It is virtually certain that the hormone is actively synthesized by the neoplastic cells but the biological significance of tumour secretion of HCG is not yet well defined. However, since HCG and other trophoblast-specific products are said to have immunosuppressive properties, it seems likely that the production of such proteins by malignant tumors, might be one method by which a tumour escapes immunological recognition and continues to grow.

Commercial preparations of HCG have been shown by many investigators to possess immunosuppressive properties on lymphocyte blastogenesis and cell-mediated immunity (1,5,9,13).

In this study we examined the effect of commercially available HCG on peritoneal macrophage activation, and the ability of HCG treated macrophages to produce prostaglandins and to alter the blastogenic response of splenic lymphocytes.

MATERIALS AND METHODS

Animals

Male or female BALB/c mice, 6 to 8 weeks old, were supplied by the Mammalian Genetics and Animal Production Section, Division of Cancer Treatment, National Cancer Institute, NIH, Bethesda, MD. The animals were housed in plastic cages and fed Purina Laboratory Chow with water ad libitum. All animals weighed at least 23 g before they were used for experimentation.

Target cells

A tissue culture strain of MBL-2 lymphoblastic leukemia cells (C57B1/6-derived) has previously been described (22). Suspension cultures were maintained in RPMI-1640 medium supplemented with 20% fetal calf serum, and 100 µg/ml gentamicin, hereafter called RPMI-FCS. Viability of the cells was determined by Trypan blue exclusion.

Drugs

Interferon (IF). Partially purified IF (SA 2 x 10^7 u/mg protein) was purchased from Dr. Kurt Paucker, Department of Microbiology, Medical College of Pennsylvania, Philadelphia, PA.

Human Chorionic gonadotropin (HCG) was purchased from Sigma Chemical Company (St. Louis, MO). The hormone was dissolved in PBS immediately before use. HCG was in the powder form, phosphate and mannitol free and its specific activity (SA) varied from 2570 to 3230 IU/mg of protein. The hormone was tested by the Limulus assay and found to be free of endotoxin. HCG, at 100 to 5000 IU/ml, was not directly cytotoxic to splenic cells or MBL-2 tumor cells when incubated for up to 72 hours. Cell viability was tested by the trypan blue dye exclusion method.

Tritiated thymidine (^{3}HTdR, 6.7 Ci/mmole), $PGF_{2\alpha}$ (^{3}HPGF$_{2\alpha}$, 120 Ci/mmole) and PGE_2 (^{3}HPGE$_2$, 140 Ci/mmole) were obtained from New England Nuclear. Rabbit $PGF_{2\alpha}$ antiserum and PGE_1 antiserum were products of Clinical

Assays and Steranti, respectively. $PGF_{2\alpha}$ and PGE_2 were the generous gifts of Dr. John Pike (Upjohn Co.) NorΨt A, KCl, and gelatin (Bloom 100) were purchased from Fisher Scientific Co.; Dextran T-70 from Pharmacia Fine Chemicals; Trizma from Sigma and Ultrafluor scintillation fluid from National Diagnostics.

Lymphocyte Preparations

Lymphocytes were obtained from BALB/c mice by aseptic removal of the spleen. The splenic populations from 6 to 8 mice were pooled in 15 ml of sterile RPMI-FCS medium and placed in 15 x 150 mm Petri dishes (Falcon, Oxnard, CA). The dishes were incubated for 2 hours in order to remove adherent macrophages. The nonadherent cells were collected and incubated at room temperature for 3 minutes with 0.11 M ammonium chloride to deplete RBC's. The nonadherent, RBC-depleted cells were resuspended in 8 ml RPMI-FCS. Two ml of the suspension was layered over 4 ml of Ficoll-Hypaque separation medium containing 12 parts of 14% Ficoll 400 (Pharmacia, Piscataway, NJ) and 5 parts 32.8% Hypaque sodium (specific grafity = 1.09; Sterling Winthrop Research Institute, Rensellaer, NY). The gradient was centrifuged at 300 xg for 30 minutes at room temperature. The interface, containing the separated lymphocytes was collected, washed three times with RPMI-1640, viability determined with Trypan blue, ana brought to a concentration of 5.0 x 10^6 viable cells/ml.

Macrophage Activation Assay

The assay for measuring the ability of agents to induce macrophage-mediated cytotoxicity has been previously described (21). Noninduced peritoneal macrophages were harvested from normal or HCG-treated BALB/c mice and purified by adherence. For in vivo macrophage activation, various groups of mice were treated i.p. with 500 IU HCG contained in a volume of 0.25 ml PBS. Mice were treated daily for a total of 2, 4, 6, 8, or 10 treatments. Control groups received PBS. Approximately 8.0 x 10^5 purified peritoneal macrophages were seeded onto 16-mm wells (Tissue Culture Cluster CB Costar, Cambridge, MA) in 1.0 ml of RPMI-FCS. MBL-2 leukemia cells, adjusted to 8.0 x 10^4 cells/ml RPMI-FCS, were added to the macrophage monolayers in 1-ml aliquots. For in vitro activation, varying doses of HCG were added to the macrophage cultures before they were overlaid with MBL-2 target cells. HCG remained in the culture medium for the duration of the experiment. Toxicity controls consisting of MBL-2 cells alone in the presence of HCG were also included in each experiment. All cultures were maintained in a humidified, 5% CO_2 in air incubator at 37°C, and viable MBL-2 cells were counted with hemocytometer. The ratio of macrophages to target cells was approximately 10:1 at the beginning of each experiment. Percent growth inhibition of MBL-2 cells due to macrophage-HCG interaction was calculated by comparison to MBL-2 cells grown in the presence of normal control macrophages.

Response to Mitogen

5.0 x 10^5 viable, nonadherent, RBC-depleted lymphocytes contained in 0.1 ml were added to each well of a Micro-test II Tissue Culture plate (3040, Falcon, Oxnard, CA). Phytohemagglutinin (PHA, Difco, Detroit, MI) in a final concentration of 5 µg/ml contained in 0.05 ml, and various concentrations of HCG contained in 0.05 ml were also added. A concentration of 5 µg/ml PHA was determined to be optimal by wide range titration versus splenic lymphocytes. In order to test the effect of in vivo HCG-treated macrophages on splenic lymphocyte response peritoneal exudate was collected from HCG-treated mice and diluted to contain 0.5, 1 or 2×10^5 macrophages per microwell. Plates were incubated for 2 hours and nonadherent cells were removed by washing. Macrophage monolayers were then overlaid with 5.0×10^5 lymphocytes. Lymphocyte:macrophage ratios were 2.5:1, 5:1 or 10:1. PHA in a final concentration of 5 µg/ml was also added. Cultures were incubated for 72 hours. Six hours before the end of the experiment ^{3}HTdR 0.5 µCi/well was added. The cells were then washed with deionized water by use of a Mash II cell harvester (Microbiological Associates, Bethesda, MD). All radioactive filters were counted in a liquid scintillation spectrometer, with Aquasol (New England Nuclear) as the scintillation fluid. Δ cpm represents the mean of six replicate cultures of mitogen stimulated minus the mean of six replicate cultures with no mitogen added. The results are expressed as percent inhibition of ^{3}HTdR incorporation or as percent of control values. The following formulas were used:

$$\% \text{ inhibition} = 1 - \frac{\text{Experimental } \Delta \text{ cpm}}{\text{Control } \Delta \text{ cpm}} \times 100 \qquad (1)$$

$$\% \text{ control values} = \frac{\text{Experimental } \Delta \text{ cpm}}{\text{Control } \Delta \text{ cpm}} \times 100 \qquad (2)$$

Determination of Prostaglandin Levels

The prostaglandins were determined by a modified procedure (23) of the radioimmunoassay (RIA) technique of Jaffe et al. (11). Briefly, the assay consisted of incubating 100 µl of the experimental samples with 50 µl rabbit antiprostaglandin $PGF_{2\alpha}$ or PGE_1, for 2 hours at room temperature, followed by the addition of 50 µl ^{3}HPGF$_{2\alpha}$ or ^{3}HPGE (8,000 cpm) with further incubation at 4°C for 12 to 16 hours (final volume 200 µl; Trizma (0.012%), NaCl/0.083%) and gelatin (0.1%); pH 7.4). The bound ^{3}H-PG was separated from the uncomplexed tracer after the addition of 0.25 ml iced Tris-NaCl-1.0% gelatin by adding 0.5 ml iced charcoal (0.5%)-dextran (0.5%) in Tris-NaCl buffer and incubating at 4°C for 20 minutes. After centrifugation (200 x g for 12 minutes) the supernatant was decanted into scintillation vials, 10 ml Ultrafluor were added, and radioactivity determined in an LS-350 (Beckman Corp., Fullerton, CA).

RESULTS

Macrophage Activation In Vitro by Human Chorionic Gonadotropin

HCG was used at concentrations from 1 to 5,000 IU/ml. Doses higher than 100 IU/ml were found to significantly transform normal resting macrophages into cytotoxic effector cells in vitro (Figure 1). The same concentrations of HCG or untreated normal macrophages alone did not significantly influence MBL-2 proliferation. Partially purified IF at 1000 IU/ml was used in parallel cultures, as a positive control, since it has been shown to be a macrophage activator (20).

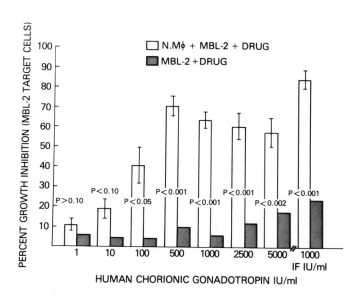

Fig. 1. Effect of various doses of HCG
on the cytotoxic activity of in vitro
treated normal macrophages (N. MØ).

HCG-treated macrophages showed accelerated spreading on plastic and
prominent vacuolization as compared to control cultures (Figure 2a and 2b).

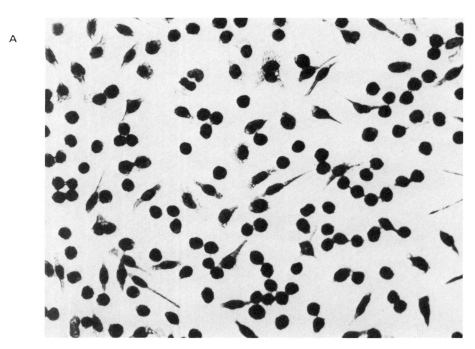

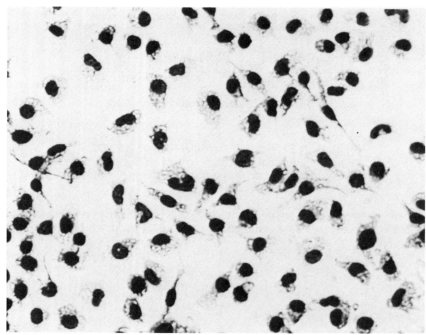

Fig. 2.   a) Normal Balb/c peritoneal macrophages after 48 hours cultured in RPMI-FCS or b) medium containing RPMI-FCS + HCG
1000 IU/ml. Note increased cell spreading and prominent
vacuolization after HCG treatment.

Macrophage Activation In Vivo by Human Chorionic Gonadotropin

HCG was similarly tested for its capacity to render macrophages cytotoxic <u>in vivo</u>. The hormone was administered daily at 500 IU/animal, for a total of 2, 4, 6, 8 or 10 treatments. Control groups were treated similarly with PBS.

Peritoneal macrophages were harvested and tested against MBL-2 cells. The results in Figure 3 show that macrophages collected from HCG-treated animals having received six or more treatments were cytotoxic for MBL-2 tumor cells. Placebo treatment lacked effect on macrophage activity on all groups tested.

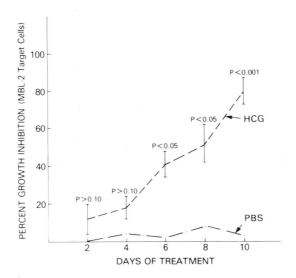

Fig. 3. <u>in vivo</u> effect of HCG on macrophage cytotoxicity.

Effect of In Vivo HCG-Activated Macrophages on Splenic Lymphocyte Mitogenic Response

Having established the <u>in vivo</u> macrophage activation after HCG treatment, we next examined its effect on lymphocyte blastogenesis. Studies were carried out using three lymphocyte:macrophage ratios for each experimental group: 10:1, 5:1, and 2.5:1. Cultures containing peritoneal macrophages and splenic lymphocytes were tested against the T-cell mitogen PHA in a final concentration of 5 µg/ml. A group where no peritoneal macrophages were added served as a control. The results in Figure 4 show a significant inhibition of lymphocyte DNA synthesis in all groups containing HCG-activated macrophages except in the lymphocyte:macrophage ratio of 10:1 of the groups HCG-2x and HCG-6x.

The group that contained macrophages from PBS-treated animals at 2.5:1 ratio also exhibited a significantly diminished response to PHA, as compared to the control containing no macrophages.

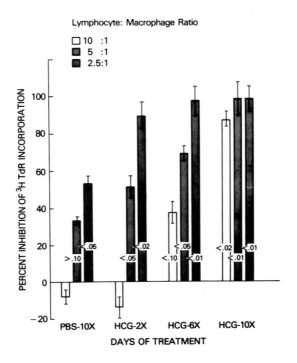

Fig. 4. Effect of *in vivo* HCG-activated macrophages on the blastogenic response of normal splenic lymphocytes.

Effect of HCG on the In Vitro Blastogenic Response of Normal Splenic Lymphocytes

Results in Figure 5 show that HCG at a concentration of 10 IU/ml significantly enhanced the ^{3}HTdR incorporation by splenic lymphocytes. However, at concentrations of HCG higher than 500 IU/ml, a dose-related supression of DNA synthesis is seen. Cultures containing HCG at a concentration of 100 IU/ml show similar activity to the normal control cultures.

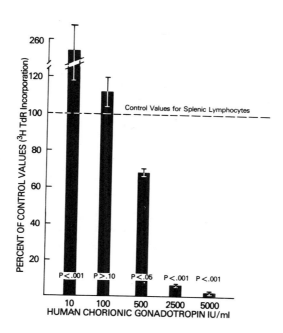

Fig. 5.   Effect of various doses of HCG on the blastogenic
response of normal splenic lymphocytes.

Prostaglandin Synthesis by In Vitro HCG-Treated Macrophages

Studies were performed to determine whether HCG-treated peritoneal
macrophage monolayers elaborated prostaglandins in culture. In these
experiments, cultures were adjusted to contain 1.0×10^6 macrophages/
16 mm well.   Three concentrations of HCG were investigated 100, 500,
2500 IU/ml contained in RPMI-FCS.   Control macrophage cultures containing only RPMI-FCS were included.   Supernatants were obtained after
16, 24, 48 hour incubation and analyzed for their concentration of PGE
and $PGF_{2\alpha}$ by radioimmunoassay.   RPMI-FCS alone was incubated for an
equal period of time and the level of prostaglandin content similarly
determined.   Results of these experiments (Table 1) demonstrate an
increased synthesis and release of both PGE and $PGF_{2\alpha}$ by HCG-treated
macrophages.   A dose-dependent increase is shown for $PGF_{2\alpha}$ and a
slight increase with the length of incubation.   PGE levels are considerably higher than control values at all concentrations of HCG tested.

TABLE 1. Prostaglandin levels from normal or HCG treated peritoneal macrophages pg/1.0 x 10^6 macrophages

Mφ+	HCG	IU/ML	Incubation Period					
			16 Hours		24 Hours		48 Hours	
			$PGF_{2\alpha}$	PGE	$PGF_{2\alpha}$	PGE	$PGF_{2\alpha}$	PGE
"	-	-	380		547		568	
				238		762		911
"	"	100	960		1511		2155	
				21492		23293		25939
"	"	500	4306		6259		5239	
				41048		38186		51123
"	"	2500	8861		9535		6560	
				45911		41337		48882
RPMI-FCS*			157		187		175	
				24		16		9

*The amount of prostaglandins contained in RPMI-FCS was subtracted from all cultures. All cultures were incubated at 37°C. Prostaglandin levels were determined by radioimmunoassay.

DISCUSSION

The results in the present study demonstrated a significant effect of HCG preparations on peritoneal macrophages. Macrophage activation, determined by cytotoxicity and morphological changes, has been manifested both in vivo and in vitro. Some activity on murine macrophages was observed at low concentrations of HCG (100 IU/ml), but the peak of activity was seen at higher concentrations. Low concentrations of HCG were found to significantly enhance splenic lymphocyte response to PHA, where high concentrations markedly inhibited lymphocyte proliferation. This biphasic response has been previously reported (14). At present there is not any explanation for this anomaly.

The immunosuppressive properties of commercial preparations of HCG have been questioned, because recent investigations using highly purified preparations of HCG failed to express significant suppression of lymphocyte proliferation. The activity of crude HCG was attributed to contaminant factors (4,8,16). However, it is important to realize that the procedures used for HCG purification invariably lead to some degradation of the attached carbohydrate moiety. After purification, the protein portion of the molecule could maintain its biologic activity as defined by rat uterine weight assay (16). However, the loss of immunologic reactivity might be related to the degradation of the carbohydrate moiety. The preparations of HCG used in this study were isolated from the urine of pregnant women and are widely used in clinical and research trials.

Most workers have utilized crude commercial preparations of HCG. Depression of antibody response to SRBC in HCG-pretreated mice (27), prolongation of skin allografts on mice treated with HCG (18) or morphologic changes of the lymphatic system after HCG administration (17) have been reported. Beling and Weksler reported that highly purified HCG preparations (S.A. 13,700 IU/mg) inhibited the response of lymphocytes from both male and female subjects to allogeneic cells in mixed lymphocyte cultures (2). Of particular interest in this study was the observation that HCG-treated macrophages elaborated and released prostaglandins and suppressed T-lymphocyte response to PHA. The suppressive effect of prostaglandins, especially of the E series on human peripheral blood lymphocytes, has previously been reported (7,24). Recently, Goodwin et al identified a population of glass adherent mononuclear cells in human peripheral blood that suppress T-cell mitogenic activity through production of prostaglandins of the E series (7). Demenkoff et al. (6) also demonstrated that canine alveolar macrophages suppressed bronchoalveolar lymphocytes through elaboration and release of prostaglandin. Similarly Metzger et al. (15) have recently reported that Corynebacterium parvum or thioglycollate-induced peritoneal macrophages obtained from C57B1/6 mice totally suppressed lymphocytes proliferation. Both hydrogen peroxide and prostaglandins were implicated in this suppression. From the results of this study, it was of particular interest to note the dual effect of HCG on the macrophage population. HCG-activated macrophages expressed both a significantly tumoricidal effect and a suppressive effect on the splenic lymphocyte blastogenesis. The latter effect appears to be due to the production of prostaglandins notably of the E series.

REFERENCES

1. Adcock, E.W., Teasdale, F., August, C.S., Cox, S., Meschia, G., Battaglia, F.C. and Naughton, M.A. (1973) Human chorionic gonadotropin: Its possible role in maternal lymphocytes suppression. Science 181, 845.

2. Beling, C.G. and Weksler, M.E. (1974) Suppression of mixed lymphocyte reactivity by human chorionic gonadotropin. Clin. Exp. Immunol. 18, 537.

3. Braunstein, G.D., Vaitukaitis, J.L., Carbone, P.P., and Ross, G.T. (1973) Ectopic production of human chorionic gonadotropin by neoplasms. Annals of Inter. Med. 78, 39.

4. Caldwell, J.L., Stites, D.P., and Fudenberg, H.H. (1975) Human chorionic gonadotropin: Effects of crude and purified preparations on lymphocyte responses to phytohemagglutinin and allogeneic stimulation. J. Immunol. 115(5), 1249.

5. Contractor, S.F. and Davies, H. (1973) Effect of human chorionic gonadotropin and human chorionic gonadotropin on PHA-induced lymphocyte transformation. Nature 243, 284.

6. Demenkoff, J.H., Ansfield, M.J., Klatreider, H.A. and Adam, E. (1980) Alveolar macrophage suppression of canine bronchoalveolar lymphocytes: The role of prostaglandin E2 in the inhibition of mitogen responses. J. Immunol. 124(3), 1365.

7.   Goodwin, J.S., Bankhurst, A.D. and Messner, R.P. (1977) Suppression of human T-cell mitogenesis by prostaglandins. J. Exp. Med. 146, 1719.

8.   Gundert, D., Merz, N.E., Hilgenfeldt, V. and Brossmer, R. (1975) Inability of higly purified preparations of human chorionic gonadotropin to inhibit the PHA-induced stimulation of lymphocytes. FEBS Lett. 53 (3), 309.

9.   Han, T. (1975) Human chorionic gonadotropin. Its inhibitory effect on cell-mediated immunity in vivo and in vitro. Immunology 29, 509.

10. Horne, C.H.W., Reid, I.N., and Milne, G.D. (1976) Prognostic significance of inappropriate production of pregnancy proteins by breast cancer. Lancet ii:279.

11. Jaffe, R.M., Smith, J.W., Newton, W.T. and Parker, C.W. (1971) Radioimmunoassay for prostaglandins. Science, 171, 494.

12. Kahn, C.R., Rosen, S.W., Weintraub, B.D., Fajaus, S.S. and Gorden, P. (1977) Ectopic production of chorionic gonadotropin and its subunits by islet-cell tumors. New Engl. J. Med., 297, 565.

13. Kaye, M.D. and Jones, W.R. (1971) Effect of human chorionic gonadotropin on in vitro lymphocyte transformation. Am. J. Obstet. Gynecol. 109, 1029.

14. Maes, R.F. and Claverie, N. (1977) The effect of preparations of HCG on lymphocyte stimulation and immune response. Immunology 33, 351.

15. Metzger, Z., Hoffeld, J.T. and Oppenheim, J.J. (1980) Macrophage-mediated suppression. I. Evidence for participation of both hydrogen peroxide and prostaglandins in suppression of murine lymphocyte proliferation. J. Immunol. 124(2), 983.

16. Muchmore, A.V. and Blaese, R.M. (1977) Immunoregulatory properties of fractions from human pregnancy urine: Evidence that human chorionic gonadotropin is not responsible. J. Immunol. 118(3), 881.

17. Nelson, J.H., Jr., and Hall, S.E. (1965) Studies on the thymo-lymphatic system in humans. ii. Morphologic changes in lymph nodes in early pregnancy and during the puerperium. A. J. Obstet. Gynecol. 93, 1133.

18. Pearse, W.H. and Kaiman, H. (1967) Human chorionic gonadotropin and skin homograft survival. Am. J. Obstet. Gynecol. 98, 572.

19. Rosen, S.W., Becker, C.E., Schlaff, S., Easton, J. and Gluck, M.C. (1968) Ectopic gonadotropin production before clinical recognition of bronchogenic carcinoma. New Engl. J. Med. 279, 640.

20. Schultz, R.M., Chirigos, M.A. and Heine, V. (1978) Functional and morphological characteristics of interferon-treated macrophages. Cell. Immunol. 35, 84.

21. Schultz, R.M., Papamatheakis, J.D. and Chirigos, M.A. (1977) Direct activation in vitro of mouse peritoneal macrophages by pyran copolymer. Cell. Immunol. 29, 403.

22. Schultz, R.M., Woods, W., Mohr, S.J., and Chirigos, M.A. (1976) Immune response of CD2F1 mice to tumor allograft during pyran copolymer-induced tumor enhancement. Cancer Res. 36, 1641.

23. Steel, L.K., Platshon, L. and Kaliver, M. (1979) Prostaglandin generation by human and guina pig lung tissue. Comparison of parenchymal and airway responses. J. Allergy Clin. Immunol. 64, 387.

24. Stockman, G.D. and Mumford, D.M. (1974) The effect of prostaglandins on the in vitro blastogenic response of human peripheral blood lymphocytes. Exp. Hemat. 2, 65.

25. Walker, R.A. (1978) Significance of α-subunit HCG demonstrated in breast carcinomas by the immunoperoxidase technique. J. Clin. Pathol. 31, 245.

26. Williams, R.R., McIntire, K.R. et al. (1977) Tumor-associated antigen levels (CEA, HCG, AFP) outdating the diagnosis of cancer in the Framingham Study. J. Natl. Cancer Inst. 58, 1547.

27. Younger, S.B., St. Pierre, R.L. and Zmizewski, G.M. (1969) Effect of human chorionic gonadotropin on antibody production. Am. J. Obstet. Gynecol. 105, 9.

Mediation of Cellular Immunity in Cancer by Immune Modifiers, edited by M. A. Chirigos et al., Raven Press, New York © 1981.

Characteristics of NK Cells and Their Possible Role *In Vivo*

Ronald B. Herberman, Tuomo Timonen, and John R. Ortaldo

Laboratory of Immunodiagnosis, National Cancer Institute, Bethesda, Maryland 20205

INTRODUCTION

The phenomenon of cytotoxicity of tumor cells and of cultured cell lines derived from tumors by lymphocytes of many normal individuals first became recognized during the course of studies attempting to examine specific cytotoxic activity of lymphocytes of tumor-bearing individuals against their own tumors or against tumors of the same histologic or etiologic type. It gradually became apparent that lymphocytes of some normal controls were actually more cytotoxic against some target cells than were the tumor-bearing individuals under study. These findings have necessitated a reevaluation of supposed disease-related cytotoxic reactivity of cancer patients, with a need to discriminate clearly between the activity of natural effector cells and of more specific immune effector cells (13).

The most extensively studied and characterized natural effector cell in man and rodents has come to be called a natural killer (NK) cell. We will summarize this information, with an emphasis on recent findings from our laboratory. It should be noted, however, that other types of natural effector cells have been found and these may also have important in vivo roles. For more details on NK cells and information on other aspects of natural cell-mediated immunity, the reader might consult recent reviews (e.g., 16) and a new comprehensive book on this subject (18).

CHARACTERISTICS OF NK CELLS

NK cells have generally been found to be nonadherent and nonphagocytic and therefore are considered to be a subpopulation of lymphocytes and not macrophages or monocytes. On the basis of initial cell separation studies, NK cells appeared to be null cells, i.e., lacking characteristic markers of either T cells or B cells. They clearly appear to be distinct from mature T cells, since high levels of NK activity have been found in nude or neonatally thymectomized mice. However, by use of more sensitive techniques, evidence has accumulated for some association of NK cells with the T cell lineage. There have also been some suggestions that NK cells may be promonocytes (for detailed discussion, see 18).

Expression of T Cell Associated Markers

In mice and humans, NK cells have been found to have several markers that suggest some relationship to T cells, possibly being early prethymic cells of the T cell lineage (summarized in 18). Each of these markers has been detected on at least a portion of NK cells and appears to be strongly associated with peripheral T cells. By use of optimal conditions for formation of rosettes with sheep erythrocytes (E rosettes), 50-80% of human NK cells were found to have low affinity receptors for E (51). As a further recent indication that human NK cells reside in the T cell lineage, treatment with specific anti-T cell sera plus complement caused virtual elimination of cytotoxic activity (21). In mice, it has been shown that treatment with high concentrations of anti-Thy 1 plus complement, or repeated treatments, eliminated most NK activity (25). In addition, it has been possible to positively select for a portion of NK cells from nude or conventional mice, using a monoclonal anti-Thy 1 antibody and the fluorescence activated cell sorter (25). Similarly, Koo and Hatzfeld (23) have reported that monoclonal antibodies to Ly 1 can react with about one-fourth of mouse NK cells. Thus, it appears that at least some human and mouse NK cells have characteristic markers of the T cell lineage.

Expression of Fc_γ Receptors and Relationship to K Cells

Another surface marker on NK cells is the $Fc_\gamma R$ (receptor for Fc portion of IgG). $Fc_\gamma R$ are readily detected on human NK cells and methods which deplete $Fc_\gamma R+$ cells result in virtual elimination of NK activity. In mice and rats, NK cells initially appeared to lack $Fc_\gamma R$. However, when more sensitive depletion procedures were used, more than half of the NK lytic units were removed (14, 28). The finding of $Fc_\gamma R$ on NK cells of each of the species studied raised questions about the relationship between NK cells and K cells mediating ADCC. However, extensive studies in our laboratory and in some others have failed to confirm that IgG is involved in natural cell-mediated cytotoxicity (18). Despite this, the NK and K cells appear to be in the same subpopulation of lymphocytes and share many characteristics. On the basis of experiments in which some target cells sensitive to NK activity were able to inhibit ADCC, it appears that NK and ADCC activities may be mediated by the same cells. It may be that the same cell can produce cytotoxic effects either by interaction with antibody-coated target cells via its $Fc_\gamma R$ or with some target cells via separate "NK receptors."

Large Granular Lymphocytes

Although several markers on mouse NK cells appear quite promising for selective depletion of cytotoxic activity (see 18), none has yet been shown to provide the basis for purification of NK cells. In contrast, some recent findings with human and rat NK cells have indicated that isolation of this effector cell population can be achieved. Timonen et al. (45) found that the majority of human lymphocytes binding to NK-sensitive target cells and thereby forming conjugates were large lymphocytes with an indented nucleus and prominent azurophilic granules in the cytoplasm (large granular lymphocytes, LGL). It has been possible to enrich for LGL on discontinuous Percoll density gradients (40, 46) and we have recently used this procedure to better characterize human NK cells (47). Most of the NK and also ADCC activity has been found in the fractions with 75-85% LGL, whereas these fractions contained only 10-20% of the input peripheral blood lymphocytes. In contrast, the fractions containing most of the small-medium lymphocytes have been virtually devoid of NK or ADCC activity. Thus this procedure consistently results in at least 5-fold enrichment of NK and ADCC activities. The possibility that the LGL are responsible for the cytotoxic activity has been supported by observations that about 50% of the LGL can form conjugates with K562 (a highly NK-sensitive target) or antibody-coated target cells and that most of these conjugate-forming LGL have the capacity to kill the attached target cells. Furthermore, almost all LGL were found to contain $Fc_\gamma R$, as measured by adherence to monolayers of immune complexes. The combination of Percoll gradient centrifugation and monolayer adsorption procedures has yielded fractions containing 90% LGL and most of the NK activity of the input population.

LGL could also be discriminated from other lymphocytes by rosetting with E. About one-half of the LGL had low affinity E receptors, forming rosettes at 4° but not at 29°, and the remainder lacked detectable receptors. In contrast, most other nylon-nonadherent lymphocytes had high affinity E receptors, rosetting at 29° as well as at 4°. This has provided the basis for an alternative procedure for further purification of NK cells (47). Removal of high affinity E-rosette forming cells from the LGL-containing Percoll fractions resulted in a subpopulation highly enriched for LGL and NK activity.

Because of reports that the natural effector cells in mice that react against monolayer target cells differ somewhat from NK cells (4, 44), it was of interest to determine whether LGL were the effector cells for cytotoxicity against human monolayer target cells as well as against the suspension K562 cell line. We have found that only LGL-enriched Percoll fractions were reactive against the whole range of targets tested (24), indicating that, in man, LGL appear to account for natural cytotoxicity against both suspension and monolayer targets.

These studies on separation of lymphocytes also have defined two morphologically distinct subpopulations of cells with $Fc_\gamma R$ and E receptors (and thus T_G cells). This was accompanied by a functional division, with only the T_G cells with LGL morphology having NK and ADCC activities. Studies are now in progress to determine the distribution between the two cell types of other immune functions that have been associated with T_G cells, particularly suppressor activity.

Rat NK cells in spleen and peripheral blood also appear to be LGL and can be enriched by a procedure similar to that used for human cells (33). In contrast, LGL have not been detectable in mouse spleens or peripheral blood and the mouse NK cell has not yet been found to have any special morphological features that would distinguish it from other lymphocytes.

The strong association between human NK cells and LGL has allowed us to perform more detailed studies on the phenotype of these effector cells and to compare it with small lymphocytic T cells. We have tested these subpopulations with a series of monoclonal antibodies (31), including those recently reported to react selectively with T cells or other cell types (20), using the fluorescence activated cell sorter. The T cell fraction gave the expected pattern of results, whereas a considerable portion of the LGL reacted with OKM1 and anti-Ia anti-

bodies and about 25% reacted with OKT8 (similar to the T cells). In
contrast, very few LGL reacted with OKT3, which reacts with a high
proportion of T cells. However, several other antibodies to T cell
associated antigens did react with an appreciable proportion of LGL.
In fact, one of these, OKT10, which has been found to react mainly with
early thymocytes, reacted with a high proportion of LGL and none of the
other peripheral blood lymphoid cell subpopulations. The explanation
for this pattern of reactivity is not clear, but this phenotype is
clearly distinct from that of typical T cells. The reactivity with
OKM1 raises the question of some relationship of LGL to monocytes, but
this antigen may be a differentiation antigen shared by cells of various lineages.

AUGMENTATION OF NK ACTIVITY BY INTERFERON (IFN)

A variety of IFN-inducers has been found to augment NK activity in
mice and inoculation of IFN itself led to boosting of activity within 3
hours (6, 7). Incubation of mouse spleen cells with poly I:C or with
IFN also has resulted in appreciable increases in NK activity. Similar
observations have been made with human NK and K cells (15-17, 49).
Administration of poly I:C to some patients resulted in increased
levels of cytotoxicity after 2 days. Incubation of human peripheral
blood lymphocytes with three different IFN preparations for 1 hour or
18 hours caused increased NK and K cell activities with most donors.

During the course of the above studies, there remained some concern
as to whether IFN was indeed the molecule responsible for augmenting
cytotoxic activity, since the antiviral substance in all of the preparations was actually less than 1-10% of the total protein. To more
definitively determine the role of IFN, we have recently had the opportunity to perform experiments with pure human leukocyte IFN (39).
Incubation of human lymphocytes with this homogeneous protein for 1
hour at 37°C resulted in substantial augmentation of NK activity, thus
confirming the role of IFN in positive regulation of NK activity (19).

The ability to separate LGL from conventional lymphocytes on Percoll
gradients and to measure binding of lymphoid cells to NK-susceptible
targets has allowed detailed examination of the interactions between
effector cells and targets and of the mechanisms for augmentation of
NK activity by IFN. One series of issues was whether only LGL formed
conjugates with K562 and whether only this subpopulation could be activated for NK activity by IFN. There have been several previous indications for pre-NK cells that can be induced by IFN (e.g., 2, 29) and
these precursors may have some characteristics that differ from those
associated with spontaneously active NK cells. Therefore, Percoll
separated fractions of LGL and of conventional lymphocytes, with or
without pretreatment by IFN, were tested for conjugate formation with
K562 (47). In addition to considerable conjugate formation by LGL,
some conventional lymphocytes also formed conjugates. However, this
was not accompanied by any detectable cytotoxic activity, even after
pretreatment with IFN. These data indicate that both active NK cells
and IFN-inducible precursors are LGL and that the conventional lymphocytes forming conjugates with K562 cells are not directly related to
NK cells. Similar results have been obtained with a variety of other
human target cells, including monolayer targets (24).

Another important question has been the mechanism for augmentation of NK activity by IFN. IFN was found to substantially increase the reactivity of LGL as well as unseparated lymphoid cells (47), indicating that IFN can act directly on NK cells and cause augmentation of activity, without the need for accessory cells. Measurements of the kinetics of cytotoxicity also indicated that augmentation by IFN could be detected during the first hour of the assay. However, such cytotoxicity experiments failed to provide insight into which step or steps in the cytotoxic process were affected by IFN. Three main possibilities were considered: a) induction on pre-NK cells of receptors for recognition of NK-susceptible targets; b) triggering of the lytic machinery of conjugate-forming inactive NK cells; and c) augmentation of the activity of already active NK cells. Measurement of conjugate formation by LGL provided a means to directly examine the first possibility. The treatment of LGL with IFN did not increase the proportion of cells forming conjugates with K562, indicating that the augmenting effects of IFN are beyond the induction of recognition receptors on LGL. To examine which of the other possibilities for IFN action were involved, we have performed experiments with the single cell agarose assay, developed by Grimm and Bonavida (10). This method allows one to directly determine the proportion of conjugate-forming cells that produce lysis of their attached targets. During the first four hours of the interaction between LGL and K562, both the rate of lysis and the proportion of active conjugate-forming cells were higher for the IFN-treated cells (48). However, with further incubation, the proportion of targets lysed by the untreated effectors approached or sometimes equalled that affected by the IFN-treated LGL. These data imply that IFN acts mainly to accelerate the rate of lysis by already active NK cells. However, since contact with target cells can induce LGL to produce IFN (41), the possibility remains that the late rise in the proportion of active NK cells in the control group was due to activation by the endogenously produced IFN. Another important result from these studies was that a high proportion of conjugate-forming LGL, often greater than 90%, were shown to have the ability to act as NK cells. Thus, not only are virtually all NK cells in the LGL population, but a substantial proportion of LGL (about 50%) can act as NK cells against one sensitive target cell. It remains to be determined whether many of the LGL that fail to bind and lyse K562 have reactivity against other NK-sensitive target cells.

When the same type of analysis was performed with human LGL and some other target cells (e.g., Gll, derived from a patient with breast cancer), a different pattern of results was obtained. After IFN pretreatment of LGL, a considerably higher proportion formed conjugates with such targets and also a higher percentage of bound target cells were killed. Thus, with some target cells, IFN can convert a portion of LGL from non-binding and/or lytically inactive cells into functional effector cells. Therefore, it appears that, depending on the target cells, the effects of IFN can be at one or more different phases of differentiation or activation of NK cells.

CYTOTOXICITY BY CULTURED T CELLS

A major limitation for detailed analysis of the characteristics and specificity of NK cells is that these cells only represent a small

portion of the lymphoid cells in the blood or spleen (probably less
than 5%). Even with the development of satisfactory isolation procedures, like the methods for enrichment of LGL, the low yield of cells
imposes serious restrictions on the studies that can be performed. It
would therefore be highly desirable to be able to propagate NK cells
and expand them to large numbers. A further potential advantage in the
growth of NK cells would be the ability to directly test our hypothesis
of polyclonality of NK cells, with differing specificities.

During the past few years, it has become possible to propagate human
or mouse T cells in the presence of T cell growth factor (26). Cultured T cells (CTC) from normal human donors were found to have considerable cytotoxic activity against a wide array of target cells (1,
3, 42, 43). Since K562 was one of the target cells that were susceptible to lysis by CTC, we have investigated the possibility that at
least some of the cytotoxicity was due to propagation of NK cells. In
detailed studies on the nature of cytotoxicity by human CTC, we have
obtained indications for four separate types of activity (30, 32): a)
cytotoxicity against K562 target cells; b) cytotoxicity against allogeneic but not autologous or histocompatible mitogen-induced lympho-
blasts; c) ADCC against antibody-coated mouse lymphoma cells; and d)
lectin-induced cytotoxicity against the mouse lymphoma cells. The
cytotoxicity against K562 and the alloblasts was distinguishable by the
augmentation of only the former activity by pretreatment of CTC with
IFN. Furthermore, in cold target inhibition experiments, unlabelled
K562 could strongly inhibit lysis of ^{51}Cr-labelled K562 but did not
appreciably affect lysis of labelled alloblasts. Conversely, unlabelled alloblasts only inhibited the lysis of labelled alloblasts. It
seems likely that the activity against alloblasts was due to poly-
clonally activated cytotoxic T cells (42, 43) and that the effectors
for K562 were of a different nature and specificity. The possibility
that the anti-K562 activity was due to NK cells was supported by the
parallel findings of reactivity against antibody-coated targets. This
appeared to be true ADCC by K cells since addition of protein A selectively blocked this reaction, as was previously demonstrated for ADCC
(22). The fourth type of cytotoxicity, in the presence of PHA, resulted in substantial cytotoxicity against the ordinarily resistant
mouse lymphoma target cell.

The finding of apparent NK activity in CTC was encouraging and was
consistent with our hypothesis of the T cell lineage of NK cells.
However, the heterogeneity of effector cells in CTC interfered with
the possible use of such cells for detailed studies of NK cells. To
circumvent this heterogeneity, we have attempted to initiate cultures
from Percoll-separated fractions of lymphocytes from normal human
donors. The LGL-containing fractions, as well as the fractions with
conventional lymphocytes, have proliferated in the presence of T cell
growth factor. The CTC from LGL fractions maintained substantial
levels of IFN-augmentable cytotoxic activity against K562 and antibody-
coated target cells. In contrast, the CTC from the fractions containing conventional lymphocytes had little or no activity against these
targets, even after pretreatment with IFN. Thus, it appears promising
that selected effector cell populations can be expanded by this procedure. We have recently initiated cultures from LGL-enriched fractions,
further purified by removal of high affinity E-rosette forming cells.
After 7-14 days, almost all of the cells in the cultures had the

morphology of LGL and high levels of cytotoxic activity were seen. It is of considerable interest that the surface phenotype of these cultured LGL was considerably different from that of fresh LGL, resembling mature T cells much more closely. The cultured cells have been positive with OKT3 and negative with OKT10 and OKM1.

In other laboratories, a few clones of mouse CTC, with cell surface characteristics of NK cells, have already been obtained (5; H. Cantor, personal communication). The clones from the two laboratories differed in specificity, supporting the concept of heterogeneity of NK cells. Clones of mouse and human CTC have also been obtained and studied in our laboratory (E. Kedar, B. Sredni, and N. Navarro, unpublished observations). Three clones of human CTC have been found to have appreciable levels of cytotoxicity against K562 and other NK-susceptible target cells. A large number of clones of mouse CTC have been obtained and most of these have had high levels of cytotoxic activity (E. Kedar, unpublished observations). Some of these clones have shown a broad range of cytotoxic activity against mouse lymphoma and monolayer target cells and also against some heterologous target cells, whereas other clones have been more restricted in their pattern of reactivity. Characterization of the phenotype of these clones is still in progress, but some have been found to contain abundant azurophilic granules (and thus resembling human and rat LGL) and markers that have been associated with mouse NK cells (asialo GM1 and Ly 5). Thus, it seems likely that some clones of CTC are derived from NK cells and that these cells will be very useful for more detailed characterization of NK cells, their specificity, and the nature of their interaction with target cells.

IN VIVO ROLE OF NK CELLS

The most important practical issue to be settled is the role of NK cells in vivo. There is increasing evidence that NK cells may play an important role in resistance against tumor growth and also in rejection of bone marrow transplants (summarized in 18).

Rapid In Vivo Clearance of Radiolabelled Tumor Cells

To obtain more direct information about the role of NK cells in rapid in vivo elimination of tumor cells, recently we have examined the correlation between levels of NK activity and the ability of mice to destroy intravenously inoculated tumors that were prelabelled with ^{125}I-iododeoxyuridine (34, 35, 38). In young mice of strains with high NK activity, there was a greater decrease in recovery of radioactivity when measured in various organs at 2-4 hours after inoculation than was seen in strains with low NK activity. In parallel with the decline of NK activity in mice after 10-12 weeks of age, in vivo clearance of intravenously inoculated tumor cells was also found to decrease (34-36). Furthermore, a variety of treatments of mice that produced augmented or decreased in vitro reactivity also resulted in similar shifts in in vivo reactivity. Thus, this in vivo assay has correlated very well with NK cell reactivity against a variety of established tumor cell lines.

As further confirmation of the role of NK cells in resistance to growth of NK-susceptible transplantable tumors, transfer of NK cells into mice with cyclophosphamide-induced depression of NK activity was

shown to significantly restore both in vivo and NK reactivities (37).
The effectiveness of the transfer correlated with the levels of NK
activity of donor cells in a variety of situations: a) NK-reactive
spleen cells were able to transfer reactivity whereas NK-unreactive
thymus cells were ineffective; b) spleen cells from young mice of high
NK strains were considerably more effective than cells from older mice
or from strains with low NK activity; c) the cells responsible for
transfer had the characteristics of NK cells, being nonadherent, nonphagocytic, expressing asialo GM1 and lacking easily detectable Thy 1
antigen; and d) cells from donors with drug-induced depression of NK
activity were unable to transfer reactivity. These results extend the
recent findings of Hanna and Fidler (11), who showed that the transfer
of NK-reactive spleen cells to cyclophosphamide-treated mice could
decrease the number of metastases developing in the lungs after challenge with NK-susceptible solid tumor cells.

A similar pattern of results was obtained when radiolabelled cells
were inoculated subcutaneously into the footpads of mice (8). Clearance correlated in several ways with the levels of NK activity in the
recipients and cells with the characteristics of NK cells were effective in local adoptive transfer. However, in contrast to NK activity
and the results with intravenously inoculated tumor cells, no decrease
in clearance was observed in older or beige mice. Those results suggest that other effector cells may also be involved in reactivity in
subcutaneous tissues [e.g., the natural cytotoxic cells described by
Stutman et al. (44)] or that in some situations local factors may augment the NK cell activity.

In Vivo Reactivity Against Normal Cells

It has been shown that NK cells can also lyse some normal cells such
as subpopulations of bone marrow and thymus cells (12, 27, 50). To
determine whether natural reactivity against normal cells could also
occur in vivo, we have tested both in vivo and in vitro reactivities
of normal mice against bone marrow cells and fetal fibroblasts (38).
As with tumor targets, young mice of high NK strains rapidly eliminated
a higher proportion of these normal cells than did older mice or those
of a low NK strain. Furthermore, both in vivo and in vitro reactivities against these targets were modulated in parallel by NK-augmenting
or depressing treatments.

Role of NK Cells Against Primary Tumors

It will be particularly important now to obtain information about
the possible in vivo role of NK cells in resistance against primary
tumors. The original formulations of the theory of immune surveillance
focused on the central role of the immune response as a natural defense
against neoplasia. Although most attention has been focused on the
relationship of thymus-dependent immunity to immune surveillance, NK
activity now has to be considered as an alternative mechanism.

One prediction of the immune surveillance hypothesis is that chemical carcinogens would cause depressed immune function, thereby impair-
ing the ability of the host to reject the transformed cells. This
postulate has been examined by many investigators in regard to the
possible role of mature T cells and humoral immunity, and conflicting

results have been obtained. In contrast, there is little information available on the effects of chemical carcinogens on NK cells. We have recently performed studies to determine the effects of urethane on NK activity (9). A/J mice, which are sensitive to the carcinogenic effects of urethane, showed depressed NK and in vivo reactivity at 7 days after treatment and later developed multiple lung adenomas. In contrast, the NK and in vivo reactivities of C57BL/6 mice, which are resistant to urethane carcinogenesis, were virtually unaffected by this treatment (E. Gorelik and R. Herberman, in preparation). Thus, carcinogenicity of urethane correlated with its ability to depress NK activity and this effect on host resistance may contribute to the development of neoplastic lesions.

REFERENCES

1. Alvarez, J.M., de Landazuri, M.O., Bonnard, G.D., and Herberman, R.B. (1978): *J. Immunol.*, 121:1270-1275.
2. Bloom, B.R., Minato, N., Neighbour, A., Reid, L., and Marcus, D. (1980): In: *Natural Cell-Mediated Immunity Against Tumors*, edited by R.B. Herberman, pp. 505-524. Academic Press, New York.
3. Bonnard, G.D., Schendel, D.J., West, W.H., Alvarez, J.M., Maca, R.D., Yasaka, K., Fine, R.L., Herberman, R.B., de Landazuri, M.O., and Morgan, D.A. (1978): In: *Human Lymphocyte Differentiation: Its Application to Human Cancer*, edited by B. Serrou and C. Rosenfeld, pp. 319-326. Elsevier/North-Holland Biomedical Press, Amsterdam.
4. Burton, R.C. (1980): In: *Natural Cell-Mediated Immunity Against Tumors*, edited by R.B. Herberman, pp. 19-35. Academic Press, New York.
5. Dennert, G. (1980): *Nature*, 287:47-49.
6. Djeu, J.Y., Heinbaugh, J.A., Holden, H.T., and Herberman, R.B. (1979): *J. Immunol.*, 122:175-181.
7. Gidlund, M., Orn, A., Wigzell, H., Senik, A., and Gresser, I. (1978): *Nature*, 223:259-261.
8. Gorelik, E., and Herberman, R.B. (1981): *Int. J. Cancer*, in press.
9. Gorelik, E., and Herberman, R.B. (1981): *J. Natl. Cancer Inst.*, in press.
10. Grimm, E., and Bonavida, B. (1979): *J. Immunol.*, 123:2861-2869.
11. Hanna, N., and Fidler, I.J. (1980): *J. Natl. Cancer Inst.*, 65:801-809
12. Hansson, M., Kärre, K., Kiessling, R., Roder, J., Anderson, B., and Häyry, P. (1979): *J. Immunol.*, 123:765-771.
13. Herberman, R.B., and Oldham, R.K. (1975): *J. Natl. Cancer Inst.*, 55:749-753.
14. Herberman, R.B., Bartram, S., Haskill, J.S., Nunn, M., Holden, H.T, and West, W.H. (1977): *J. Immunol.*, 119:322-326.
15. Herberman, R.B., Djeu, J.Y., Ortaldo, J.R., Holden, H.T., West, W.H., and Bonnard, G.D. (1978): *Cancer Treat. Rep.*, 62:1893-1896.
16. Herberman, R.B., Djeu, J.Y., Kay, H.D., Ortaldo, J.R., Riccardi, C., Bonnard, G.D., Holden, H.T., Fagnani, R., Santoni, A., and Puccetti, P. (1979): *Immunol. Rev.*, 44:43-70.
17. Herberman, R.B., Ortaldo, J.R., and Bonnard, G.D. (1979): *Nature*, 227:221-223.

18. Herberman, R.B., editor (1980): <u>Natural Cell-Mediated Immunity Against Tumors</u>. Academic Press, New York.
19. Herberman, R.B., Ortaldo, J.R., Djeu, J.Y., Holden, H.T., Jett, J., Lang, N.P., and Pestka, S. (1980): <u>Ann. N.Y. Acad. Sci.</u>, 350:63-71.
20. Hoffman, R.A., Kung, P.C., Hansen, W.P., and Goldstein, G. (1980): <u>Proc. Natl. Acad. Sci. USA</u>, 77:4914-4917.
21. Kaplan, J., and Callewaert, D.M. (1978): <u>J. Natl. Cancer Inst.</u>, 60:961-964.
22. Kay, H.D., Bonnard, G.D., and Herberman, R.B. (1979): <u>J. Immunol.</u>, 122:675-685.
23. Koo, G.C., and Hatzfeld, A. (1980): In: <u>Natural Cell-Mediated Immunity Against Tumors</u>, edited by R.B. Herberman, pp. 105-116. Academic Press, New York.
24. Landazuri, M.O., Lopez-Botet, M., Ortaldo, J.R., Timonen, T., and Herberman, R.B. (1981): Submitted for publication.
25. Mattes, M.J., Sharrow, S.O., Herberman, R.B., and Holden, H.T. (1979): <u>J. Immunol.</u>, 123:2851-2860.
26. Morgan, D.A., Ruscetti, F.W., and Gallo, R.C. (1976): <u>Science</u>, 193:1007-1008.
27. Nunn, M.E., Herberman, R.B., and Holden, H.T. (1977): <u>Int. J. Cancer</u>, 20:381-387.
28. Oehler, J.R., Lindsay, L.R., Nunn, M.E., and Herberman, R.B. (1978): <u>Int. J. Cancer</u>, 21:204-209.
29. Oehler, J.R., Lindsay, L.R., Nunn, M.E., Holden, H.T., and Herberman, R.B. (1978): <u>Int. J. Cancer</u>, 21:210-220.
30. Ortaldo, J.R. (1980): Submitted for publication.
31. Ortaldo, J.R., Sharrow, S.O., Timonen, T., and Herberman, R.B. (1981): Submitted for publication.
32. Ortaldo, J.R., Timonen, T., and Bonnard, G.D. (1981): <u>Behring Inst. Mitt.</u>, in press.
33. Reynolds, C.W., Timonen, T., and Herberman, R.B. (1981): Submitted for publication.
34. Riccardi, C., Puccetti, P., Santoni, A., and Herberman, R.B. (1979): <u>J. Natl. Cancer Inst.</u>, 63:1041-1045.
35. Riccardi, C., Santoni, A., Barlozzari, T., and Herberman, R.B. (1980): In: <u>Natural Cell-Mediated Immunity Against Tumors</u>, edited by R.B. Herberman, pp. 1121-1139. Academic Press, New York.
36. Riccardi, C., Santoni, A., Barlozzari, T., Puccetti, P., and Herberman, R.B. (1980): <u>Int. J. Cancer</u>, 25:475-486.
37. Riccardi, C., Barlozzari, T., Santoni, A., Herberman, R.B., and Cesarini, C. (1981): <u>J. Immunol.</u>, in press.
38. Riccardi, C., Santoni, A., Barlozzari, T., and Herberman, R.B. (1980): <u>Cell. Immunol.</u>, in press.
39. Rubinstein, M., Rubinstein, S., Familletti, P.C., Miller, R.S., Waldman, A.A., and Pestka, S. (1979): <u>Proc. Natl. Acad. Sci. USA</u>, 76:640-644.
40. Saksela, E., and Timonen, T. (1980): In: <u>Natural Cell-Mediated Immunity Against Tumors</u>, edited by R.B. Herberman, pp. 173-185. Academic Press, New York.
41. Saksela, E., Timonen, T., Virtanen, I., and Cantell, K. (1980): In: <u>Natural Cell-Mediated Immunity Against Tumors</u>, edited by R.B. Herberman, pp. 645-653. Academic Press, New York.

42. Schendel, D.J., Wank, R., and Bonnard, G.D. (1980): Scand. J. Immunol., 11:99-107.

43. Schendel, D.J., Wank, R., and Bonnard, G.D. (1981): Behring Inst. Mitt., in press.

44. Stutman, O., Figarella, E.F., Paige, C.J., and Lattime, E.C. (1980): In: Natural Cell-Mediated Immunity Against Tumors, edited by R.B. Herberman, pp. 187-229. Academic Press, New York.

45. Timonen, T., Saksela, E., Ranki, A., and Hayry, P. (1979): Cell. Immunol., 48:133-148.

46. Timonen, T., and Saksela, E. (1980): J. Immunol. Methods, 36:285-291.

47. Timonen, T., Ortaldo, J.R., and Herberman, R.B. (1981): J. Exp. Med., in press.

48. Timonen, T., Ortaldo, J.R., and Herberman, R.B. (1981): In preparation.

49. Trinchieri, G., and Santoli, D. (1978): J. Exp. Med., 147:1314-1333.

50. Welsh, R.M., Zinkernagel, R.M., and Hallenbeck, L. (1979): J. Immunol., 122:475-481.

51. West, W.H., Cannon, G.B., Kay, H.D., Bonnard, G.D., and Herberman, R.B. (1977): J. Immunol., 118:355-361.

Mediation of Cellular Immunity in Cancer by Immune Modifiers, edited by M. A. Chirigos et al., Raven Press, New York © 1981.

Activation of Natural Killer Cells by Interferon and by Allogeneic Stimulation

D. Santoli, B. Perussia, and G. Trinchieri

The Wistar Institute of Anatomy and Biology, Philadelphia, Pennsylvania 19104

Lymphocytes obtained from the peripheral blood (PBL) of normal healthy donors, with no known or deliberate sensitization, are cytotoxic in vitro against unsensitized and IgG antibody-sensitized target cells. These two types of cytotoxic activity are referred to as spontaneous and antibody-dependent cell-mediated cytotoxicity (SLMC and ADCC) (1). The effector cells are functionally defined as Natural Killer (NK) and Killer (K) cells, respectively (1, 21). Both activities are mediated by cells that are negative for surface immunoglobulin, C3b receptors and DR antigen, but positive for IgG-Fc receptors (FcR) (10, 12, 18, 21). Saksela and Timonen (14) have shown by adsorption-elution on target cell-coated plastic beads and by density gradient separation, that the NK cells have the morphology of large granular lymphocytes. Several studies have been performed to determine whether or not NK and K cells are in the T cell lineage. Cells that are able to form rosettes with sheep erythrocytes (E-RFC) were found to contain up to 50% of both cytotoxic activities, indicating that a proportion of NK and K cells have receptors for sheep erythrocytes (12). The rosetting population contains a small proportion of FcR-positive cells which is responsible for the NK and K cytotoxic activities. This cell population, known as T_G, has been recently shown to be nonreactive with monoclonal antibody OKT3 specific for a common human T-cell antigen (8). In another study, NK and K cells were shown to be reactive with monoclonal antibody OKM1, which reacts with monocytes, granulocytes and a small proportion of lymphocytes (2). This finding suggests that the cytotoxic cells might belong to the myelo-monocytic lineage.

It is now well established that interferon (IFN) plays an important role in the modulation of NK activity. We have shown that when lymphocytes are incubated with most tumor-derived or virus-infected cells, high levels of IFN are released in the supernatant within a few hours of incubation (11, 15, 17). In human peripheral blood, the "null" lymphocytes bearing FcR are responsible for IFN production in these mixed cultures. The same cell population contains most of the activity

of the NK and K cells. IFN exerts a rapid enhancing effect on the
cytotoxicity mediated by NK cells (11, 16, 18). Lymphocytes that have
been treated with IFN display an increased cytotoxicity within a few
hours after treatment, with a maximum at about 24 hr. In the cultures
of lymphocytes with IFN-inducing cell lines, an increase in the rate of
cytotoxicity is concomitant with the appearance of antiviral activity
in the supernatant. When fresh lymphocytes are tested as effector
cells against IFN-inducing target cells, the enhancing effect of the
IFN released in the culture medium is responsible for up to 90% of the
total cytotoxicity observed. As shown in the analysis of cytotoxicity
at the single-cell level, IFN acts mainly by increasing the kinetics of
killing (20), and probably allows each effector cell to lyse a higher
number of target cells in the same time interval. When NK cell activity is removed by absorption on fibroblasts, IFN treatment endows with
cytotoxic ability a population of cells ("pre-NK") that were originally
inactive (13). However, results of single cell cytotoxic assays in
agarose suggest the possibility that IFN conveys cytotoxic ability to
"pre-NK" cells that originally could only bind to the target cells but
were not able to lyse them (19).

The in vitro augmentation of NK activity by IFN may reflect the
mechanism and sequence of events by which NK cells are rendered more
efficient in vivo in response to a stimulus such as a tumor or a viral
infection. However, IFN is only able to enhance the cytotoxicity of
the lymphocyte subpopulations that originally contain NK activity (11,
16). Those subpopulations that do not contain NK cells (B cells,
FcR-negative "null" cells and FcR-negative T cells) do not acquire
cytotoxic activity when exposed to IFN.

In the present study we used mixed lymphocyte cultures (MLC) to ana-
lyze the possibility of generating cytotoxic cells from inactive
precursors. The NK and K cell cytotoxic activities gradually disappear
when the cells are cultured in vitro for a period of several days. If,
however, lymphocytes are activated during the culture period, they are
cytotoxic against targets that have no known antigenic relationship to
the stimulus. In human MLC, different kinds of effector cells are
generated: cytotoxic T lymphocytes (CTL), which specifically destroy
target cells carrying the sensitizing alloantigens, and non-specific
cytotoxic cells, which mediate NK-like and K-like cytotoxicity (3, 7).
The characterization of MLC-activated killer cells and their mechanism
of lysis is necessary to discriminate between specific and non-specific
cytotoxic effects and to reveal any similarities or differences between
in vitro induced (either MLC- or IFN-activated) NK cells and those that
occur spontaneously.

In order to study the generation of cytotoxic cells, in the present
analysis we used purified FcR-negative E-RFC as responders in the MLC.
Such cells lack both SLMC and ADCC activities when freshly isolated
(10, 12). Non-E-RFC were used as stimulators after γ irradiation
(4,500 rad). The same unsensitized lymphocyte subpopulations were also
cultured in parallel with the MLC for 6 days. Lymphocyte subpopulations were tested for their ability to form E rosettes, as well as EA7S
and EA19S rosettes with sensitized ox erythrocytes (OE) (10, 12).
Monoclonal antibodies reactive with T cells (OKT3) (2, 8), with monocytes and granulocytes (B13.4.1), and with DR antigens (B33.1.1) (6)
were used in an indirect immunofluorescence assay to detect surface
markers of lymphocyte fractions. Lymphocytes were tested for all these

markers on day 6 after the onset of the MLC. Likewise, cytotoxic assays were performed immediately after separation of PBL fractions and after 6 days of sensitization in MLC. ADCC and SLMC assays have been extensively described previously (9, 10, 12, 16, 18). The target for ADCC in our study was the murine mastocytoma cell line P815Y, sensitized with anti-P815Y rabbit antibodies; the target for SLMC was the NK-sensitive human erythroleukemia line K562, which lacks HLA-A, B, C and DR antigens. Specific CTL activity was measured in the cell-mediated lympholysis (CML) assay on day 6 against PHA blasts autologous to the stimulator cells. In the CML assay, lysis of PHA blasts autologous to the responder-effector cells was variable but always significant. Although the nature of this auto-killing is not understood, it appears to be mediated by cells with characteristics similar to those of the CTL responsible for specific allogeneic lysis (22). Cytotoxic assays were performed by incubating various dilutions of effector cells with ^{51}Cr-labeled target cells for 4 hr at 37°C. Results concerning the generation of cytotoxic cells from non-cytotoxic precursors (FcR-negative E-RFC) are depicted in Fig. 1. On day 0, FcR-negative E-RFC were completely inactive against both K562 and antibody-coated P815Y cells. After stimulation in MLC, however, they became very efficient against the same targets. The same responder cells cultured in the absence of stimulator cells were non-cytotoxic. Cytotoxic effector cells were also generated in autologous MLC in which FcR-negative E-RFC were cultured with autologous γ-irradiated non-E-RFC. These effector cells were several-fold less efficient, however, than the ones generated after allosensitization. The non-E-RFC used as stimulator had high ADCC and SLMC activities on day 0, but only slight activity after irradiation and none at all after 6 more days in culture. These data suggest that the cytotoxic cells generated in MLC are newly generated from precursors contained in the responder FcR-negative E-RFC population and do not derive from stimulator cells that might have escaped inactivation.

In some experiments unfractionated PBL and FcR-negative E-RFC were used as responders in two parallel sets of MLC. After 6 days of culture, the cells were fractionated into E-RFC and non-E-RFC populations. Separation was repeated twice in order to improve purification. When FcR-negative E-RFC were used as responders, only 1% of the cells were recovered in the non-E-RFC fraction (Table 1), and E-RFC mediated both specific and nonspecific cytotoxicity (Fig. 2). Similarly, the data obtained with antibodies to specific surface antigens (Table 1) indicate that the large majority of effector cells generated in MLC from a pure T cell population maintains the surface markers of T cells. Moreover, these cytotoxic cells can be lysed by anti-T cell monoclonal antibodies and complement (data not shown). In contrast, when unfractionated PBL were used as responders, two kinds of effector cells were obtained: E-RFC, which mediated NK- and K-like activities as well as CML, and the non-E-RFC, which lysed K562 and antibody-sensitized P815 but not allogeneic or autologous PHA blasts (Fig. 2). These results suggest that the NK- and K-like cytotoxicity mediated by MLC-activated killer cells is due to two separate effector cell populations that differ in their ability to form rosettes with sheep erythrocytes. Lysis of PHA, in contrast, is mediated only by E-RFC. Thus, analysis can be restricted to the E-RFC effector population through the use of pure T cells as responders.

TABLE 1. Surface markers of PBL and MLC fractions

Day	Lymphocyte fraction	% Recovery	% E-RFC	% OKT3[a]	% EA7S-RFC	% SIg[b]	% B13.4.1[c]	% B33.1.1[d]
0	PBL		66.3	72	5	7	18	18
	FcR-negative E-RFC	75.0	75.0	98	<1	<1	<1	1
6	ABx1[e], unfractionated	100	78.1	84	5.6	<1	2	40
	ABx1, E-RFC	67.4	91.5	90	<1		<1	24
	ABx1, non-E-RFC	7.9	20.4		4			99
	ABx2[f], unfractionated	100	96	92	1.4	<1	<1	30
	ABx2, E-RFC	75.4	94.7	90	2.9		<1	28
	ABx2, non-E-RFC	1.1	62.7		11.5		<1	18

[a]Anti-T cell monoclonal antibody.
[b]Surface immunoglobulin-positive cells as detected with fluorescein-labeled rabbit F(ab')2 anti-human F(ab')2.
[c]Monoclonal antibody reactive with monocytes and granulocytes.
[d]Monoclonal antibody reactive with DR antigens.
[e]Responders = unfractionated PBL.
[f]Responders = FcR-negative E-RFC.

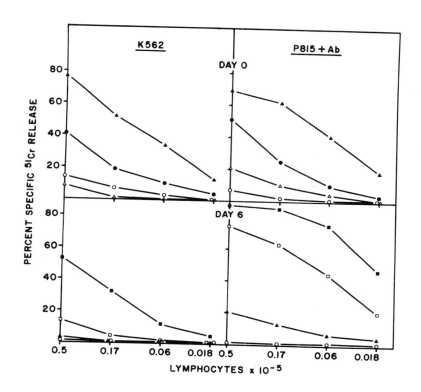

FIG 1.   Generation of NK-like and K-like cells in MLC from non-cytotoxic precursors.   Four-hr cytotoxic assays were performed against
^{51}Cr-labeled K562 cells and antibody-sensitized P815Y to test SLMC and
ADCC, respectively.   The effector cells from donor A on day O were:
freshly purified E-RFC (●), FcR-negative E-RFC (o), non-E-RFC (▲), and
γ-irradiated non-E-RFC (△).   MLC were set up on day O using FcR-negative E-RFC as responders and non-E-RFC as stimulators.   The effector
cells on day 6 after the onset of the MLC were: the allogeneic MLC ABx
(■), the autologous MLC AAx (□), the FcR-negative E-RFC of donor A
cultured alone (o) and the non-E-RFC of donor A cultured alone (▲).

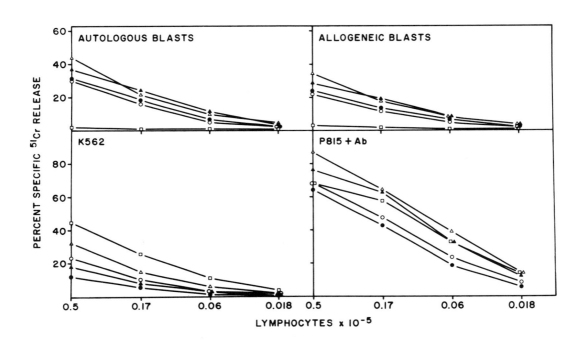

FIG. 2. Separation of different populations of effector cells responsible for CML, NK-like, and K-like cytotoxic activities, after allosensitization. Two parallel sets of MLC (ABx1 and ABx2) were set up in which unfractionated PBL and FcR-negative E-RFC were used as responders, respectively. Six days after the onset of the two MLC, the cultures were separated into pure E-RFC and non-E-RFC populations. Four-hr cytotoxic assays against K562, sensitized P815Y and autologous and allogeneic blasts were done with the following effector cells: ABx1 (o), ABx1, E-RFC (●), ABx1, non-E-RFC (□), ABx2 (△) and ABx2, E-RFC (▲).

Several differences can be demonstrated between freshly separated NK and K cells and MLC-activated cytotoxic T cells. Fresh NK and K cells are FcR-positive, whereas we were not able to detect FcR on the MLC-activated T cells using the EA7S rosetting technique. Both SLMC and ADCC activities of fresh lymphocytes are abolished following depletion of FcR-positive cells, or when tested in the presence of immune complexes which induce modulation of the FcR (4). In the present experiments, depletion of FcR-bearing cells on EA7S monolayers did not affect or only slightly affected the ability of MLC-activated killers to mediate specific and non-specific lysis (Table 2). When cytotoxicity was performed directly in microplates containing EA7S monolayers, fresh K and NK cells were greatly inhibited whereas MLC-activated killers were inhibited to a significantly less extent. The comparison between the inhibition of lysis of PHA blasts by fresh PBL and CTL was not shown in Table 2 as such targets are only slightly sensitive or completely insensitive to lysis by fresh lymphocytes. The overall results suggest that FcR are present on MLC-activated cytotoxic T cells but are not detectable because of their very low affinity. It seems unlikely that these cells lack FcR and mediate lysis of antibody-sensitized targets with a mechanism different from that described for K cells.

A characteristic of fresh NK cells but not of K cells is their sensitivity to trypsin (4). Pronase, in contrast, depletes both K and NK cell functions. MLC-generated killers and fresh cells (10^7/ ml) were treated for 30 min at 37°C with 1 mg/ml of these enzymes and the effects compared (Table 2). Unlike fresh NK cells, the activated NK-like cells were not sensitive to trypsin treatment. Specific cytotoxicity was greatly enhanced following treatment with trypsin. Pronase abolished the ADCC and SLMC activities of both fresh and activated killers and also CML activity of activated lymphocytes.

Treatment of fresh NK cells and of MLC-generated NK-like T cells with IFN resulted in a similar enhancement of cytotoxic efficiency. In addition to enhancing NK cell activity, IFN can interact with target cells and induce up to 98% protection of these cells against the cytotoxicity mediated either by fresh or IFN-stimulated human lymphocytes (16). The protective effect of IFN on the target cells is specific for the cytotoxicity mediated by NK cells. IFN-treated and untreated fibroblasts are lysed with equal efficiency by antibody-dependent cytotoxic cells, PHA-induced effector cells, CTL and antibody and complement. In these experiments, IFN treatment of fibroblasts protected them from lysis by both fresh NK and MLC-activated killer cells.

Cold target competition assays were also performed. When various concentrations of unlabeled K562 cells were added to the effectors and ^{51}Cr-labeled K562 targets, fresh NK and MLC-activated cells were inhibited in a dose-dependent manner. Cytotoxic assays against ^{51}Cr-labeled K562 were also performed in which the effector cells were preincubated with cold K562 cells at 37°C for 4 hr. Fresh NK cells become inactivated after interaction with cold K562 in the absence of IFN induction (5, 20). Our results show that MLC-activated killers are also inactivated after a 4-hr incubation with cold K562 cells.

In summary, differences and similarities can be observed between fresh and MLC-activated killer cells. Although additional studies are needed to further characterize activated killers and their mechanism of lysis, our data show tht the MLC is a good system for generating cyto-

TABLE 2. Cytotoxicity mediated by fresh and MLC-activated effector cells

Target	Effector	Depletion of FcR-positive cells on EA7S monolayers	Interaction with EA7S immune complexes	Trypsin treatment	Pronase treatment
K562	PBL	6.4 ± 1.3[a]	46 ± 15.4	6.3 ± 4.3[a]	3.6 ± 1.5
	MLC	88 ± 23.9	79.8 ± 12.3	70.8 ± 23.6	10.6 ± 1.4
P815 + Ab	PBL	9.6 ± 5.1	27.3 ± 9.3	84.4 ± 19.5	29.5 ± 36.1
	MLC	75.6 ± 19.1	58.4 ± 8.7	102.6 ± 32.0	16.6 ± 2.3
Autologous blasts	MLC	81.6 ± 28.2	89.8 ± 17.7	1288.0 ± 1999.5	46.3 ± 40.6
Allogeneic blasts	MLC	84.5 ± 10.3	102.4 ± 29.0	421.6 ± 326.6	21.9 ± 0.4

[a]Data are given as mean percentage ± S.D. of cytotoxicity (measured as lytic units/10^8 cells) as compared to control assays.

toxic cells. Furthermore, the MLC may represent, like the modulation of NK cell activity mediated by IFN, an *in vitro* model for the study of the regulation of cell-mediated defense mechanisms.

Supported in part by NIH grants NS 11036-08, CA 10815, CA 20833 and by ACS grant IN-143.

REFERENCES

1. Jondal, M., and Pross, H. (1975): *Int. J. Cancer*, 15:596-605.
2. Kay, H.D., and Horwitz, D.A. (1980): *J. Clin. Invest.*, 66:847-851.
3. Miggiano, V.C., Bernoco, D., Lightbody, J., Trinchieri, G. and Ceppellini, R. (1972): *Transpl. Proc.*, IV:231-237.
4. Perussia, B., Trinchieri, G., and Cerottini, J.C. (1979): *J. Immunol.*, 123:681-687.
5. Perussia, B., and Trinchieri, G. (1981): *J. Immunol.* (in press).
6. Perussia, B., Lebman, D., Ip, S., Rovera, G., and Trinchieri, G. (1981): *Proc. Natl. Acad. Sci. USA* (submitted).
7. Poros, A., and Klein, E. (1978): *Cell Immunol.*, 41:240-255.
8. Reinherz, E.L., Cooper, M.D., and Schlossman, S.F. (1980): *J. Exp. Med.*, 151:969-974.
9. Santoli, D., Trinchieri, G., Zmijewski, C., and Koprowski, H. (1976): *J. Immunol.*, 117:765-770.
10. Santoli, D., Trinchieri, G., and Lief, F. (1978): *J. Immunol.*, 121:526-531.
11. Santoli, D., Trinchieri, G., and Koprowski, H. (1978): *J. Immunol.*, 121:532-538.
12. Santoli, D., Trinchieri, G., Moretta, L., Zmijewski, C.M., and Koprowski, H. (1978): *Clin. Exp. Immunol.*, 33:309-318.
13. Saksela, E., Timonen, T., and Kantell, K. (1979): *Scand. J. Immunol.*, 10:257-266.
14. Saksela, E., and Timonen, T. (1980): In: *Regulatory Functions of Interferons*, edited by J. Vilcek, I. Gresser, and T.C. Merigan. Annals of the New York Academy of Sciences, 350:102-111.
15. Trinchieri, G., Santoli, D., and Knowles, B.B. (1977): *Nature* 270:611-613.
16. Trinchieri, G., and Santoli, D. (1978): *J. Exp. Med.* 147:1314-1333.
17. Trinchieri, G., Santoli, D., Dee, R.R., and Knowles, B.B. (1978): *J. Exp. Med.* 147:1299-1313.
18. Trinchieri, G., Santoli, D., and Koprowski, H. ((1978): *J. Immunol.*, 120:1843-1855.
19. Trinchieri, G., Perussia, B., and Santoli, D. (1980): In: *Natural Cell-Mediated Immunity Against Tumors*, edited by R. Herberman, pp. 655-670. Academic Press, New York.
20. Trinchieri, G., Santoli, D., Granato, D., and Perussia, B. (1981): *Fed. Proc.* (in press).
21. West, W.H., Cannon, G.B., Kay, H.D., Bonnard, G.D., and Herberman, R.B. (1977): *J. Immunol.*, 118:355-361.
22. Zarling, J.M., Bach, F.H., and Kung, P.C. (1981): *J. Immunol.*, 126:375-378.

*Mediation of Cellular Immunity in Cancer by
Immune Modifiers*, edited by M. A. Chirigos
et al., Raven Press, New York © 1981.

Target Cell Lysis by Cloned Cell Lines with Natural Killer Activity

Gunther Dennert

*Department of Cancer Biology, The Salk Institute for Biological Studies,
San Diego, California 92138*

ABSTRACT

Permanent cell lines with natural killer (NK) activity were initiated
from mouse spleen cells in the presence of conditioned media. One of
the cell lines was cloned by limiting dilution and assayed on several
mouse and human NK sensitive targets in order to determine whether
target specificities segregate upon cloning. Results showed that
target specificities of the cloned lines were identical to the specificities of NK cells in normal spleen. It is therefore likely that NK
cells recognize identical target structures on all NK sensitive targets.
Cold target inhibition assays revealed that there exist several classes
of targets distinguishable by their effectiveness in inhibiting cytotoxicity. One shows little or no inhibition and presumably lacks the
target structures; another shows intermediate inhibition, while the
third exerts inhibition like YAC-1 which serves as labeled target in
these assays. Cells which exert good or intermediate inhibition and
therefore may express target structures are lysed to various degrees by
NK effectors while targets which do not inhibit show no or little lysis.
In the presence of Concanavalin A (Con A), NK effectors may cause increased target lysis both to targets which are lysable or are not
lysable in the absence of Con A. This shows that cells lacking target
structures can be lysed by NK cells under certain experimental conditions. It is concluded that lysis of NK targets is a function of two
variables: Effector binding to the target and sensitivity of the
target to lysis. Cell surface marker analysis of NK cells reveals that
they are Thy 1.2^+, Lyt 1^-2^-, $T200^+$, asialo $GM1^+$, asialo $GM2^+$, which
distinguishes them from specific cytolytic thymus derived lymphocytes.

INTRODUCTION

Recently it has been possible to establish *in vitro* as permanent cell
lines thymus derived lymphocytes which retain effector cell function
(2, 7). While this will greatly enhance our understanding of T lymphocytes, many other important cell types in the immune system are neither
well characterized nor have they been established as permanent cell
lines. One of these cell types is the natural killer (NK) cell which may

play an important role in immunosurveillance of neoplasia (8, 15). NK cells lyse certain tumor target cells and hence may carry specific receptors able to bind to target antigens (11, 16, 17). But neither the nature of these hypothetical receptors nor the determinants to which they may bind have yet been elucidated. Other gaps in our knowledge on NK cells concern their cell surface markers and *in vivo* activity. As a first step towards investigating these questions we have established permanent lines of NK cells *in vitro,* cloned them and determined their target specificity and some of their cell surface markers.

RESULTS

Cloning of NK Cell Lines

Spleen cells of normal or nu/nu Balb/c mice cultured in tissue culture medium supplemented with media conditioned by lymphocytes in the presence of Con A (ConACM) maintain NK activity (3, 4, 5). After establishment of the culture, the cytotoxicity on YAC-1 cells increases dramatically over the first two or four weeks, suggesting that a predominant proliferation of NK cells in these cultures occurred. In

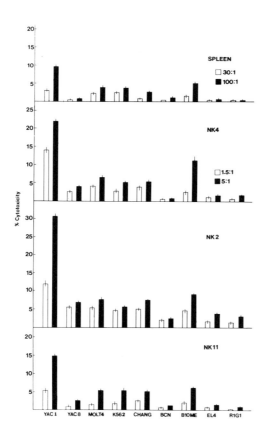

FIG. 1. Cytolytic specificity of two NK cell lines. NK 2 and NK 4 were derived from Balb/c nu/nu and NK 11 from normal Balb/c spleen cells. Attacker to target ratios were 30:1 and 100:1 for spleen cells and 1.5:1 and 5:1 for the NK cell lines. The 5 hr timepoint is given. The cytotoxicity assay using ^{51}Cr labeled targets has been described (3, 5). The following targets were used: YAC-1 (H-2^a) thymic lymphoma and its NK resistant derivative YAC-8 (kindly provided by Drs. R. Kiessling and M. Hansson, Karolinska Institute, Stockholm, Sweden), Chang, Molt 4 and K 562, human cell lines, BCN (H-2^d), fibroblast and its NK sensitive derivative B10ME (kindly provided by Drs. P. Patek, J. Collins and M. Cohn, Salk Institute), EL4 (H-2^b) thymic lymphoma, Rl.G.1 (H-2^k), thymic lymphoma.

comparison to fresh normal spleen cells, NK cultures established for two or three weeks exerted about twenty-fold higher lytic activity on YAC-1 targets. When assayed on a panel of different targets (Fig. 1), high cytolytic activity is seen on YAC-1 and lower activity is seen on all others (5). There was always very low or no activity on Rl.G.1, EL4 and BCN, somewhat higher activity on YAC-8, Molt 4, K562 and Chang, and usually rather high activity on B10ME. YAC-8 is a relatively NK resistant derivative of YAC-1; so is BCN, the relatively NK resistant parent of B10ME (1). Several interesting points emerged from this comparison of independent NK lines (5). The relative sensitivity of the targets to NK killing is the same regardless of the effector cell population employed, i. e., whether fresh spleen cells or various NK lines were used. The level of cytolytic activity on a given target is variable between experiments. Apparently this variability is a reflection of both the growth condition of the effector cells at the time of assay as well as that of the target cells.

To study whether target recognition structures are expressed clonally on NK cells, cell lines were cloned at limiting dilution in microtiter plates (3, 5). This could be accomplished with some but not all cell lines by initially subculturing them at 1000 cells per well followed by subculturing at 100 or 10 cells per well and finally at 1 cell per well.

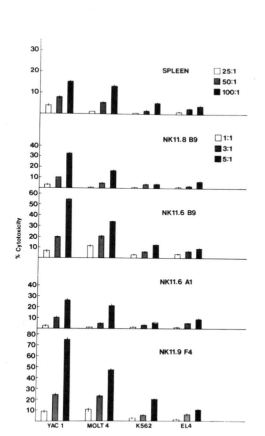

Cell line NK 11 was cloned at 1 cell per well and individual isolates tested on YAC-1, Molt 4, K562 and EL4. Figure 2 shows representative results of four out of a total of six clones which all showed lysis identical in specificity to that of normal spleen cells. It is therefore obvious that if there are specific receptors for human and mouse target antigens on NK effectors, they are not clonally distributed.

FIG. 2. Cytolygic specificity of two cloned NK sublines. Sublines were cloned at 1 cell per well and isolates were grown up and assayed for cytotoxicity at ratios of 1:1, 2:1 and 5:1 in a 7 hr assay. Spleen effector cells were used at ratios of 25:1, 50:1, 100:1

NK Lysis is a Function of Target Binding and Target Lysability

There are two possible explanations for the failure of NK effector cells to lyse certain targets. The target may not have a target structure to which the effector can bind or, although binding is accomplished the target may not be lysed. In order to study which targets have the structures which allow binding, cold target inhibition assays were done using YAC-1 as labeled target. In Fig. 3 it is seen that Chang targets inhibit lysis as well as YAC-1, while Raji and S49 show only about half as efficient inhibition as YAC-1. In contrast, Rl.G.1, EL4 and P815 show inhibition which is less than one-fourth of that of YAC-1.

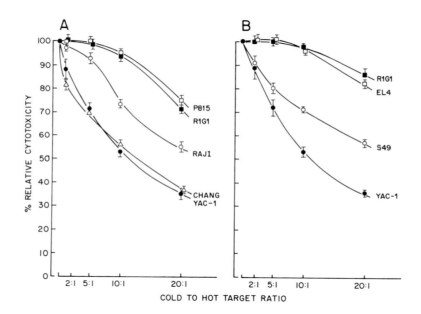

FIG. 3. Cold target inhibition assay of YAC-1 killing by various unlabeled targets. Attacker to target ratio was 10:1 for the labeled YAC-1 targets and a five hour timepoint was taken. Cytotoxicity in the absence of cold targets was 33% in A and 31% in B, which were expressed at 100% relative cytotoxicity. The cold to hot target ratios are indicated on the abscissa. Clone NK 11.6D6 was used for this experiment. Besides some of the targets mentioned in Fig. 1, the human cell line Raji, the H-2^d thymic lymphoma S49 and the H-2^d mastocytoma P815 were tested as cold targets.

In Fig. 4 it is seen that YAC-1, Chang, S49 and Raji are targets which are lysed to various degrees by NK cells, while Rl.G.1, EL4 and P815 show little or no lysis. One could therefore postulate that the former four targets possess structures to which the effector cell can bind while the latter three do not and consequently are not lysed. This interpretation however does not take into account possible differences of lysability in these targets. For instance, lysis of Raji is relatively poor and both P815 and EL4 show some low lysis. Hence, the question is whether the difference of lysis between all these targets is solely a function of expression of target structures or not. In order to examine this question, target lysis was also determined in the presence of Con A in order to couple the effectors to the targets (Fig. 4). Results showed that addition of Con A stimulated lysis with all targets, however, to varying degrees. There was very high lysis induced in YAC-1, EL4 and P815. This showed that these three targets are among the most sensitive targets and would suggest that the lack of lysis of EL4 and P815 in the absence of Con A is in fact due to the lack of the structures to which the effector can bind. Quite in contrast, Rl.G.1 is not lysed to any great extent when in the presence of Con A, suggesting that this target not only lacks target structures but also is relatively resistant to lysis. The three cell lines, Chang, S49 and Raji, do not show much enhanced lysis in the presence of Con A. These three cell lines therefore appear to belong to the category of NK targets which possess target structures but are relatively more resistant to lysis than YAC-1. NK lysis therefore appears to be the result of at least two variables, target binding and target lysability (5).

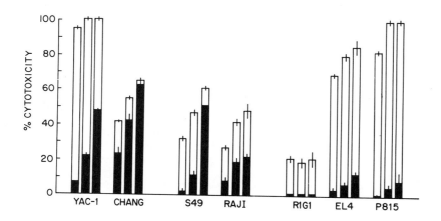

FIG. 4. Ability of NK 11.6.D6 to lyse YAC-1, Chang, S49, Raji, Rl.G.1, EL4 and P815 in the absence (black bars) or presence of 4 µg/ml Con A (white bars). Spontaneous ^{51}Cr release from targets was determined in the presence of 4 µg/ml Con A, although Con A did not increase spontaneous ^{51}Cr release. The 5 hr timepoint is given at the a/t ratios of 1:1, 3:1, 10:1 (from left to right).

Cell Surface Markers of NK Cells

The surface antigenic phenotype of NK cells has been a somewhat controversial issue (6, 9, 10, 12, 13, 14), and it was therefore of interest to determine the cell surface antigens of our NK cell lines. This was done by using monoclonal antibody in combination with flow microfluorometry (FMF), ^{14}C galactose labeling and thin-layer chromatography, as well as functional assays (5 and Table 1).

TABLE 1. Cell surface markers of NK clones

	NK[d]	TK[e]	
Thy 1.2	+	+	FMF[a]
T200	+	+	FMF
Lyt 1	−	+	FMF
Lyt 2	−	−	FMF
Asialo GM1	+	±	^{14}C gal labeling TLC[b], orcinol staining
Asialo GM2	+	−	^{14}C gal labeling TLC, orcinol staining
Fc	−	−	ADCC[c] on EL4

[a]Flow microfluorometry
[b]Thin layer chromatography
[c]Antibody dependent cell mediated cytotoxicity
[d]Various NK lines and clones were tested.
[e]T killer line C.C3.11.75 was tested as control. This T killer line is specific for IA antigens and is therefore Lyt 1^+2^- as opposed to lines which are K/D specific which tend to be Lyt 1^-2^+ (5).

FMF analysis revealed that the NK cells are Thy 1.2^+, $T200^+$, Lyt 1^-2^-, which sets them apart from functional thymus derived lymphocytes (T cells) with helper or killer activity (5). Glycosphingolipid analysis revealed that asialo GM1 and asialo GM2 were detectable on NK cells by both autoradiography and orcinol staining (5). In contrast, T killer cells expressed very little asialo GM1, detectable only by autoradiography and no asialo GM2. Assay for Fc receptors was done by employing antibody dependent cell mediated cytotoxicity assays on EL4 targets. Although EL4 targets are very efficiently lysed by NK cells in the presence of Con A (Fig. 4), no ADCC activity with this target could be observed (5). This showed that NK cells do not express Fc receptors detectable in an ADCC assay.

DISCUSSION

Cloned NK cell lines were used to study the question whether NK cells possess specific receptors and whether these receptors are clonally distributed. Our results clearly show that target specificities do not segregate upon cloning (3, 5). This could either suggest that NK cells do not possess antigen receptors or that NK cells recognize identical structures on NK sensitive targets. Still another possibility would be that NK effectors possess a multitude of receptors, each with its individual specificity. Our experiments are consistent with all three possibilities and do not distinguish between them. In particular, it should be emphasized that inhibition of lysis in the cold target inhibition assay does "per se" not prove that distinct antigenic determinants are recognized by the effector cells nor that these antigenic determinants are shared between the targets which inhibit. It is quite possible that the target effector binding is caused by different cell surface structures and hence could be referred to as stickiness of the target. Our experiments suggest that the binding of effectors to targets, regardless of whether it involves specific receptors or not, is a prerequisite for lysis and that there are striking differences between the lysability of targets.

The failure to uncover evidence for clonally distributed receptors on NK cells brings up the more general question of heterogeneity of NK effector cells. For instance, it is possible that there exist additional NK cell types which in contrast to our cell lines express ADCC activity (9, 14). It is possible that these latter NK cells belong to a Thy-1$^-$ NK population (13), which may exist in addition to the Thy 1$^+$ NK population (3,9,12,13). It is therefore still an open question whether NK activity is also carried out by other yet to be characterized cell types. The presence of Thy 1 antigen on NK cells raises the question of relationship of NK effector cells and T killer cells. NK cells can be distinguished from T killer cells by their lack of Lyt 1 and Lyt 2 antigen and their expression of considerable amounts of asialo GM1 and asialo GM2 (5).

Many questions pertaining to NK cells such as the presence of receptors and mechanism of cytolysis are still unresolved. But with now available cloned NK cell lines they may be much more amenable to analysis. For instance, exploration of the *in vivo* effects of NK cells on tumor growth and Fl hybrid resistance to parental marrow grafts can now be attempted. For this purpose it will be important to know how stable our NK lines are. Since our NK lines have been in culture for a relatively short time, no statement with regard to their stability can be made. It has been noticed, however, that some sublines may show decreased cytolytic activities over periods of some months while others do not. Recloning of sublines may therefore be necessary in some cases.

This work was supported by grants CA 15581 and CA 19334 from the National Institutes of Health.

REFERENCES

1. Collins, J. C., Patek, P. Q., and Cohn, M. (1980): J. Exp. Med. (in press).

2. Dennert, G., and DeRose, M. (1976): J. Immunol. 116:1601-1606.

3. Dennert, G. (1980): Nature 287:47-49.

4. Dennert, G., and Hyman, R. (1980): Europ. J. Immunol. 10:583-589.

5. Dennert, G., Yogeeswaran, G., and Yamagata, S. (1980): J. Exp. Med. (in press).

6. Gidlund, J., Haller, O., Orn, A., Ojo, E., Stern, P., and Wigzell, H. (1980): In: Natural Cell Mediated Immunity to Tumors, edited by R. B. Herberman, Academic Press, New York.

7. Gillis, S., and Smith, D. A. (1977): Nature 268:154-156.

8. Herberman, R. B., and Holden, H. T. (1978): Adv. in Cancer Res. 27:306-376.

9. Herberman, R. B., Djeu, J. Y., Kay, H. D., Ortaldo, J. R., Riccardi, C., Bonnard, G. D., Holden, H. T., Fagnani, R., Santori, A., and Puccett, P. (1979): Immunol. Rev. 44:43-70.

10. Kasai, J., Leclerc, J. C., Shen, F. W., and Cantor, H. (1979): Immunogenetics 8:153-159.

11. Koide, Y., and Takasugi, M. (1978): Europ. J. Immunol. 8:818-822.

12. Koo, G. C., Jacobson, J. B., Hämmerling, G. J., and Hämmerling, U. (1980): J. Immunol. 125:1003-1006.

13. Mattes, M. J., Sharrow, S. O., Herberman, R. B., and Holden, H. T. (1979): J. Immunol. 123:2851-2860.

14. Ojo, E., and Wigzell, H. (1978): Scand, J. Immunol. 7:297-306.

15. Roder, J. C., and Kiessling, R. (1978): Scand. J. Immunol. 8:135-144.

16. Roder, J. C., Ahrlund Richter, L., and Jondal, M. (1979): J. Exp. Med. 150:471-481.

17. Roder, J. C., Rosen, A., Fenyo, E. M., and Troy, F. A. (1979): Proc. Nat. Acad. Sci. 76:1405-1409.

Mediation of Cellular Immunity in Cancer by
Immune Modifiers, edited by M. A. Chirigos
et al., Raven Press, New York © 1981.

Augmentation of Natural Killer Cell Activity and Induction of Interferon by Tumor Cells and Other Biological Response Modifiers

J. Y. Djeu, *T. Timonen, and *R. B. Herberman

*Food and Drug Administration, Bureau of Biologics, Division of Virology and *National Cancer Institute, Laboratory of Immunodiagnosis, Bethesda, Maryland 20205*

Natural killer (NK) cells are a class of lymphocytes that are capable of spontaneously lysing tumor cells and they are present in man, rat, mouse and a range of other species (1). This activity is readily enhanced by a variety of biological agents. The best studied of these modifiers is interferon (2-5), but double-stranded RNA, viruses (2,6, 7), bacteria (8,9), and tumor cells (10,11) all have the ability to augment NK activity. In the past few years we have addressed ourselves to 3 questions concerning the augmentation of NK activity, namely, 1) Do these biological modifiers augment NK activity via their common ability to induce interferon (IFN)? 2) What is the source of IFN in response to these agents and can NK cells produce IFN? 3) What is the mechanism by which IFN augments NK activity?

In order to answer these queries, highly purified subclasses of lymphocytes, particularly NK cells, are required and for this purpose we have employed a discontinuous Percoll gradient that was developed by Timonen and Saksela (12). Peripheral blood lymphocytes were obtained by Ficoll-Hypaque density gradient centrifugation of lymphoid cell concentrates from the Platelet-pheresis Center at the National Institutes of Health, Bethesda, Md. Nonadherent cells, enriched in NK and T cells, were prepared by removal of adherent cells on Petri dishes for 45 min at 37°C and subsequent incubation on nylon wool columns for 30 min at 37°C. These cells were then placed on a 7 step-discontinuous Percoll density gradient that varied in 2.5% concentrations from 40% to 55% Percoll. After centrifugation at 550 g for 30 min, the fractions were collected and incubated overnight at 37°C with various biological agents. The following day, the supernatants were collected and tested for the presence of antiviral activity against vesicular stomatitis virus in human foreskin fibroblasts, and the lymphocytes were collected and assayed for NK activity against ^{51}Cr-labelled K562 tumor cells.

TABLE 1.   Separation of NK cells by discontinuous Percoll gradient
                                centrifugation

Effector cell	% Cytotoxicity[a]	% Cell recovery	% Large granular lymphocytes (LGL)	% Small lymphocytes
Cell input	15.4		18.0	78.0
Fraction 1	0.5	2.0	1.0	0.0
2	28.8	6.2	74.0	5.0
3	35.9	9.4	91.0	6.0
4	12.1	20.9	22.0	61.0
5	1.8	19.3	2.0	73.0
6	0.2	27.4	0.0	96.0
7	0.4	30.4	0.0	99.0

[a] Effector/target ratio of 10/1.

Table 1 shows a typical profile of cells separated by this technique. NK activity peaked between Fractions 2 and 3 which were
primarily made up of large granular lymphocytes (LGL), which have
azurophilic granules scattered throughout the cytoplasm. No activity
was seen in the denser Fractions 5-7, which were comprised mainly of
small, mature T cells. LGL which were associated with NK activity
constituted only 10-15% of the total nonadherent cell input.

TABLE 2.   Induction of interferon and augmentation of NK activity
                        by poly I:C and mitogens

| Effector cell | % Cytotoxicity[a] (units of IFN/ml)[b] after 18 hr culture with: | | | |
	None	Poly I:C	SEA	Con A
Cell input	18.5 (0)	31.8 (>625)	29.2 (0)	21.7 (0)
Fraction 1	-3.6 (0)	-0.8 (>625)	-0.7 (0)	-0.8 (0)
2	12.5 (0)	22.8 (>625)	23.7 (25)	19.1 (5)
3	33.5 (0)	49.8 (>625)	50.9 (125)	51.4 (125)
4	21.3 (0)	18.5 (>625)	28.1 (5)	24.5 (0)
5	4.3 (0)	2.9 (>625)	8.5 (0)	7.3 (0)
6	2.1 (0)	2.6 (>625)	4.0 (0)	3.7 (0)
7	1.9 (0)	2.7 (>625)	2.8 (0)	2.9 (0)

[a] Effector/target ratio of 10/1.
[b] Interferon titer in the supernatant of cell cultures.

Each fraction, along with the original cell input was tested for IFN
production and NK activity after 18 hr incubation with poly I:C, or the
mitogens, staphyloccocal enterotoxin A (SEA) and Concanavalin A (Con
A). As shown in Table 2, all fractions responded to poly I:C by IFN
production but only Fractions 2-3, containing LGL, showed spontaneous
NK activity that was boosted in the presence of poly I:C. In contrast,
SEA and Con A induced IFN and enhanced NK activity only in Fractions
2-3.

TABLE 3. Induction of interferon and augmentation of NK activity by viruses

Effector cell	% Cytotoxicity[a] (units of IFN/ml)[b] after 18 hr culture with:		
	None	Herpes simplex 1	Influenza A/PC
Cell input	11.4 (0)	22.5 (251)	21.8 (251)
Fraction 1	0.4 (0)	1.0 (30)	3.5 (625)
2	7.3 (0)	19.6 (251)	21.7 (>625)
3	25.5 (0)	39.9 (25)	36.5 (50)
4	9.2 (0)	.17.1 (10)	13.4 (0)
5	3.4 (0)	7.2 (0)	0.5 (0)
6	1.2 (0)	0.4 (0)	0.1 (0)
7	1.4 (0)	0.6 (0)	0.2 (0)

[a] Effector/target ratio of 10/1.
[b] Interferon titer in the supernatant of cell cultures.

In response to viruses, herpes simplex I and influenza A/Port Chalmers, again, the earlier fractions produced significant levels of IFN and NK activity but the later fractions had neither activities (Table 3). Bacteria, such as Bacterium Calmette-Guerin (BCG) and Corynebacterium parvum (C. parvum) also induced IFN and enhanced NK activity which were restricted to the fractions that contained LGL (Table 4). Similarly, tumor cells, such as K562, MOLT-4, G-11

TABLE 4. Induction of interferon and augmentation of NK activity by bacteria

Effector cell	% Cytotoxicity[a] (units of IFN/ml)[b] after 18 hr culture with:		
	None	BCG	C. parvum
Cell input	10.6 (0)	8.0 (0)	17.2 (125)
Fraction 1	0.2 (0)	0.9 (10)	1.1 (5)
2	7.9 (0)	27.8 (50)	25.6 (220)
3	21.2 (0)	29.4 (50)	32.1 (50)
4	8.7 (0)	16.4 (0)	31.9 (10)
5	6.4 (0)	6.4 (0)	5.1 (0)
6	1.3 (0)	0.1 (0)	0.4 (0)
7	0.8 (0)	0.4 (0)	0.6 (0)

[a] Effector/target ratio of 10/1.
[b] Interferon titer in the supernatant of cell cultures.

and T-24, enhanced the two functions in the LGL-containing fractions (Table 5). All these biological agents, with the exception of poly

TABLE 5. Induction of interferon and augmentation of NK activity
by tumor cells

| Effector cell | None | % Cytotoxicity[a] (units of IFN/ml)[b] after 18 hr culture with: | | | |
		K562	MOLT	G-11	T-24
Cell input	16.4 (0)	21.6 (25)	25.5 (50)	22.8 (50)	19.9 (10)
Fraction 1	1.1 (0)	0.9 (0)	1.3 (0)	0.3 (0)	0.4 (0)
2	12.6 (0)	31.1 (200)	26.3 (50)	19.9 (25)	18.3 (25)
3	24.8 (0)	38.0 (625)	35.9 (251)	39.3 (125)	32.8 (200)
4	5.8 (0)	15.5 (5)	10.4 (0)	17.9 (10)	2.9 (0)
5	1.2 (0)	1.4 (0)	2.3 (0)	0.8 (0)	0.3 (0)
6	0.4 (0)	0.9 (0)	0.7 (0)	0.9 (0)	0.5 (0)
7	0.5 (0)	0.7 (0)	0.8 (0)	0.4 (0)	0.7 (0)

[a] Effector/target ratio of 10/1.
[b] Interferon titer in the supernatant of cell cultures.

I:C, did not induce IFN in Fractions 5-7 which contained highly-
purified T cells. It is possible that T cells may produce IFN, particularly in response to mitogens, after longer incubation with these
agents, but at 18 hr, only NK cells appear to respond by IFN production.

These results suggest that NK cells have multiple natural host
defense functions, being able to produce IFN in response to a variety
of biological agents as well as to lyse a wide range of target cells.
It also appears that NK cells are capable of rapid, positive self-
regulation, by producing IFN which in turn can augment their cytolytic activity.

TABLE 6. Enhancement of NK activity and IFN production by mouse
tumor cells

| Recipient | Intraperitoneal inoculation with: | % Cytotoxicity[a] (units of IFN/ml serum) | | |
		1 Day	2 Days	3 Days
BALB/c	none	3.3 (<5)	2.9 (<5)	4.1 (<5)
	medium	2.4 (<5)	2.6 (<5)	4.6 (<5)
	RL♂1	18.4 (400)	15.8 (2000)	5.9 (<5)
	RBL-5	18.7 (500)	17.6 (1000)	5.2 (<5)
	EL-4 G+	15.9 (120)	18.8 (1250)	16.1 (133)
	RL♂1 (pact.)[b]	18.2 (500)	16.1 (2000)	2.5 (<5)
BALB/c	none	1.8 (<5)	2.4 (<5)	2.6 (<5)
	medium	1.8 (<5)	2.4 (<5)	2.8 (<5)
	RL♂1	24.5 (2500)	19.4 (1260)	4.8 (<5)
	RBL-5	16.8 (4000)	25.4 (3160)	12.9 (<5)
	EL-4 G+	20.4 (630)	18.3 (2000)	3.5 (<5)

[a] Effector/target ratio of 200/1.
[b] RL♂1 tumor cells were incubated with 10^{-5}M pactamycin for 45
min at $37°C$ to inhibit protein synthesis, before they were inoculated into mice.

Another area of interest has been the characterization of the IFN induced during the augmentation of NK activity. In the murine system, the same biological agents mentioned above were also capable of boosting NK activity and stimulating IFN (8). In particular, tumor cells, both syngeneic and allogeneic (11), could induce the two functions in mice as early as 24 hr after in vivo administration (Table 6). These could also be achieved in athymic nude mice, consistent with the source of IFN being NK cells. The inoculated tumor cells did not produce the IFN since they could be inhibited in protein synthesis by pactamycin and still maintained their ability to induce IFN in host mice. Characterization of the tumor-induced IFN revealed a similarity

TABLE 7. Characterization of tumor induced IFN

Treatment	Units of IF/ml serum		
	NDV-IFN[a]	RLo1-IFN	RBL-5 IFN
none	56000	5600	6300
56°C, 1 hr	<10	310	250
Antiviral activity on HeLa cells	<10	<10	<10
pH 3.0	50000	<10	<10
pH 6.0		4700	5500
pH 9.0		5000	4790
Incubation of L929 cells with IFN:			
1 hr	50000	<10	<10
4 hr	50000	400	2500
8 hr		5000	5500
12 hr		5000	6300

[a] Serum IFN collected from mice inoculated with Newcastle Disease virus.

to gamma IFN in that it was heat and pH labile (Table 7). In addition, it required prolonged incubation with indicator cells to convey protection against virus challenge, as has been described for gamma IFN. Further analysis of the tumor-induced IFN will require the examination of its sensitivity to antisera against the various known types of IFN.

Studies on the mechanism of augmentation of NK activity have shown that IFN bound to NK cells at 4° and 37°C within 5-10 minutes (13). After this brief exposure to IFN, lymphocytes underwent a temperature dependent stage whereby they developed increased lytic activity in the absence of IFN. This increase in activity was also dependent on new RNA and protein synthesis, as shown by sensitivity of the IFN-treated lymphocytes to actinomycin D, emetine and puromycin. Transcription and translation events occurred early and were not required beyond 4-6 hr after exposure to IFN. Therefore, stable proteins were made after IFN treatment which then could mediate NK activity. These proteins are most likely receptors for target cells or lytic enzymes involved in cytolysis, as has been postulated previously (12). Both types of proteins could lead to increased number of NK cells and/or increased lytic efficiency of already active NK cells. Further analysis will be needed to determine whether IFN induces the differentiation of pre-NK cells to active cells or it simply enhances the lytic machinery of NK cells without the increase in the number of NK cells.

REFERENCES

1. Herberman, R.B. (1980): <u>Natural cell-mediated immunity against Tumors</u>. Academic Press, New York.
2. Gidlund, A., Orn, A., Wigzell, H., Senik, A., and Gresser, I. (1978). <u>Nature</u>, 273:759-761.
3. Djeu, J.Y., Heinbaugh, J.A., Holden, H.T., and Herberman, R.B. (1979): <u>J. Immunol</u>. 122:175-181.
4. Trinchieri, G., and Santoli, D. (1978): J. Exp. Med. 147:1314-1333.
5. Herberman, R.B., Ortaldo, J.R., and Bonnard, G.D. (1979): Nature 277:221-223.
6. Welsh, R.M., and Zinkernagel, R.M. (1977): Nature 268:646-648.
7. Quinnan, G.V., and Manischewitz, J.E. (1979): J. Exp. Med. 150:1549-1554.
8. Herberman, R.B., Nunn, M.E., Holden, H.T., Staal, S., and Djeu, J.Y. (1977): Int. J. Cancer 19:555-564.
9. Tracey, D.E., Wolfe, S.A., Durdik, J.M., and Henney, C.S. (1977): J. Immunol. 119:1145-1151.
10. Trinchieri, G., Santoli, D., Dee, R.R., and Knowles, R.B. (1978). Exp. Med. 147:1299-1313.
11. Djeu, J.Y., Huang, K.Y., and Herberman, R.B. (1980). J. Exp. Med. 151:781-789.
12. Timonen, T. and Saksela, E. (1980): J. Immunol. Methods 36:285-291.
13. Djeu, J.Y., Stocks, N., Holden, H.T., and Herberman, R.B. (1981): Cell. Immunol. In press.

Mediation of Cellular Immunity in Cancer by
Immune Modifiers, edited by M. A. Chirigos
et al., Raven Press, New York © 1981.

Enhancement of Human Cytotoxic T Cell Responses and NK Cell Activity by Purified Fibroblast Interferon and Polyribonucleotide Inducers of Interferon'

Joyce M. Zarling

Immunobiology Research Center, Department of Laboratory Medicine and Pathology, University of Minnesota, Minneapolis, Minnesota 55455

Anti-tumor effects of interferon (IF) and IF inducers have been demonstrated in several animal tumor systems as previously reviewed (14) and there is mounting evidence indicating that IF may be effective against certain human tumors (34,44). With tumors of viral etiology where there is continuous production of virus, inhibition of virus replication may contribute to IF's anti-tumor effects. With other neoplasia the mechanisms of the anti-tumor effects are not clear, however direct anti-proliferative effects as well as immunomodulatory effects of IF-containing preparations have been demonstrated. For example, leukocyte-IF containing preparations were found to enhance the in vitro generation of human cytotoxic T lymphocytes (CTLs) (22) and several IF-containing preparations have been shown to augment mouse and human natural killer (NK) cell activity in vitro (6,11,21, 47). Recently, both human leukocyte and fibroblast IF have been reported to augment human NK cell activity in patients (8,25,39). Since both T cells specifically immune to tumor associated antigens as well as NK cells can contribute to tumor cell growth inhibition in animals, it is possible that IF or its inducers could be of immunotherapeutic value in cancer patients in whom the tumor cell load has been reduced by conventional therapy, if the tumor cells express either target antigens for CTLs or determinants against which activated NK cells can be directed. Support for the contention that human malignant cells may express target antigens against which autologous CTLs can be directed derives partially from our studies showing that CTLs can be generated in vitro against autologous leukemia cells (52,54). Data reviewed herein also show that fresh human leukemia cells can be lysed by activated NK cells.

The aims of the studies discussed in the present chapter, reviewed from our recent publications (51-57), were focused on assessing the effects of highly purified human fibroblast interferon (HFIF) and polyribonucleotide inducers of IF on the generation of human CTLs and

The experimental work discussed in this chapter was supported by NIH grants CA 20409, CA 26738, CA 14520, CA 14801, CA 15502 and GM 16066. This is Paper no. 260 from the Immunobiology Research Center. J.Zarling is a Scholar of the Leukemia Society of America.

augmentation of NK cell activity. Briefly summarized, our results show that first, highly purified HFIF suppresses proliferative T cell responses yet markedly augments cytotoxic T cell responses; second, HFIF as well as polyinosinic:polycytidylic acid ($rI_n \cdot rI_n$) and its non-toxic analogues can augment human NK cell activity; third, activated NK cells lyse not only NK-sensitive leukemia cell lines but can also lyse fresh human leukemia cells that have not been adapted to tissue culture whereas they do not lyse normal lymphocytes or Con A induced blasts. Finally, evidence is presented that CTLs and NK cells, heretofore difficult to distinguish between, can be differentiated by reactivity with various monoclonal antibodies.

AUGMENTATION OF HUMAN CTL RESPONSES BY PURIFIED FIBROBLAST INTERFERON (HFIF)

It was reported that the addition of virus induced human leukocyte IF to mixed leukocyte cultures (MLC) resulted in enhanced CTL responses to alloantigens (22). We asked whether highly purified fibroblast IF induced by $rI_n \cdot rC_n$, which lacks products of virus infection and other lymphokines that can be present in leukocyte IF-containing preparations (45), could augment CTL responses. Results of a typical experiment are shown in Table I. The addition of HFIF (100-125 U/ml) at the onset of MLC resulted in decreased proliferative responses as evidenced by a decrease in cell recovery and also in a decrease in ^{3}H-thymidine incorporation (57), however significantly higher cytotoxic responses were detected against the allogeneic target cells derived from the stimulating cell donors. The addition of HFIF to wells containing responding cells alone did not result in cytotoxicity against autologous or allogeneic target cells and HFIF did not render allo-stimulated cells cytotoxic for autologous target cells (57).

TABLE I.   Suppression of proliferative responses and enhancement of cytotoxic T cell responses by fibroblast interferon[a]

MLC culture	-HFIF	+HFIF	-HFIF	+HFIF
	% cell recovery		% ^{51}Cr release	
AB_x	520	200	66.7	88.8
BA_x	700	400	24.2	38.0
CD_x	300	120	66.0	82.7
DC_x	140	70	22.0	38.0
EF_x	480	220	50.3	73.9

[a]Lymphocytes (0.5×10^6) from individuals A through E were cultured in microtiter wells with 1×10^6 x-irradiated (2500R) allogeneic lymphocytes with or without HFIF (100-125 U/ml). On day 7 after the onset of MLC, 1×10^4 ^{51}Cr labeled target cells from the stimulating cell donors were added to each well and the ^{51}Cr release assay was terminated after 6 hr. The HFIF was prepared and purified to a specific activity of 2×10^7 U/mg protein as previously detailed (5,18,23,24). (Modified from Zarling, et al., 1978, with permission from the Journal of Immunology.)

At least two explanations could be put forth to account for the findings that IF increases CTL responses. IF may decrease the generation of alloantigen-induced suppressor cells that may regulate the level of cytotoxic responses generated. Alternatively, IF may directly increase the responsiveness of cytotoxic T cell precursors, perhaps by increasing the interaction between receptors on the responding and stimulating cells.

The observation that $rI_n \cdot rC_n$ induced human fibroblast IF, which was purified to an extremely high specific activity (2×10^7 U/mg protein), augments the generation of CTLs is similar to that of Heron et al. (22) who showed that less pure virus-induced leukocyte IF (specific activity, 1×10^6 U/mg protein) increased human CTL responses. Thus, although virus-induced leukocyte IF and $rI_n \cdot rC_n$ induced fibroblast IF differ with regards to physicochemical and biological properties (7,17,26,43), it is apparent that both types of IF effect T cell cytotoxic responses to alloantigens. The possibility that IF can likewise augment CTL responses to tumor associated antigens expressed on autologous malignant cells is exciting, however experimental verification of this hypothesis remains to be presented.

ENHANCEMENT OF NK CELL ACTIVITY BY HFIF AND POLYRIBONUCLEOTIDES

A considerable amount of evidence has been presented in recent years which implicates NK cells as playing a center role in prevention of tumor growth by cell lines as well as possibly spontaneous tumors. First, a correlation exists between the level of NK cell activity of lymphocytes from different mice, as measured by in vitro cytotoxicity assays against tumor cell lines, and resistance to tumor cell challenges in vivo (16,19,30,40). Second, the mutant beige mice and humans with Chediak Higashi Syndrome have extremely low NK cell activity (15,28,41, 46) and have a higher incidence of lymphomas than do normal mice or humans. Third, several agents including $rI_n \cdot rC_n$, Bacille Calmette-Guerin (BCG), statolon, many viruses and certain tumor cells augment NK cell activity and can increase resistance to tumor growth (6,11,24,39,49). Since these agents all induce IF, it has been posulated that they may augment NK cell activity through IF which is induced. Evidence to support this contention derives from findings that IF-containing preparations can augment both mouse and human NK cell activity (6,8, 11,21,25,39,47). In this section, results of our recently reported studies are presented which indicate that highly purified fibroblast IF as well as $rI_n \cdot rC_n$ and its non-toxic analogue, $rI_n \cdot r(C_{12}, U)_n$ augment human NK cell activity.

Results in Table II show that treatment of human mononuclear cells overnight with HFIF (150 U/ml) augments cytotoxicity against NK-sensitive K562 leukemia cells by lymphocytes isolated from individuals with both low and high native NK cell levels. With individual D, it can be seen that HFIF treated cells were approximately 4 fold more cytotoxic than untreated cells in that 4 fold more untreated effector cells were required to cause the same amount of cytotoxicity as HFIF treated cells. With over 30 individuals tested, we have found that HFIF treatment of lymphocytes increases NK cell activity by 2.5 to 5 fold and that treatment with HFIF for as few as 30 minutes results in marked augmentation of NK cell activity (52).

Table II. Augmentation of human NK cell activity by HFIF[a]

Individual	Effector:target cell ratio	% ^{51}Cr release from K562 cells	
		-HFIF	+HFIF
A	40:1	6.1	17.7
B	40:1	31.0	50.0
D	100:1	32.2	63.7
	25:1	12.5	30.5

[a]Lymphocytes cultured for 16 hr with or without HFIF (150 U/ml) were washed and tested for cytotoxicity against K562 cells in a 6 hr ^{51}Cr release assay. (Modified from Zarling, et al., 1979, with permission from the Journal of Immunology.)

Interferon would seem to be an ideal immunotherapeutic agent for treatment of cancer patients since, as discussed above, it augments CTL responses and cytotoxic activity of NK cells, both of which may inhibit tumor growth in vivo. However, IF is presently limited for widespread clinical use because of its scarcity and its extreme cost for preparation and purification. We have thus asked whether relatively inexpensive and readily synthesized polyribonucleotide inducers of IF would augment NK cell activity. The results shown in Table III indicate that treatment with $rI_n \cdot rC_n$ for 4 hr results in approximately a 2.5 fold increase in NK cell activity against K562 cells. In contrast; treatment with $rI_n \cdot rC_n$ for 1 hr did not increase NK cell activity whereas treatment with HFIF for as few as 30 minutes increases NK cell activity (52). This finding supports the contention that $rI_n \cdot rC_n$ increases NK cell activity through IF which is induced since several hours are required for polyribonucleotides to trigger and induce IF biosynthesis (13).

TABLE III. Augmentation of human NK cell activity by $rI_n \cdot rC_n$[a]

Treatment time	Effector:target cell ratio	% ^{51}Cr release from K562 cells ± S.D.	
		$-rI_n \cdot rC_n$	$+rI_n \cdot rC_n$
1 hr	10:1	47.1 ± 4.8	45.3 ± 2.7
	3:1	23.4 ± 2.0	19.3 ± 2.0
4 hr	10:1	46.1 ± 4.4	62.0 ± 4.8
	3:1	24.3 ± 1.9	39.5 ± 2.2

[a]Lymphocytes cultured with or without $rI_n \cdot rC_n$ (120 ug/ml) for 1 or 4 hr were washed and compared for cytotoxicity against K562 cells in a 4 hr ^{51}Cr release assay. (Modified from Zarling, et al., 1980, with permission from the Journal of Immunology.)

Although the IF inducer $rI_n \cdot rC_n$ is inexpensive to synthesize, its clinical applications are constrained since it causes several adverse effects including fever, coagulation defects, reduced hemopoesis (3,10,35,48); further, $rI_n \cdot rC_n$ is immunogenic (56). Several structural mismatched analogues of $rI_n \cdot rC_n$ have been synthesized by Dr. Paul Ts'o, Dr. William Carter and their colleagues which induce IF yet do not cause the toxic effects ascribed to $rI_n \cdot rC_n$ (3,4,12,35,48). One such clinical promising analogue is $rI_n \cdot r(C_{12},U)_n$ which triggers IF production but is degraded before it induces toxic effects. Experiments were undertaken to determine whether $rI_n \cdot r(C_{12},U)_n$ would augment NK cell activity as well as does $rI_n \cdot rC_n$. Results in Table IV show that $rI_n \cdot rC_n$ increased NK cell activity in all individuals tested with a range of 1.5 to 4 fold increases. Likewise, the non-toxic analogue $rI_n \cdot r(C_{12},U)_n$ augmented NK cell activity with a range of 1.4 to 2.7 fold. In contrast, we have found that an analogue of $rI_n \cdot rC_n$ which fails to induce interferon, namely $rI_n \cdot mC_n$, also fails to augment NK cell activity (56). Thus, it appears that the ability of a polyribonucleotide to induce IF is a prerequisite for its ability to augment NK cell activity. However, it is clear that the toxic effects of polyribonucleotides can be separated from effects on NK cells since $rI_n \cdot r(C_{12},U)_n$ and another non-toxic analogue, $rI_n \cdot r(C_{29},G)_n$, (56) are nearly as efficacious as $rI_n \cdot rC_n$ in augmenting NK cell activity.

TABLE IV. <u>Comparative ability of $rI_n \cdot rC_n$ and its non-toxic analogue $rI_n \cdot r(C_{12},U)_n$ to augment NK cell activity[a]</u>

Cells from individual	% of control cytotoxicity mediated by treated cells	
	Cells pretreated with:	
	$rI_n \cdot rC_n$	$rI_n \cdot r(C_{12},U)_n$
A	235	166
B	247	235
C	400	272
D	204	167
F	185	143
G	226	224
H	154	248
I	331	172

[a]Lymphocytes from individuals A through I, cultured alone or with $rI_n \cdot rC_n$ or $rI_n \cdot r(C_{12},U)_n$ (125 ug/ml) for 16 hr were washed and compared for their ability to lyse K562 cells in a 4 hr ^{51}Cr release assay. The values shown are the percent of control lysis mediated by treated cells, determined by comparing the number of untreated (control) effector cells with the number of treated cells required to cause 35% ^{51}Cr release. (Modified from Zarling, et al., 1980, with permission from the Journal of Immunology.)

ABILITY OF ACTIVATED NK CELLS TO LYSE FRESH HUMAN LEUKEMIA CELLS

With regard to the potential clinical usefulness of attempting to augment NK cell activity in cancer patients, it would be essential that the patients' malignant cells be susceptible to lysis by activated NK cells. Most studies involved in assessment of NK cell activity in vitro and the role of NK cells in vivo in inhibiting tumor growth have employed tumor cell lines which are highly susceptible to lysis by NK cells. Whether susceptibility to lysis by activated NK cells is restricted to certain tumor cell lines or can include fresh malignant cells that have not been established as cell lines is an important question when considering the rationale for attempting to boost NK

TABLE V. Ability of HFIF treated lymphocytes to lyse normal lymphocytes, Con A blasts and fresh leukemia cells[a]

% ^{51}Cr released from various target cells by HFIF treated lymphocytes

HFIF treated effector cells from individual	A's Con A blasts	A's lymphocytes	B's Con A blasts	B's lympyocytes
A	-12.2	-5.0	-5.4	-5.7
B	- 6.0	-3.4	0.1	-3.4

	AML cells from patient no.									CML cells from patient no.		
	1	2	3	4	5	6	7	8	9	14	15	16
I	1.4	19.0	15.5	11.6	7.1							
K						21.2	3.2	16.2	15.3			
P										24.0	40.7	40.6

[a]Lymphocytes, cultured for 16 hr with HFIF (150-200 U/ml) were compared with untreated cells for their ability to lyse ^{51}Cr labeled autologous and allogeneic normal lymphocytes, Con A blasts and allogeneic acute myelogenous leukemia cells (AML) and chronic myelogenous leukemia cells (CML) from several patients at an effector to target cell ratio of 150:1 in 7 hr ^{51}Cr release assays. The leukemic cells were thawed 24 hr prior to labeling with ^{51}Cr. Cells cultured without HFIF were not cytotoxic for any of the targets tested. HFIF augmented NK cell activity against K562 target cells in all individuals tested. (Modified from Zarling, et al., 1979, with permission from the Journal of Immunology.)

cell activity in cancer patients. We and others (36,42,52) have found that fresh human leukemia cells are rarely lysed by fresh human peripheral blood mononuclear cells; however, the possibility remained that they may be susceptible to lysis by activated NK cells. We thus asked whether activation of human NK cells with HFIF would render the cells cytotoxic for fresh human leukemia cells that have not been established as cell lines or adapted to tissue culture. Results of an experiment shown in Table V indicate that leukemia cells from many patients with acute myelogenous leukemia (AML) or chronic myelogenous leukemia (CML) can be lysed by HFIF activated NK cells from normal individuals, while these same leukemic cells were not lysed by untreated mononuclear cells (54). In addition, we have found that cells from certain patients with chronic lymphocytic leukemia can also be lysed by IF activated NK cells (51,52). Mantovani et al. have similarly shown that fresh ovarian carcinoma cells can be lysed by IF activated NK cells (33). Thus, not only tumor cell lines, but also certain malignant cells that have not been adapted to tissue culture, can be lysed by activated NK cells.

Another clinically important question is whether normal cells are lysed by activated NK cells. In contrast to our observations that leukemia cells from many patients can be lysed by HFIF treated lymphocytes are results shown in Table V indicating that neither autologous nor allogeneic lymphocytes or Con A blasts are lysed by activated NK cells. In addition, in preliminary experiments we have found that neither autologous nor allogeneic bone marrow cells are lysed in ^{51}Cr release assays by HFIF treated lymphocytes; further, activated NK cells did not inhibit either erythroid or myeloid colony formation by bone marrow cells (51).

A critical question that has not yet been resolved is whether IF or IF inducers will render patients' lymphocytes cytotoxic for autologous malignant cells. In this regard, it should be emphasized here that whereas IF augmented NK cell activity against K562 cells in all individuals tested, IF treatment of some individuals' cells did not render them cytotoxic for fresh human leukemia cells (51,52). The failure to activate lymphocytes to lyse fresh human leukemia cells in certain individuals cannot be explained at the present time. However, it may prove worthwhile to ascertain whether in vitro treatment with IF or IF inducers of lymphocytes from patients in remission would result in acquisition of cytotoxic potential against autologous malignant cells. Such in vitro data may be of value in predicting the likelihood that IF treatment of a particular cancer patient would activate NK cells which could then contribute to tumor cell eradication in vivo.

PHENOTYPIC DISTINCTION BETWEEN CTLs AND NK CELLS

Natural killer cells were so called because they spontaneously lyse tumor cells without overt immunization of the host. If lymphocytes from cancer patients, before or after treatment with IF or IF inducers, were found to be cytotoxic for autologous malignant cells, it could not be assumed a priori that cytotoxicity was mediated by NK cells since the tumor cells may express tumor associated antigens against which CTLs may be directed. Further, as discussed above, IF increases CTL responses and augments NK cell activity so it is possible that either type of effector cell may be increased in cytotoxic activity following IF therapy.

   The difficulty in distinguishing CTLs from NK cells became apparent upon the demonstrations that both T cells and NK cells can form rosettes with sheep red blood cells (E) (50) and react with xenogeneic anti-human T cell serum (25). One way that has proven useful for distinguishing CTLs from NK cells has been to determine whether depletion of cells expressing receptors for the Fc portion of IgG (referred to as FcR+ cells) results in a loss in cytotoxic activity (50,52). Adsorbtion of lymphocytes to E monolayers coated with anti-E IgG results in depletion of NK cell activity. Likewise, as shown in Table VI, depletion of FcR+ cells from HFIF or $rI_n \cdot rC_n$ treated lymphocytes results in marked diminuition of cytotoxicity against K562 cells. In contrast, absorption of CTLs generated in MLC to such antibody coated E monolayers fails to decrease cytotoxicity against allogeneic normal lymphocyte targets. Thus, fresh NK cells and NK cells augmented in cytotoxic activity by IF or polyribonucleotides can be distinguished from CTLs by virtue of their expression of Fc receptors. Under certain conditions however, NK-like cells which lyse NK-sensitive target cells appear to lack Fc receptors (9). Thus, the failure to deplete cytotoxic activity following removal of FcR+ cells can not be taken as conclusive evidence that cytotoxicity is mediated by CTLs.

TABLE VI.   Differential effects of Fc receptor cell-depletion on NK, augmented NK and CTL activities[a]

Effector cells	% ^{51}Cr release	
	before FcR+ cell depletion	after FcR+ cell depletion
	K562 targets	
A alone 16 hr[a]	37.1	3.1
A + HFIF 16 hr	75.3	17.0
B alone 16 hr	43.8	1.1
B + $rI_n \cdot rC_n$ 16 hr	72.6	9.2
	B's lymphocyte targets	
AB_x day 7[b]	67.9	65.8

[a]Lymphocytes from individuals A and B were cultured alone or overnight with HFIF (200 U/ml) or $rI_n \cdot rC_n$ (100 ug/ml) and tested for cytotoxicity against K562 cells before and after depletion of cells bearing receptors for the Fc portion of IgG (FcR+ cells) as previously described (29).

[b]Lymphocytes from individual A were stimulated for 7 days in MLC with x-irradiated cells from individual B and the CTLs were tested for their ability to lyse ^{51}Cr labeled cells from individual B before and after FcR+ cell depletion. (Modified from Zarling, et al., 1979 and 1980, with permission from the Journal of Immunology.)

Recently I have undertaken studies in collaboration with Dr. Patrick Kung, who has developed several monoclonal antibodies reactive with subsets of human mononuclear cells, to determine whether reactivity with monoclonal antibodies can discriminate NK and NK-like cells from CTLs. All of the antibodies used were produced by immunizing mice with peripheral E rosetting human lymphocytes, fusing the immune spleen cells with a mouse myeloma and obtaining the ascites fluid from

TABLE VII Differential effects of monoclonal antibody treatment on NK, NK-like and CTL activities

Effector Cells	Effector cell treatment Total LU recovered against K562 targets			
	Control ascites + C'	OKT8 + C'	OKT3 + C'	OKM1 + C'
A alone 16 hr[a]	44.6	47.6	42.8	<11.5
A + $rI_n \cdot rC_n$ 16 hr[a]	106.2	128.6	201.3	<23.8
A pool$_x$ day 7[b]	25.7	30.5	51.5	

	Total LU recovered against allogeneic lymphocytes		
A pool$_x$ day 7[b]	143	<.9	<.3

[a]Ten x 10^6 mononuclear cells, cultured for 16 hr with or without $rI_n \cdot rC_n$ (100 ug/ml) were washed and treated for 1 hr at 4°C with control ascites fluid or monoclonal anti-T cell antibodies OKT3 or OKT8 at a final dilution of 1:100 or monoclonal antibody OKM1 (reactive with monocytes in a low percentage of non-adherent mononuclear cells) at a final dilution of 1:10. Non-toxic rabbit complement (C') was then added at a dilution of 1:2 followed by a 1 hr incubation at 37°C. Dead cells were removed by ficoll-hypaque sedimentation and the live cells were washed and tested for cytotoxicity against ^{51}Cr labeled K562 cells. One lytic unit (LU) was defined as the number of effector cells required to cause 35% ^{51}Cr release from 8 x 10^3 target cells. Total LU recovered after treating 10^7 cells was calculated as follows: LU/10^6 cells x no. viable cells recovered. The number of viable cells recovered after treatment of 10^7 cells with OKT3, OKT8, control ascites and OKM1 plus C' was 3.0, 5.0, 9.3 and 8.2 x 10^6 or 3.1, 3.6, 9.3 and 8.5 x 10^6 for untreated or $rI_n \cdot rC_n$ treated effector cells, respectively.

[b]Lymphocytes from individual A, after 7 days stimulation with x-irradiated pooled allogeneic normal cells, were treated with control ascites, OKT3 or OKT8 plus C' as detailed above and were tested for their ability to lyse K562 cells and normal allogeneic lymphocytes. One LU was defined as the number of effector cells required to cause 40% or 15% ^{51}Cr release from 8,000 K562 cells or allogeneic lymphocytes, respectively. Total LU recovered were calculated as shown above. The number of viable cells recovered after treating 10^7 A pool$_x$ effector cells with control ascites, OKT3 or OKT8 plus C' was 5.7, 1.4 and 4.4 x 10^6, respectively.

mice bearing hybridoma cells producing the relevant antibodies (for review, see 30). The control ascites was from mice bearing the parental myeloma cell line. Monoclonal antibody OKT3 reacts with approximately 95% of E rosetting cells (29), OKT8 reacts with subset of T cells which includes cytotoxic and suppressor cells (30) and OKM1 is reactive with monocytes and a small percentage of non-adherent mononuclear cells (1,36). We have recently reported that treatment of cells with these monoclonal antibodies and complement (C') can distinguish CTLs from NK cells (53). Results of a representative experiment are shown in Table VII. Treatment of fresh mononuclear cells or $rI_n \cdot rC_n$ activated cells with OKT3 or OKT8 and C' did not decrease cytotoxicity against K562 cells, as shown by findings that the total lytic units (LU) recovered after such treatment were not lower than after treatment with control ascites and C'. Similarly, lysis of the HLA^- NK-sensitive K562 cells by NK-like cells generated in MLC is not decreased by treatment of the effector cells with OKT3 or OKT8 and C'. In contrast, effector cells generated in MLC which lyse allogeneic normal cells (that are lysed by CTLs but not be NK-like cells) are diminished in cytotoxic activity following treatment with OKT3 or OKT8 and C'. Thus, CTLs are $OKT3^+$, $OKT8^+$ whereas NK cells, $rI_n \cdot rC_n$ activated NK cells and NK-like cells generated in MLC are $OKT3^-$, $OKT8^-$.

Whereas treatment with OKT3 or OKT8 does not decrease NK cell activity, treatment of fresh lymphocytes or $rI_n \cdot rC_n$ activated lymphocytes with OKM1 and C' reduces cytotoxic activity against K562 cells by more than 75%. Although the majority of NK cell activity can be decreased by treatment with OKM1 and C', we failed to decrease MLC generated NK-like cell activity with OKM1 (53) and have found minimal or no $OKM1^+$ cells by immunofluorescence present in MLCs on day 6. Thus, NK-like cells are either derived from OKM1- precursor cells or are derived from OKM1+ cells which then fail to continue to express this marker.

We have recently found that treatment with OKT11a which reacts with 100% peripheral E rosetting cells as well as thymocytes, but not with B cells or monocytes (Verbi et al., in preparation), markedly depletes NK cells as well as MLC generated NK-like cells and CTLs (Ziegler et al., submitted for publication). It appears from preliminary double immunofluorescence studies that only a very low proportion of OKM1+ cells are also OKT11a+ (Kung, personal communication) suggesting that there are at least two phenotypically distinguishable populations of NK cells; one is OKT3-, OKT8-, OKT11a-, OKM1+ and the other is OKT3-, OKT8-, OKT11a+, $OKM1^-$.

In summary, since treatment with monoclonal anti-T cell antibodies, OKT3 or OKT8, and C' totally ablates CTL activity but does not decrease cytotoxic activity of either fresh NK cells, $rI_n \cdot rC_n$ or IF activated NK cells or NK-like cells generated in MLC, it should be possible to ascertain whether effector cells cytotoxic for malignant cells, that are activated in vitro or in vivo following treatment with IF or IF inducers, are CTLs which may be directed against tumor associated antigens or activated NK cells. Additionally, treatment of effector cells with OKM1 or OKT11a and C' will provide additional information concerning the nature of anti-tumor effector cells.

CONCLUDING REMARKS

The following conclusions can be drawn from the results discussed in this chapter:

a.) Highly purified human fibroblast interferon (HFIF) augments the generation of CTLs to alloantigens. It is tempting to speculate that IF treatment of cancer patients may likewise augment CTL responses to tumor associated antigens which may be expressed on autologous malignant cells.

b.) HFIF enhances human NK cell activity against NK sensitive target cells. In addition, fresh human leukemia cells that have not been adapted to tissue culture are not lysed by untreated lymphocytes but are susceptible to lysis by IF treated cells from some, but not all, normal individuals. Whether activated NK cells are cytotoxic for autologous malignant cells has yet to be ascertained.

c.) The interferon inducer $rI_n \cdot rC_n$ augments NK cell activity and the temporal requirements for enhancement of NK cell activity are consistant with the hypothesis that IF induction is required for the effect on NK cells. Further support for this contention derives from our findings that mismatched structural analogues of $rI_n \cdot rC_n$ including $rI_n \cdot r(C_{12},U)_n$ and $rI_n \cdot r(C_{29},G)_n$ which induce IF, but not $rI \cdot mC_n$ which fails to induce IF, augment NK cell activity. Since structural analogues of $rI_n \cdot rC_n$ which lack the toxic effects ascribed to $rI_n \cdot rC_n$ augment NK cell activity, it is clear that polyribonucleotides' augmentation of NK cell activity can be separated from their induction of toxic effects. If it can be shown that activated NK cells can lyse autologous malignant cells, then non-toxic polyribonucleotides may be more clinically useful than IF for activating NK cells to lyse autologous malignant cells since polyribonucleotides are infinitely less expensive than IF and could be more available on a widespread basis for immunotherapy trials.

d.) Monoclonal antibodies OKT3 or OKT8 with C' deplete CTLs but do not lyse NK cells, $rI_n \cdot rC_n$ activated NK cells nor NK-like cells generated in MLC. In contrast, treatment with OKM1 and C' deplete the majority of NK cells. These monoclonal antibodies are thus useful for distinguishing CTLs from NK and NK-like cells and these antibodies will facilitate studies involved in determining the nature of effector cells cytotoxic for malignant cells that may be detected after treatment with IF or IF inducers.

Acknowledgements

I am indebted to Drs. William Carter, James Greene, Paul Ts'o and Patrick Kung for their collaborations. The technical assistance of M.S. Dierckins and E. Sevenich and secretarial assistance of J. Ritter and M. Bump are gratefully acknowledged.

REFERENCES

1. Breard, J., Reinherz, E.L., Kung, P.C., Goldstein, G., and Schlossman, S.F. (1980): J. Immunol., 124:1943.
2. Carter, W.A., and DeClercq, E. (1974): Science, 186:1172.

3. Carter, W.A., O'Malley, J.A., Beeson, M., Cunnington, P.,
    Kelvin, A., Vere-Hodge, A., Alderfer, J.L., and Ts'o, P.O.P.
    (1976): Molec. Pharm., 12:440.
4. Carter, W.A., Pitha, P.M., Marshall, L.W., Tazawa, I., Tazawa, S.,
    and Ts'o, P.O.P. (1972): J. Mol. Biol., 70:567.
5. Davey, M.W., Sulkowski, E., and Carter, W.A. (1976):
    Biochemistry, 15:704.
6. Djeu, J.Y., Heinbaugh, J.A., Holden, H.T., and Herberman, R.B.
    (1979): J. Immunol., 122:175.
7. Edy, V.G., Billiau, A., and DeSomer, P. (1976): J. Gen. Virol.,
    31:251.
8. Einhorn, S., Blomgren, H., and Strander, H. (1978): Acta Med.
    Scand., 20:477.
9. Eremin, O., Ashby, J., and Plumb, D. (1978): J. Immunol. Methods,
    24:251.
10. Freeman, A.I., Al-Bussam, N., O'Malley, J.A., Stutzman, L.,
    Bjornsson, S., and Carter, W.A. (1977): J. Med. Virol., 1:79.
11. Gidlund, M., Orn, A., Wigzell, H., Senik, A., and Gresser, I.
    (1978): Nature, 273:759.
12. Greene, J.J., Alderfer, J.L., Tazawa, I., Tazawa, S., Ts'o, P.O.P.,
    O'Malley, J.A., and Carter, W.A. (1978): Biochemistry,
    17:4214.
13. Greene, J.J., Dreffenbach, C.W., and Ts'o, P.O.P. (1978): Nature,
    271:81.
14. Gresser, I. (1977): In: Cancer. A Comprehensive Treatise,
    edited by F. Becker, p. 521. Plenum Press, New York.
15. Haliotis, T., Roder, J., Klein, M., Ortaldo, J., Fauci, A.S., and
    Herberman, R.B. (1980): J. Exp. Med., 151:1039.
16. Haller, O., Hansson, M., Kiessling, R., and Wigzell, H. (1977):
    Nature 270:609.
17. Havell, E.A., Berman, B., Ogburn, C.A., Berg, K., Paucker, K.,
    and Vilcek, J. (1975): Proc. Natl. Acad. Sci., 72:2185.
18. Havell, E.A., and Vilcek, J. (1972): Antimicrob. Agents
    Chemother., 2:476.
19. Herberman, R.B., Djeu, J.Y., Kay, H.D., Ortaldo, J.R.,
    Riccardi, C., Bonnard, G.D., Holden, H.T., Fagnani, R.,
    Santoni, A., and Puccetti, P. (1978): Immunol. Rev., 44:43.
20. Herberman, R.B., Nunn, M.E., Holden, H.T., Staal, S., and
    Djeu, J.Y. (1977): Int. J. Cancer, 19:555.
21. Herberman, R.R., Ortaldo, J.R., and Bonnard, G.D. (1979): Nature,
    277:221.
22. Heron, I., Berg, K., and Cantell, K. (1976): J. Immunol.,
    117:1370.
23. Horoszewicz, J.S., Karakousis, C., Leong, S., Holyoke, E., Ito, M.,
    Buffest, R.F., and Carter, W.A. (1978): Cancer Treatment
    Rep., 62:1897.
24. Horoszewicz, J.S., Leong, S.S., Ito, M., Di Berardino, L.A., and
    Carter, W.A. (1978): Infect. Immun., 19:720.
25. Huddlestone, J.R., Merigan, T.C., and Oldstone, M.B.A. (1979):
    Nature, 282:417.
26. Jankowski, W.J., Davey, M.W., O'Malley, J.A., Sulkowski, E., and
    Carter, W.A. (1975): J. Virol., 16:1124.
27. Kaplan, J., and Callewaert, D.M. (1978): J. Natl. Cancer Inst.,
    60:961.
28. Karre, K., Klein, G.O., Kiessling, R., Klein, G., and Roder, J.C.
    (1980): Nature, 284:624.

29. Kedar, E.M., Ortiz de Landazuri, M., and Bonavida, B. (1974): J. Immunol., 112:1231.
30. Kiessling, R., Petrányi, G.G., Klein, G., and Wigzell, H. (1975): Int. J. Cancer, 15:933.
31. Kung, P.C., Goldstein, G., Reinherz, E.L., and Schlossman, S.F. (1979): Science, 206:347.
32. Kung, P.C., Talle, M.A., DeMaria, M.E., Butler, M.S., Lifter, I., and Goldstein, G. (1980): Trans. Proc., 12:141.
33. Mantovani, A., Allavana, P., Valente, P., and Belloni, C. (1980): Proc. Am. Cancer Res., 21:204.
34. Merigan, T.C., Sikora, K., Breeden, J.H., Levy, R., and Rosenberg, S.A. (1978): New Engl. J. Med., 299:1449.
35. O'Malley, J.A., Leong, S.S., Horoszewicz, J.S., Carter, W.A., Alderfer, J.L., and Ts'o, P.O.P. (1979): Molec. Pharm., 15:140.
36. Ortaldo, J., Oldham, R.K., Cannon, G.L., and Herberman, R.B. (1977): J. Natl. Cancer Inst., 59:77.
37. Pitha, P.M., Marshall, L.W., and Carter, W.A. (1972): J. Gen. Virol., 15:89.
38. Reinherz, E.L., Moretta, L., Roper, M., Breard, J.M., Mingari, M.C., Cooper, M.D., and Schlossman, S.F. (1980): J. Exp. Med., 151:969.
39. Reithmuller, G., Pape, G.R., Hadam, M.R., and Saal, J.G. (1980): In: Natural Cell-Mediated Immunity Against Tumors, edited by R.B. Herberman, p. 633. Academic Press, New York.
40. Riccardi, C., Santoni, A., Barlozzari, T., and Herberman, R.B. (1980): In: Natural Cell-Mediated Immunity Against Tumors, edited by R.B. Herberman, p. 1121. Academic Press, New York.
41. Roder, J.C., Haliotis, T., Klein, M., Korec, S., Jett, J.R., Ortaldo, J., Herberman, R.B., Katz, P., and Fauci, A.S. (1980): Nature, 284:553.
42. Rosenberg, E.B., Herberman, R.B., Levine, P.H., Halterman, R.H., McCoy, J.L., and Wunderlich, J.R. (1972): Int. J. Cancer, 9:648.
43. Stewart, W.E. II, and Desmyter, J. (1975): Virology, 67:68.
44. Strander, H. (1977): Blut, 35:277.
45. Strander, H., Cantell, K., Carlström, G., and Jakobsson, P.A. (1973): J. Natl. Cancer Inst., 51:733.
46. Talmadge, J.E., Meyers, K.M., Prieur, D.J., and Starkey, J.R. (1980): Nature, 284:622.
47. Trinchieri, G., Santoli, D., Dee, R.R., and Knowles, B.B. (1978): J. Exp. Med., 147:1299.
48. Ts'o, P.O.P., Alderfer, J.L., Levy, J., Marshall, L.W., O'Malley, J., Horoszewicz, J.S., and Carter, W.A. (1976): Molec. Pharm., 12:299.
49. Welsh, R.M., and Kiessling, R.W. (1980): In: Natural Cell-Mediated Immunity Against Tumors, edited by R.B. Herberman, p. 671. Academic Press, New York.
50. West, W.H., Cannon, G.B., Kay, H.D., Bonnard, G.D., and Herberman, R.B. (1977): J. of Immunol., 118:355.
51. Zarling, J.M. (1980): In: Natural Cell-Mediated Immunity Against Tumors, edited by R.B. Herberman, p. 687.
52. Zarling, J.M., Eskra, L., Borden, E.C., Horoszewicz, J., and Carter, W.A. (1979): J. Immunol., 123:63.
53. Zarling, J.M., and Kung, P.C. (1980): Nature, 288:394.
54. Zarling, J.M., Raich, P.C., McKeough, M., and Bach, F.H. (1976): Nature, 262:691.

55. Zarling, J.M., Robins, H.I., Raich, P.C., Bach, F.H., and Bach, M.L. (1978): Nature, 274:269.
56. Zarling, J.M., Schlais, J., Eskra, L., Greene, J., Ts'o, P.O.P., and Carter, W.A. (1980): J. Immunol., 124:1852.
57. Zarling, J.M., Sosman, J., Eskra, L., Borden, E.C., Horoszewicz, J.S., and Carter, W.A. (1978): J. Immunol., 121:2002.

Mediation of Cellular Immunity in Cancer by Immune Modifiers, edited by M. A. Chirigos et al., Raven Press, New York © 1981.

Tumor-Associated Macrophages and Lymphoid Cells in Human Ovarian Carcinoma: Modulation of Their Tumoricidal Capacity by Immunopharmacologic Agents

A. Mantovani, G. Peri, N. Polentarutti, P. Allavena, M. Introna, *C. Sessa, and *C. Mangioni

*Istituto di Ricerche Farmacologiche "Mario Negri," 62-20157 Milan, Italy; *Clinica Ostetrica e Ginecologica, Università di Milano, Milan, Italy*

INTRODUCTION

Cells of the macrophage and lymphoid series infiltrate experimental and human tumors (3,6,7). The role played by tumor-associated host cells in the regulation of tumor growth has been the object of controversy (25). It is conceivable that the isolation and characterization of host cells from tumors should provide evidence relevant to a better understanding of the tumor-host relationship of the tumor site, but little information is available on lymphocytes and macrophages in human neoplasms.

Ovarian carcinoma frequently spreads in the peritoneal cavity and ascites occurs. Ovarian ascitic tumors provide an easily accessible source of lymphocytes, macrophages and tumor cells in suspension and we have developed methods to isolate and characterize tumor-associated macrophages (TAM), tumor-associated lymphoid cells (TAL) and neoplastic cells from this anatomical site (15,20,21). More recently, we have investigated host cells purified from solid ovarian tumors (17). In the present report, we summarize data on the in vitro modulation of the tumoricidal activity of human TAM and TAL. Moreover we will present results on the effect of i.p. C.parvum on cytotoxicity of macrophages and natural killer (NK) cells isolated from ovarian carcinomatous ascites.

IN VITRO MODULATION OF THE TUMORICIDAL ACTIVITY OF TAM IN HUMAN OVARIAN CANCER

Peripheral blood monocytes obtained from patients with advanced ovarian epithelial tumors had somewhat impaired cytolytic capacity against TU5 tumor cells and impaired capacity to mature in vitro into macrophages (17, 19-21); a wide overlap with control values was observed. Similarly, TAM from ascitic ovarian tumors showed cytotoxicity levels similar to or lower than peritoneal exudate macrophages from control subjects undergoing surgery for benign non infectious gynecological diseases (20,21).

More recently, we have studied the responsiveness of TAM from ascitic and solid ovarian tumors to stimuli which have been shown to augment monocyte or macrophage-mediated tumoricidal activity. It has been demonstrated that in vitro exposure to interferon (IF) from fibroblasts, leukocytes and lymphoblastoid cells, to lymphokine supernatants and to endotoxin enhances the tumoricidal activity of human monocytes or macrophages (1,2,13,16,18,28). Expression of baseline and stimulated cytotoxicity was a function of the maturation stage of the mononuclear phagocytes, epithelioid and giant cells being anergic, and of the anatomical site of origin, alveolar macrophages being relatively inefficient effectors (16,19). Indirect evidence suggested the hypothesis that IF and lymphokines supernatants (LK) activated human mononuclear phagocytes through at least partially distinct biological pathways (16,18,19). It was therefore of interest to evaluate the effect of various stimuli on the tumoricidal activity of TAM. So far we have investigated TAM from 27 ascitic tumors and results of a typical experiment with endotoxin are presented in Table 1. IF, LK and endotoxin augmented the tumoricidal activity of TAM to an extent comparable to control peritoneal exudate macrophages. In a more limited series of experiments TAM from solid ovarian tumors were investigated and Table 2 shows findings with 4 preparations which could be tested in parallel with ascites TAM from the same patient. While in 2 patients (No. 2 and 21) TAM from the ascitic and solid tumor had similar baseline cytotoxicity and similar responsiveness to stimuli in 2 other subjects (No. 27 and 29) macrophages from the solid neoplasm showed defective cytotoxicity compared to those from the carcinomatous ascites from the same subject. The defective responsiveness to activation of TAM from solid tumors is not attributable to the disaggregation procedures (mincing and exposure to collagenase) because the cytotoxicity of TAM from effusions which were treated in the same way was not affected.

In experiments discussed so far cytotoxicity of macrophages was measured against the TU5 line, because adherent effector cells against this tumor had been extensively characterized (18,19). In an effort to obtain data more relevant to the actual in vivo conditions, in a series of experiments primary cultures from ovarian tumors, consisting primarily of carcinoma cells, were used as targets (21). When unstimulated normal

TABLE 1. Effect of endotoxin on the tumoricidal activity of tumor-associated macrophages

Macrophages from	Endotoxin (ug/ml)				
	$-$	0.01	0.1	1	10
Control peritoneal exudate	44.8+2.8	51.2+3.2[a]	54.7+4.9[a]	55.5+3.3[a]	58.3+0.9
Carcinomatous ascites	34.9+1.7	35.2+3.1	40.5+3.4[a]	41.6+5.0[a]	42.7+4.7[a]

Cytolytic activity was measured as $/^3H/$ thymidine release from TU5 target cells at an attacker to target (A:T) ratio of 20:1 as described (16-21). Endotoxin was from Salmonella typhosa (W.)
Results are percentage of specific lysis.
[a]Significantly above background lysis of macrophages alone, p < 0.01.

TABLE 2. Responsiveness of macrophages from solid ovarian carcinoma to IF and lymphokines

Patient No.	Macrophages from	Percentage of specific lysis ± S.D.		
		−	IF	Lymphokines
2	Ascites	23.2 ± 2.1	44.0 ± 2.4[a]	NT[b]
	Solid tumor	24.6 ± 3.8	46.3 ± 2.2[a]	NT[b]
21	Ascites	12.7 ± 5.3	16.7 ± 0.6[a]	17.1 ± 2.6
	Solid tumor	10.3 ± 0.5	14.9 ± 0.4[a]	14.3 ± 1.0
27	Ascites	17.2 ± 1.3	68.7 ± 2.1[a]	43.1 ± 2.1[a]
	Solid tumor	3.6 ± .0.8	4.1 ± 0.7	8.6 ± 1.5[a]
29	Ascites	11.1 ± 1.0	59.5 ± 8.1[a]	NT[b]
	Solid tumor	9.8 ± 0.3	13.9 ± 0.1[a]	NT[b]

Cytolytic activity of macrophages from ascites or solid tumor was tested against TU5 (see Table 1). IF concentration was 1000 units/ml (16) and lymphokines were diluted 1/3 (18).
[a] $p < 0.05$ compared to unstimulated effectors
[b] Not tested.

macrophages or TAM were used as effectors, primary ovarian carcinoma cultures appeared heterogeneous in their susceptibility to macrophage cytotoxicity, a minority of the patients yielding tumor cells resistant to cytolysis (21). Stimulation by macrophages of the proliferative capacity of resistant primary cultures was observed (21). More recently, we have studied the susceptibility of primary ovarian carcinoma cultures to activated macrophage cytotoxicity. As illustrated by the examples given in Table 3, while carcinoma cells from patient No. 5 were consistently killed by IF or LK-stimulated macrophages, no augmentation of cytolysis was detected with tumor No. 3. The mechanisms underlying the heterogeneity of the susceptibility of different primary ovarian carcinoma cultures and, specifically, the failure to observe augmented lysis of tumor cells from some patients after stimulation of effectors by various agents, remain elusive. It can be speculated that, within the tumor, subpopulations of cells endowed with different susceptibility to macrophages exist, and their relative representation in a given primary

TABLE 3. Susceptibility to macrophage cytotoxicity of primary ovarian carcinoma cultures

Target cells	Specific lysis (%)		
	−	IF	Lymphokines
TU5	27	56[a]	54[a]
Ovarian carcinoma No. 5	23	33[a]	48[a]
Ovarian carcinoma No. 3	18	15	9

The experimental conditions were as in Table 1 and 2.
[a] $p < 0.01$ compared to unstimulated effectors.

culture determines the outcome of the interaction with normal or activated macrophages. Churchill et al. (4) have recently presented preliminary evidence that the susceptibility of various tumor cell lines to
macrophages is related to sialic acid content. It remains to be elucidated whether this plays a role in determining the susceptibility to
macrophage cytotoxicity of ovarian carcinoma cells.

IN VITRO MODULATION OF THE TUMORICIDAL ACTIVITY OF TAL IN HUMAN OVARIAN CANCER

Lymphoid cells infiltrating human tumors were generally reported to
have little NK activity (30,32,33). TAL from ascitic ovarian tumor had
low, but significant NK activity against K562 (15). Preliminary evidence for the existence, in part of the patients, of suppressor cells,
was obtained (5,15). IF enhances NK activity (see for review 11), but
it was not known whether tumor-associated lymphoid cells are responsive
to this stimulus. As shown by the experiments in Table 4, IF augmented
NK activity against K562 of TAL from ascitic ovarian tumors. Interestingly enough, stimulation of NK by IF was also observed with TAL
preparations (No. 4 and 6 in Table 4) which, when mixed with peripheral
blood lymphocytes, inhibited NK activity (58 and 19% inhibition for preparation No. 4 and No. 6).

In an effort to elucidate further lymphocyte-tumor cell interactions
in human ovarian carcinoma, in a series of experiments fresh tumor cells
purified from 27 ascitic and 3 solid tumors as previously described (15),
were used as targets in a 4 or 20 h ^{51}Cr release assay. Freshly purified
ovarian carcinoma cells were relatively resistant to lysis by normal
unstimulated peripheral blood lymphocytes (PBL), although low, but significant, killing was occasionally observed particularly after 20 h of
incubation, as previously reported in a preliminary series of subjects
(15). PBL and TAL from ovarian tumors had cytolytic activity levels
against autologous cancer cells which did not exceed that of control
normal subjects: only one PBL preparation had high levels of killing of
autologous (36.2 and 42.9 % specific lysis after 4 and 20 h) but not of
allogeneic (<5% lysis) ovarian carcinoma cells.

In a series of experiments, the effect of IF on cytotoxicity of PBL
and TAL against autologous or allogeneic fresh carcinoma cells was
investigated: Table 5 shows two typical experiments in which IF enhanced
cytotoxicity of PBL and TAL against fresh autologous carcinoma cells and
Table 6 summarizes results of this study. IF enhanced the cytotoxicity
of normal PBL against ovarian carcinoma cells in a 4 and 20 h assay;

TABLE 4. Effect of IF on NK activity (K562) of TAL

Effector cells	IF	
	−	+
Normal PBL	48	65[a]
TAL No. 4	15	31[a]
No. 6	17	58[a]
No. 19	51	60[a]

TAL were preincubated with IF (1000 units/ml) for 18 h
[a] $p < 0.01$

TABLE 5. Effect of IF on cytotoxicity of PBL and TAL against ovarian carcinoma No. 3

Effector cells[a]	IF	Specificy lysis (% ± S.D.)	
		4h	20 h
Normal PBL	−	6.2 + 3.9	-15.7 + 2.6
	+	22.6 + 5.8[c]	22.6 + 6.4[c]
PBL (autologous)	−	6.2 + 0.8	7.2 + 1.1
	+	11.3 + 0.8[b]	12.1 + 3.3[b]
TAL (autologous)	−	.4.0 + 1.9	8.8 + 2.4
	+	7.3 + 1.5[b]	22.6 + 5.1[c]
PBL (allogeneic ov. cancer)	−	-4.9 + 1.5	-11.8 + 4.3
	+	7.5 + 1.5[c]	11.5 + 3.8[c]
TAL (allogeneic ov. cancer)	−	1.4 + 3.3	0.3 + 1.8
	+	8.8 + 2.3[c]	16.0 + 5.5[c]

[a]Effector cells (1-2x10^6/ml) were preincubated for 18 h with fibroblast IF (1000 units/ml, HEM) as previously described (15).
Results are mean (+ S.D.) specific ^{51}Cr release after 4 or 20 h (15).
[b]$p < 0.05$ compared to effector cells incubated without IF
[c]$p < 0.01$ compared to effector cells incubated without IF

TABLE 6. Augmentation by IF of cell-mediated lysis of fresh ovarian carcinoma cells

Effector cells[a]	Carcinomas with increased lysis/total		Absolute increase in lysis[b]	
	4h	20h	4h	20h
Normal PBL	11/19	12/18	7.6 (5-17)	8.9 (5-42)
Patient PBL (autologous)	3/13[c]	8/14	10.3 (5-15)	6.7 (5-11)
Patient PBL (allogeneic)	2/11[c]	4/11	9.3 (6-12)	11.3 (7-23)
TAL (autologous)	3/9	5/9	6.0 (5-7)	6.8 (5-13)
TAL (allogeneic)	3/5	3/5	5.3 (5-7)	9.6 (5-16)

[a]Effector cells (1-2x10^6/ml) were preincubated with IF (1000 units/ml) for 1-20h. Lysis was measured in a 4 or 20 h ^{51}Cr release assay as previously described (15).
[b]Results are mean absolute increase in lysis (with range in parenthesis) of IF stimulated effectors above unstimulated lymphocytes. Only experiments (see Fig. 4-8) in which IF caused a significant (p 0.05) augmentation of lysis were used to calculate the mean.
[c]$p < 0.05$ compared to normal PBL tested at 4 h, Fisher's exact test.

stimulation by IF was less frequently observed with ovarian cancer PBL
and TAL in a 4 h assay, but, after 20 h, effector cells from tumor-
bearing subjects showed IF-boosted cytotoxicity against carcinoma cells
similar to controls. IF enhanced the cytotoxicity of ovarian cancer PBL
and TAL against both autologous and allogeneic carcinoma cells. Thus,
PBL and TAL are rarely cytotoxic against ^{51}Cr labelled fresh autologous
carcinoma cells, but in vitro exposure to IF enhances killing of ovarian
tumor cells.

Vanky et al. (31) have recently reported in a heterogeneous series
of human neoplasms that IF augmented killing of allogeneic but not
autologous cancer cells, and, on this basis, they speculated that alloantigens may play a role in natural killing (31). Data obtained with
human ovarian carcinoma briefly summarized here appear at variance with
previous observations by Vanky et al. (31). While differences in the
experimental protocols could account for the apparent discrepancy between
data reported here and those of Vanky et al. (31), it is possible that
these divergent findings are the expression of a different immunobiology
of the tumors investigated. In this context, it is of interest that
mature NK cells were reported to kill allogeneic but not autologous
fibroblasts, but, after stimulation of effectors, killing was detected
against both autologous and allogeneic targets (29).

In part of the ovarian cancer patients, IF enhanced the cytotoxicity
of PBL and TAL against autologous carcinoma cells. In addition to
stimulating NK lysis (11), IF was reported to enhance specific T cell-
mediated cytotoxicity (14) and one might speculated that IF-boosted
cytolysis of autologous carcinoma cells is mediated by mature T cells.
Characterization of IF-boosted effector cells capable of lysing autologous fresh ovarian carcinoma cells should elucidate the nature of this
reactivity.

EFFECT OF I.P. C.PARVUM ON THE TUMORICIDAL ACTIVITY OF TAM AND TAL FROM ASCITIC OVARIAN TUMORS

Formation of ascites, requiring frequent paracenteses, is a cumber-
some complication of advanced ovarian tumors resistant to chemotherapy.
Webb et al. (34) reported that intraperitoneal administration of C.parvum
caused a dramatic reduction of ascites formation in patients with
various tumors including ovarian carcinoma. We have confirmed these
clinical findings in a series of 8 ovarian cancer patients resistant to
first and second line chemotherapy, whose peritoneal effusions required
repeated, frequent paracenteses. C.parvum (Coparvax, Wellcome Research
Laboratories, Beckenham, England) was given i.p. at a dose of 14 mg in
200 ml saline during a 1 h infusion. This treatment was repeated on
day 7 (14 mg) and 28 (7 mg). Clinical findings confirmed previous
observations (34) and will only be briefly summarize here to provide a
framework for the presentation of laboratory studies. Toxicity included:
gastrointestinal pain (8/8 subjects); nausea and vomiting (7/8); fever
(5/8); dyspnea and hypotension (1/8) requiring hydrocortisone. Two
patients showed a complete disappearance of the ascitic effusion after 2
C.parvum administrations and one after the first dose of this agent.
They have remained free of ascites for 2,6 and 13^{+} months. In two
subjects definite evidence of marked reduction of the effusion was
obtained, but peritoneal fluid did not disappear. Three patients received no appreciable benefit from C.parvum treatment. In none of the
subjects was any indication obtained for an effect of C.parvum on solid

tumor masses. In agreement with previous observations (34). Cytological examination of cell smears from ascites revealed a decrease of the percentage of tumor cells as early as 7 days after the first treatment, an increase in polymorphs and, to a lesser extent, in macrophages.

In rodents, systemic administration (i.v. or i.p.) of this agent enhances macrophage-mediated cytotoxicity (see for instance ref. 9 and 24) and NK activity (8,12,22,23). In murine systems, there is evidence that the antitumor activity of i.v. or i.p. C.parvum is related, at least in part, to stimulation of macrophage and/or NK cell function (26,35). It was therefore of interest to evaluate whether the limited, but signi-ficant, antitumor activity of i.p. C.parvum in human ovarian carcino-matous ascites was related to stimulation of these tumor-associated effector mechanisms.

In 4 patients (Fig. 1,2) TAL were separated and tested for NK activ-ity against K562 as previously described (15) at different times after entering the C.parvum protocol. In agreement with previous data, 3 of 4 patients had very low pretreatment NK activity in TAL, and no stimula-tion of cytotoxicity by C.parvum was observed. TAL from a 4th subject had NK cytotoxicity in the range of normal PBL (RCI = 0.8) and cytolytic activity was markedly decreased following i.p. injection of C.parvum (Fig. 1 and 2).

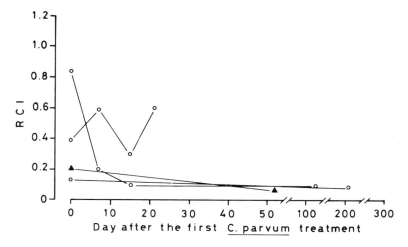

FIG. 1. NK activity against K562 of TAL after i.p. treatment with C.parvum. Cytotoxicity is presented as relative cytotoxicity index (RCI) calculated rela-tive to control PBL as previously described (15). The o and Δ symbols indicate patients responsive or unresponsive to C.parvum (in terms of reduction of ascites) respectively.

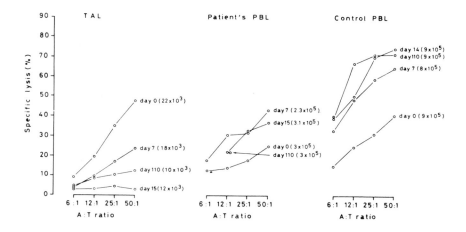

FIG. 2. NK activity of TAL from patient No. 1 tested on different
days after C.parvum treatment. Numbers in parenthesis indicate
the recoveries of lymphoid cells (per ml) from ascites or blood.
Values for control PBL are means of at least 2 donors.

The effect of i.p. C.parvum on the tumoricidal activity of TAM was
investigated in 6 patients (Fig. 3). No evidence of augmentation of
macrophage-mediated cytotoxicity was obtained throughout the 110 days
observation period. In all 4 subjects in whom macrophage-mediated cytotoxicity was measured between day 14 and 21 after the first C.parvum
administration, a marked depression of the tumoricidal potential of TAM
was observed at these times, specific lysis being 7.6 ± 1.8 (mean $\pm$ S.D.)
compared to a pretreatment value of 25.5 ± 5.5 (p $<$ 0.01). Subsequent
evaluations 48 to 110 days after starting C.parvum therapy showed cytolytic activity levels similar to pretreatment values. The drop of cytotoxicity consistently observed between day 14 and 21 was not attributable to a failure of the assay to detect cytolysis on those particular
occasions, as peripheral blood monocytes from the same patients or from
normal donors tested in parallel on the same days showed no decrease in
cytolysis values. Macrophages cytotoxicity at different A:T ratios for
one of these subjects is presented in Fig. 4. Specific lysis at an A:T
ratio of 20:1 was 32% on day 0 and declined to 5 and 4% on day 14 and 21.
This decrease of macrophage cytotoxicity was not related to alterations
in the sensitivity of the assay, because no such changes were detected
with blood monocytes from the same subject or from normal donors tested
in parallel on the same days (Fig. 4).
  Intraperitoneal administration of C.parvum has been shown repeatedly
to cause a long lasting stimulation of macrophage cytotoxicity in rodents
(see for instance 9,24). Human PBL exposed in vitro to C.parvum produce
IF (27,28), an agent capable to enhance human macrophage cytotoxicity
(13,16,18,19). Moreover, supernatants generated by coculture of human
PBL with anaerobic coryneforms augmented the cytolytic activity of human

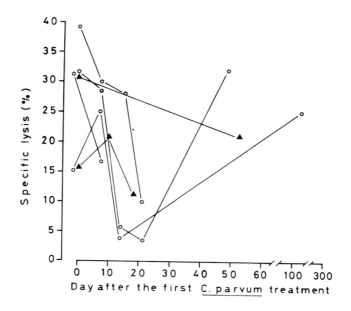

FIG. 3.   Tumoricidal activity of TAM against the TU5 line (16,21) after i.p. C.parvum.   The A:T ratio was 20:1

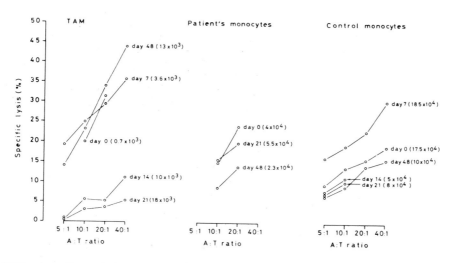

FIG. 4.   Tumoricidal activity of TAM from patient No. 5 tested on different days after the first C.parvum treatment.   Numbers in parenthesis indicate the recoveries of mononuclear phagocytes per ml of blood or ascites.   Cytotoxicity and recovery values for control monocytes, tested in parallel, are means of at least 2 normal donors, except for day 7 when only one volunteer was tested for monocyte-mediated cytolysis.

monocytes and inhibited their migration (18,28). On the basis of these data, intraperitoneal injection of C.parvum in human ovarian ascites was expected to stimulate the tumoricidal activity of TAM. This prediction was not verified in the present study. 14-21 days after the first C.parvum treatment, a significant decrease of the tumoricidal activity of TAM was consistently observed, cytotoxicity returning to pretreatment values at later times. No such changes were observed with peripheral blood monocytes from the same patients. The mechanism(s) responsible for inhibition of ascites macrophage cytotoxicity by C.parvum remains to be elucidated, but it is noteworthy that, while this work in humans was in progress, Haskill and coworkers (10) reported a similar inhibition of the direct and antibody-dependent cytotoxic activity of TAM from a murine carcinoma following intratumor administration of C.parvum.

CONCLUDING REMARKS

Human ovarian carcinomatous ascites is an easily accessible source of tumor cells, macrophages and lymphoid cells in suspension. The tumoricidal capacity of tumor-associated NK cells and macrophages can be quantitated using cell lines as targets and we have shown that the expression of cytotoxicity can be modulated by in vitro exposure to agents such as IF, lymphokine supernatants or endotoxin. Since ascites can be easily obtained and this is frequently done for therapeutic purposes in advanced ovarian cancer, we have been able to investigate the effect of i.p. C.parvum on host defense mechanisms at an anatomical site directly involved by neoplasia. We had previously used a similar approach to study the effect of chemotherapy on intratumor macrophage-mediated cytotoxicity (19). These studies indicate that ovarian ascites can be invaluable to assess the effects of therapeutic agents on host defense mechanisms at an anatomical site directly involved by neoplasia. The potential importance of such an approach is suggested by findings with C.parvum, inasmuchas a marked stimulation of the cytotoxicity of TAM and, possibly, NK cells was expected on the basis data in rodents, but it was not detected in human ovarian asictes treated i.p. with this agent.

While the expression of cytotoxicity of TAM and TAL can be modulated in vitro by various agents, ovarian carcinoma cells, tested either immediately after purification or as primary cultures, are in part relatively resistant to the killing mechanisms investigated in the present study. It appears conceivable that resistance or susceptibility of the relevant neoplastic cells can be one critical determinant of the actual in vivo role of NK cells and macrophages in the regulation of the growth of these tumors.

Experiments with TAM from the ascitic and solid ovarian tumors from the same patient tested in parallel indicated that, at least in part of the subjects, solid tumor macrophages had defective cytotoxicity compared to effector cells purified from the effusion. Therefore although ovarian ascites is a unique easily accessible source of TAM and TAL, it must be stressed that tumor-associated effector cells isolated from this peculiar anatomical site need not be representative of host cells within the solid neoplasms.

ACKNOWLEDGMENT

This work was supported by Grant RO1 CA 26824 from the National Cancer Institute and by finalized project "Control of neoplastic growth" (contract No. 79.00643.96) from CNR, Rome, Italy.

REFERENCES

1. Cameron, D.J., and Churchill, W.H. (1979): J.Clin.Invest., 63:977-984.
2. Cameron, D.J., and Churchill, W.H. (1980): J.Immunol., 124:708-712.
3. Carr, I. (1977) In: The Macrophage and Cancer, edited by K.James, B.McBride, and A.Stuart, pp.364-374. University of Edinburgh, Edinburgh.
4. Churchill, W.H., and Cameron, D.J. (1980): In: 4th.International Congress of Immunology, Paris July 21-26,1980, abstract 10.2.02.
5. Eremin, O. (1980) : In: Natural Cell-Mediated Immunity Against Tumors, edited by R.B. Herberman, pp.1011-1029. Academic Press, New York.
6. Evans, R. (1972) : Transplantation,14:468-473.
7. Evans, R. (1976) : In:The Macrophage in Neoplasia, edited by M.A. Fink, pp.27-42. Academic Press, New York.
8. Flexman, J.P., and Shellam, G.B. (1980): Br.J.Cancer, 42:41-51.
9. Ghaffar, A., Cullen, R.T., and Woodruff, M.F.A. (1975): Br.J.Cancer, 31:15-22.
10. Haskill, S., Ritter, F., and Becker, S. (1980): J.Immunol., 125: 454-458.
11. Herberman, R.B., Djeu, J.Y., Kay, H.D., Ortaldo, J.R., Riccardi,C., Bonnard, G.D., Holden, H.T., Fagnani, R., Santoni, A., and Puccetti, P. (1979): Immunol.Rev. 44:43-70.
12. Herberman, R.B., Nunn, M.E., Holden, H.T., Staal, S., and Djeu, J.Y. (1977): Int.J.Cancer,19: 555-564.
13. Jett, J., Mantovani, A., and Herberman, R.B. (1980). Cell.Immunol., 54:425-434.
14. Lindahl, P., Leary, P., and Gresser, I. (1972): Proc.Natl.Acad.Sci. USA, 69:721-725.
15. Mantovani, A., Allavena, P., Sessa, C., Bolis, G., and Mangioni, C. (1980a): Int.J.Cancer, 25:573-582.
16. Mantovani, A., Bar Shavit, Z., Peri, G., Polentarutti, N., Bordignon, C., Sessa, C., and Mangioni, C. (1980b): Clin.Exp.Immunol., 39:776-784.
17. Mantovani, A.,Bordignon, C., Biondi, A., Introna, M., and Allavena,P. (1981) In: Movement,Metabolism.Microbicidal and Tumoricidal Activity of Phagocytes, edited by P.Patriarca, and F.Rossi, Plenum Press, New York, in press.
18. Mantovani, A., Dean, J.H., Jerrells, T.R., and Herberman, R.B.(1980c): Int.J.Cancer, 25:691-699.
19. Mantovani, A., Peri, G., Polentarutti, N., Allavena, P., Bordignon, C., Sessa, C., and Mangioni, C. (1980): In: Natural Cell-Mediated
20. Mantovani, A., Peri, G., Polentarutti, N., Bolis, G., Mangioni,C., and Spreafico, F. (1979): Int.J.Cancer, 23:157-164.
21. Mantovani, A., Polentarutti, N., Peri, G., Bar Shavit, Z., Vecchi,A., Bolis, G., and Mangioni, C. (1980d): J.Natl.Cancer Inst., 64:1307-1315.
22. Oehler, J.R., Lindsay, L.R., Nunn, M.E., Holden, H.T., and Herberman, R.B.(1978): Int.J.Cancer, 21:210-218.

23. Ojo, E., Haller, O., Kimura, A., and Wigzell, H. (1978): Int.J.Cancer Cancer, 21:444-451.
24. Olivotto, M., and Bomford, R. (1974): Int.J.Cancer, 13: 478-488.
25. Prehn, R.T. (1977): J.Natl.Cancer Inst., 59:1043-1049.
26. Scott, M.T. (1974): Semin.Oncol. 1:367-378.
27. Sugiyama, M., and Epstein, L.B. (1978): Cancer Res., 38:4467-4473.
28. Tagliabue, A., Mantovani, Boraschi, D., and Herberman, R.B. (1980): Eur.J.Immunol., 10:542-546.
29. Tarkkanen, J., Timonen, T., and Saksela, E. (1980): Scand.J.Immunol., 11:383-390.
30. Tötterman, T.H., Häyry,P., Saksela, E., Timonen,T., and Eklund, B. Eur.J.Immunol., 8:872-875.
31. Vanky, F.T., Argov, S.A., Einhorn, S.A., and Klein, E. (1980): J.Exp.Med., 151:1151-1165 (1980).
32. Vose, B.M., Vanky, F., Argov, S., and Klein, E. (1977a): Eur.J. Immunol., 7:753-757.
33. Vose, B.M., Vanky, F., and Klein, E. (1977b): Int.J.Cancer, 24:895-902.
34. Webb, H.E., Oaten, S.W., and Pike, C.P. (1978): Br.Med.J., 1:338-340.
35. Woodruff, M.F.A., and Warner, N.L. (1977): J.Natl.Cancer.Inst., 58:111-116.

Mediation of Cellular Immunity in Cancer by
Immune Modifiers, edited by M. A. Chirigos
et al., Raven Press, New York © 1981.

Enhanced Human NK Cell Activity Following Treatment with Interferon *In Vitro* and *In Vivo*

S. Einhorn, H. Blomgren, H. Strander, and M. Troye

Radiumhemmet, Karolinska Hospital and Department of Immunology, University of Stockholm, Stockholm, Sweden

INTRODUCTION

Interferon (IFN) preparations have been found to exert a multiplicity of effects on the immune system (1). In some cases IFN preparations suppress functions of lymphoid cells, whereas in others they augment the action of the immune system. In several cases, the effects on the immune system that have been observed using more or less impure IFN preparations have also been found using completely purified IFN, showing IFN and not contaminants in the preparations, to be responsible for the effects (2,3,4,5).

Clinical trials with human leukocyte IFN as therapy for various tumor diseases were started in 1969 at the Karolinska Hospital and later at other clinics throughout the world. In some diseases, e.g. Hodgkin's and non-Hodgkin's lymphoma, myeloma, mammary carcinoma, acute and chronic leukemia, ovarian carcinoma and juvenile laryngeal papilloma, antitumor effects, expressed as partial and in some cases as complete remissions, have been observed (6). Although the number of tumor types observed to respond to IFN therapy are increasing, this therapy has to date not been shown to be superior to conventional treatment for any malignant disease.

Although IFN has been shown to exert antitumor effects in animals (7) and in man the mechanisms behind these effects are not known. One of several possible mechanisms is a direct effect on the tumor cells in which their multiplication is inhibited. Another is that IFN acts indirectly, e.g. by augmenting a possible antitumor defence of the immune system. To furhter investigate the latter possibility studies have been initiated with the aim of investigating whether the immune system of tumor patients is affected by IFN therapy and whether effects seen are correlated to those observed following IFN treatment *in vitro*. In this paper we present some data on the effects of IFN treatment *in vitro* and *in vivo* on the natural killer (NK) activity of peripheral lymphocytes. Some of the data discussed have been previously published (2,8,9,10,11).

MATERIALS AND METHODS

Patient material

The material consist of 68 patients with a variety of diseases; myeloma, osteosarcoma, melanoma, ovarian carcinoma, small cell carcinoma of the lung, thyroid carcinoma, carcinoma of the colon, myocarditis, larynge-

al papilloma and cancer of the prostate. All patients received daily in-
tramuscular injections of 3 million IFN units during the time of the study.

IFN preparations

The leukocyte IFN (IFN-α) preparations were derived from human peripheral blood leukocytes exposed to Sendai virus as previously described
(12). Most patients received partially purified IFN with a specific activity of 1 x 10^6 units/mg of protein (13), whereas the others (3 patients)
received concentrated IFN with a specific activity of 2 x 10^4 units/mg of
protein. Partially purified IFN was used for the *in vitro* experiments.

In some *in vitro* experiments completely pure fibroblast IFN (IFN-β)
was used. This IFN-β was kindly provided by Dr E. Knight Jr. and was
produced and purified as previously described (14). Aminoacid analysis
of this preparation, containing 2 x 10^8 units/mg of protein, has shown
it to contain no polypeptides except IFN (14).

Cytotoxic assay using unfractionated lymphocytes

The cytotoxic assay was performed as previously described (2,8,9,10,
11). Lymphoid cells were separated from heparinized venous blood by centrifugation on Ficoll-Isopaque (15). The cells were then washed twice by
centrifugation in medium. When assesed after crystal violet staining,
approximately 90% of the cells were classified as lymphocytes. If not
otherwise stated Chang-cells, from human liver, were used as targets.
One million of these cells suspended in 0.5 ml of medium were labelled
with ^{51}Cr. 10.000 labelled were then transferred to tubes together with
various numbers of lymphocytes giving lymphocyte to target cell ratios
of 25, 50 and 100:1 after which the volume was adjusted with medium to
0.6 ml. To some of the tubes IFN was added at a final concentration of 30
units/ml. Spontaneous isotope release was determined in tubes containing
target cells and medium only. The cells were incubated for 4 hours at
37°C after which the radioactivity of 0.2 ml of the supernatant and of
the remaining 0.4 ml was determined using a gammacounter. A cytotoxic
index was calculated according to the formula:

$$\frac{\text{\% release with lymphocytes - \% spontaneous release}}{100 - \text{\% spontaneous release}}$$

Cytotoxicity assay using fractionated lymphocytes

Lymphocytes from heparinized peripheral blood were isolated and purified by gelatin sedimentation, followed by treatment with carbonyl iron
and Ficoll-Isopaque centrifugation. For details see Perlmann et al (16).

Separation of lymphocytes. Briefly, 1 ml of lymphocytes (1.6×10^7/ml)
were rosetted with 1 ml untreated 2% SRBC in RPMI 1640 (TCM) supplemen-
ed with glutamine, penicillin, streptomycin and 5% heat-inactivated fetal bovine serum (FBS). The mixture was incubated for 5 minutes at 37°C,
centrifugated at 100 xg for 5 minutes and then incubated on ice for 1 h.
Thereafter, the pellets were gently suspended and rosetting and nonrosetting cells were separated by Ficoll-Isopaque (FIP) density gradient centrifugation. SRBC attaced to lymphocytes were lysed by brief exposure
to hypotonic TMC (2:1). Cells forming rosettes with SRBC under these
conditions will be termed high avidity E-cells.

From the nonrosetting fraction low avidity E-cells were separated under optimal conditions - that is, using neuraminidase (NANAase)treated SRBC, concentrated FBS and incubation at 4°C over night. The NANAase treated SRBC were prepared as previously described (17). The rosetting cells (termed low avidity E-cells) and the nonrosetting cells (termed non-E-cells) were separated on a FIP gradient and SRBC were removed from the low avidity E-cell fraction as described above.

Cytotoxic assay. The NK activity of the lymphocyte fractions was analysed in a short term ^{51}Cr-release assay (4 hours of incubation) with target cells from the myeloid cell line K562 as described previously (18). Target cells were labelled with ^{51}Cr after which the assay was performed in tubes containing 5×10^3 target cells and 3×10^5 or 1.5×10^5 lymphocytes (lymphocyte/target cell ratios 60:1 and 30:1, of which only 30:1 is presented). The cells were incubated for 4 hours at 37°C after which the release was determined in a gamma counter. Cytotoxicity was expressed as above.

Surface markers. 1) Lymphocytes forming spontaneous rosettes with SRBC (E-rosettes) were assayed by rosetting with NANAase-treated SRBC (ratio 1:25) in concentrated FBS over night (15). 2) Lymphocytes carrying Fc receptors for IgG (FcR$^+$) were determined by rosette formation with bovine erythrocytes (E_b) coated with the IgG fraction of rabbit anti E_b (ratio 1:35) (EA-rosettes) (19).

RESULTS

In vitro studies

Pretreatment of lymphocytes with IFN *in vitro* augmented their NK activity (8). An augmented NK activity was also observed when IFN was added to the assay. To ascertain that this effect on NK activity was due to IFN and not to contaminants in the preparations, the influence of completely pure IFN-β on NK activity was measured. As can be seen in table 1. pure IFN-β as well as partially purified IFN-α enhanced NK activity, showing IFN to be the factor in human IFN preparations responsible for this effect (2).

TABLE 1. Effect of preincubating lymphocytes for 1 hour in medium only or in medium containing 100 units/ml of partially purified IFN-α or pure IFN-β on NK activity against Chang and K562 cells.

Target	Lymphocyte: target cell ratio	Preincubation		
		medium	IFN-α	pure IFN-β
Chang	50:1	0.06	0.17	0.21
"	100:1	0.06	0.24	0.30
K 562	50:1	0.27	0.34	0.37
"	100:1	0.34	0.48	0.45

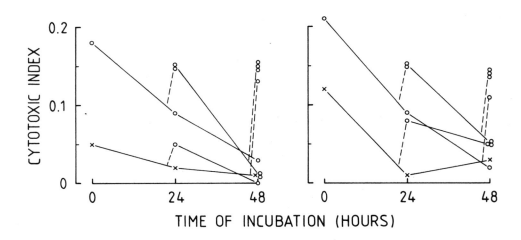

FIGURE 1. Effect of IFN treatment (1000 units/ml during 1 h) on the NK activity of lymphocytes incubated at 37°C for various times. X = untreated lymphocytes, O = lymphocytes treated with IFN once, 8 = lymphocytes treated with IFN twice, 8 = lymphocytes treated with IFN three times. Two experiments using lymphoid cell preparations containing phagocytic cells (left) and depleted of phagocytic cells (right) are presented. Lymphocyte: target cell ratio 100:1.

During *in vivo* therapy with IFN the patient's lymphocytes are repeatedly stimulated by IFN (daily injections). To study whether once stimulated lymphocytes can be restimulated with IFN, lymphocytes were incubated *in vitro* for 48 hours, during which time the lymphocytes were pulsed with IFN 1, 2 or 3 times (1 hour of incubation with IFN and subsequent washing of the lymphocytes). As can be seen in Fig. 1, once IFN stimulated lymphocytes can be restimulated with IFN at least two times.

TABLE 2. Effect of IFN on target cell sensitivity to NK activity of lymphocytes. K562 cells were incubated for 24 hours in medium only or in medium containing 100 units/ml of partially purified IFN-α or pure IFN-β prior to testing their susceptibility to killing.

Lymphocyte: target cell ratio		Preincubation		
		medium	IFN-α	pure IFN-β
Exp. 1	50:1	0.18	0.13	0.10
	100:1	0.33	0.24	0.24
Exp. 2	100:1	0.31	0.26	0.25

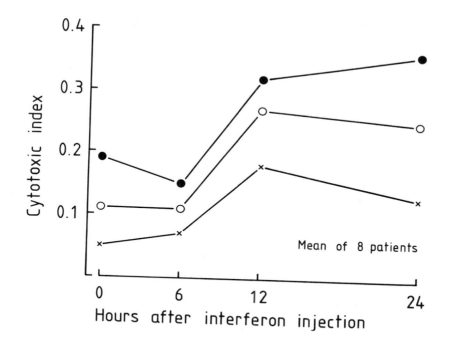

<u>FIGURE 2.</u>   Mean NK activity of 8 patients lymphocytes as measured prior to and 6, 12 and 24 hours following the first injection of IFN. Lymphocyte: target cell ratios 25:1 (x–x), 50:1 (o–o) and 100:1 (●–●) were used.

Treatment of Chang-cells with IFN prior to the NK assay inhibits their subseptibility to killing (10). This is in agreement with the findings by Trichieri and Santoli (20). To ascertain that the decreased susceptibility of target cells to killing is due to IFN and not to contaminants in the preparations, k562 cells were incubated with partially purified IFN-α or completely pure IFN-β for 24 hours prior to testing their sensitivity to NK. As can be seen in Table 2, partially purified IFN-α as well as pure IFN-α diminished the susceptibility of k562 cells to killing.

In vivo studies

In 8 patients the NK activity was measured before and 6, 12 and 24 hours after receiving their first injection of IFN. The mean NK activity of these patients lymphocytes was essentially unaltered at 6 hours, but was increased 12 and 24 hours following the IFN injection (Fig. 2). To date, the NK activity of 68 patients lymphocytes has been tested prior to and 24 hours following their first injection of IFN. With few exceptions the NK activity of their lymphocytes was augmented after IFN administration (Fig. 3).

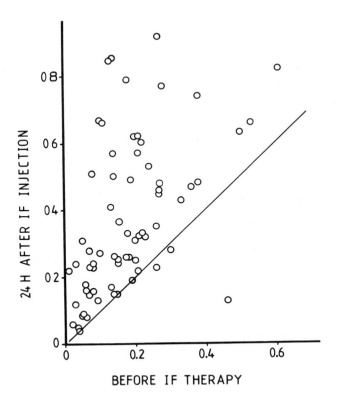

FIGURE 3. NK activity of 68 patients lymphocytes, tested before and 24 h after the first injection of IFN. A lymphocyte: target cell ratio of 50:1 is presented. Symbols above the diagonal line denote an increase in NK activity after IFN injection as compared to values obtained before IFN injection.

In some patients the NK activity was followed during prolonged IFN therapy, up to one year. With few exceptions the NK activity of the patients lymphocytes remained elevated during the time of IFN therapy. Fig. 4 shows the cytotoxic activity of 21 patients lymphocytes, as measured prior to and after 3 months of IFN therapy.

Prior to IFN injection addition of IFN to the assay *in vitro* caused an enhancement of NK activity. This IFN induced enhancement of NK activity *in vitro* was essentially similar for tumor patients as compared to that of healthy donors (Table 3). Already 6 hours after the first IFN injection the ability of IFN to augment NK activity *in vitro* was diminished (Fig. 5). Also 12, 18, 24 and 48 hours following IFN injection the ability of IFN to enhanced NK activity *in vitro* was diminished in most patients. During prolonged IFN therapy, up to 9 months, the capacity of IFN to augment NK activity *in vitro* was reduced (Fig 6).

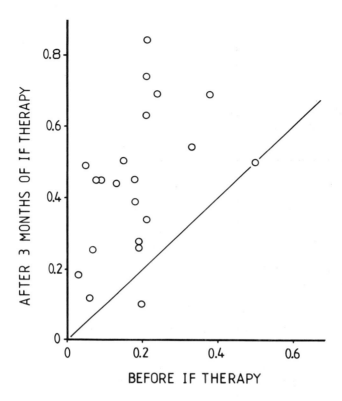

FIGURE 4. NK activity of 21 patients lymphocytes, tested before and after three months of IFN therapy. A lymphocyte: target cell ratio of 50:1 is presented. Symbols above the diagonal line denote an increase in NK activity during IFN therapy as compared to values obtained before IFN therapy.

TABLE 3. IFN induced enhancement of NK activity *in vitro*. Comparison between tumor patients and a group of healthy donors. Mean ± S.E. are presented.

| Donors | No | Lymphocyte: target cell ratio | | |
		25:1	50:1	100:1
Patients	39	0.10 ± 0.01	0.13 ± 0.01	0.15 ± 0.02
Healthy donors	22	0.10 ± 0.01	0.12 ± 0.01	0.15 ± 0.01

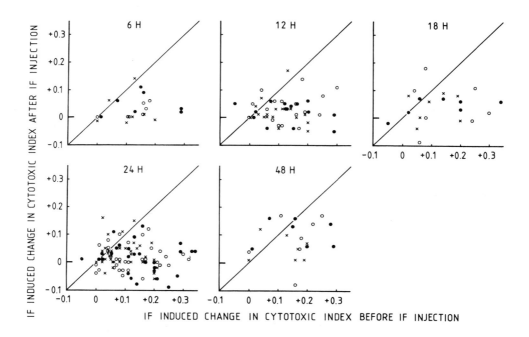

FIGURE 5. *Ability of IFN (30 units/ ml) to enhance NK activity in vitro. Enhancement before and 6, 12, 18, 24 and 48 hours after the first IFN injection. Lymphocyte: target cell ratios 25:1 (x), 50:1 (o) and 100:1 (●) were used. Symbols below the diagonal line denote a decreased ability of IFN to enhance NK activity in vitro after IFN injection as compared to values obtained before IFN injection.*

In an attempt to further characterize the cells responsible for the enhancement of NK activity *in vivo* the lymphocytes of 10 tumor patients were fractionated by rosetting with SRBC and tested for NK activity before and 24 hours following the first injection of IFN. In these experiments K652 cells served as targets. As can be seen in Table 4, the NK activity of unfractionated lymphocytes against K562 increased following IFN injection. A statistically significant increase in NK activity was seen in the fraction enriched for high avidity E-cells. In the lymphocyte fraction depleted of high avidity E-cells the numerical increase was essentially similar as for high avidity E-cells, although the increase was not statistically significant. In 6 patients, the fraction depleted of high avidity E-cells was further separated into a lymphocyte fraction enriched for low avidity E-cells and a fraction depleted of E-cells. The IFN injection caused essentially similar increments in NK activity in these two fractions (Table 4)..

In this study the proportion of lymphocytes expressing SRBC-(E-rosettes and Fc-(EA-rosettes) receptors was also measured prior to and 24 h following the IFN injection for the different fractions. The only significant change in the proportion of lymphocytes expressing the different receptors was observed in the fraction enriched for non-high avidity E-cells in which the number of E-rosettes increased (p< 0.01). An in-

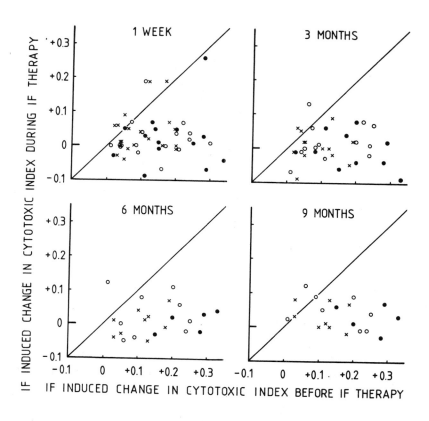

FIGURE 6. *Ability of IFN (30 units/ml) to enhance NK activity in vitro. Enhancement before and after one week, 3 months, 6 months and 9 months of IFN-therapy. Lymphocyte: target cell ratios 25:1 (x), 50:1 (o) and 100:1 (o) were used. Symbols below the diagonal line denote a decreased ability of IFN to enhance NK activity in vitro during IFN therapy as compared to values obtained before IFN therapy.*

crease in the proportion of lymphocytes expressing receptors for SRBC has previously been reported in tumor patients following an injection of IFN (21).

DISCUSSION

Treatment of human lymphocytes with IFN *in vitro* causes an increase in their NK activity (8,20). This enhancement is due to a direct effect on the lymphocytes rather than on the target cells, since treatment of the latter cells rather reduces their susceptibility to killing (10,20). The finding that treatment of tumor cells with IFN *in vitro* reduced their susceptibility to NK lysis might bear relevance for the clinical situation in which the tumor cells of patients are in contact with IFN *in vivo*. The IFN induced enhancement of NK killing as well as the redu-

TABLE 4. Change in NK activity and the proportion of lymphocytes forming E- and EA-rosettes as measured prior to and 24 hours following the first injection of IFN. Comparison between different fractions obtained by rosetting with SRBC. Mean ± S.E. are presented.

	Unfractionated	Depleted of high avidity E-cells	High avidity E-cells	Low avidity E-cells	Non-E-cells
NK					
Prior to inj.	18.5±4.0	25.7±4.7	9.4±2.9	12.3±3.4	21.6±9.0
Change	+14.1±4.2 (p<0.01)	+ 6.1±4.4	+7.3±3.2 (p<0.05)	+11.5±5.8	+14.3±5.7
% E-rosettes					
Prior to inj.	77.7±3.6	36.5±4.8	78.2±1.9	69.8±2.9	13.5±3.0
Change	0±1.7	+ 7.8±2.2 (p<0.01)	+ 0.7±2.3	+ 1.3±2.8	+ 1.3±1.4
% EA-rosettes					
Prior to inj.	21.1±2.5	62.5±5.1	20.8±6.1	40.3±2.0	45.0±5.2
Change	+ 1.3±2.5	- 5.9±3.1	+ 0.4±1.3	- 0.3±5.3	- 1.7±1.5
Number of patients	10	10	10	6	6

ced susceptibility of target cells to killing is due to IFN and not to contaminants in the preparations since pure IFN-β is capable of excerting these effects (2) (Tables 1 and 2).

In vivo administration of human IFN-α to tumor patients caused an increase in their NK activity. The augmentation of NK activity ususlly appeared 12-24 hours after the first injection and during prolonged IFN therapy the NK activity was maintained at an elevated level for at least one year. The finding that lymphocytes can be restimulated with IFN several times was also confirmed *in vitro* (Fig. 1).

Prior to IFN therapy, addition of IFN to the assay *in vitro* induced an increase in the NK activity. This increase was essentially similar for tumor patients as compared to a control group consisting of 22 healthy donors. During IFN therapy the ability of IFN to enhance NK activity *in vitro* was reduced, indicating similarities in the mechanism by which IFN enhances NK activity *in vitro* and *in vivo*.

NK cells have been characterized as Fc-receptor carrying lymphocytes, some of which express low avidity receptors for SRBC (22). In an attempt to further characterize the cells responsible for the *in vivo* induced enhancement of NK activity, lymphocytes were separated according to their avidity for SRBC prior to and 24 hours after the patients received their first IFN injection. Although the NK activity differed between the various fractions the IFN induced enhancement of NK activity *in vivo* did not seem to differ to any major extent between the different fractions (Table 4).

The NK activity of peripheral lymphocytes increased in tumor patients during IFN therapy. This can be of clinical relevans only if the antitumor effect of IFN is, at least in part, mediated by the immune system and if NK activity plays a role in the hosts defence against tumors. Results from animal experiments suggest that NK activity may play a role in tumor immunity (23). No conclusive trial have been performed in man. Of interest in this context is a study by Vånky et al. (24). Fresh tumor cells from solid tumors were rarely found to be sensitive to the cytotoxic activity of allogeneic lymphocytes. In autologous combinations, however cytotoxicity could be detected in 28% of the cases. In several cases IFN treatment of the lymphocytes induced cytotoxicity against allogeneic targets. IFN treatment of the lymphocytes had, however, no effect on their cytotoxic activity against autologous tumor cells.

ACKNOWLEDGEMENTS

The excellent technical assistance of Mrs. Elisabet Anderbring, Mrs. Waltraut Szczerba and Mrs. Margareta Karlsson is gratefully acknowledged. Our thanks are due to Drs. Kari Cantell and Ernest Knight Jr. for their generous supply of IFN. This study was supported by grants from the Swedish Cancer Society and the Cancer Society of Stockholm.

REFERENCES

1. Epstein, L. (1977): In: Interferons and their actions, ed. W.E. Stewart, p. 91. CRB Press, Cleveland, Ohio.

2. Einhorn, S. (1980): J. Clin. Lab. Immunol., 3:35.

3. Einhorn, S., Blomgren, H., and Troye, M. (1980): Cell. Immunol., 56:374.

4. Heron, I., Hökland, M., Garotta, G., and Berg, K. (1979) Conference on regulatory functions of interferons. Abstract.

5. Jarstrand, C., and Einhorn, S. (1980) J. Clin. Lab. Immunol., Submitted for publication.

6. Strander, H., and Einhorn, S. (1981) British Medical Journal., Submitted for publication.

7. Gresser, I. (1977): In: Cancer - a comprehensive treatise (Chemother. vol. 5), ed. by F. Becker, p. 525. New York: Plenum Publ. Corp.

8. Einhorn, S., Blomgren, H., and Strander, H. (1978) Int. J. Cancer, 22:405-412.

9. Einhorn, S., Blomgren, H., and Strander, H. (1978) Acta Med. Scand., 204:477.

10. Einhorn, S., Blomgren, H., and Strander, H. (1979) Cancer Letters, 7:1.

11. Einhorn, S., Blomgren, H., Strander, H. (1980) Int. J. Cancer, 26:419

12. Mogensen, K.E., and Cantell, K. (1977) Pharmacol. Therapeut., 1:369.

13. Cantell, K., and Hirvonen, S. (1978) J. Gen. Virol., 39:541.

14. Knight, E. Jr., Hunkapiller, N.W., Korant, D.D., Hardy, R.W.F., and Hood, L.E. (1980) Science, 207:525.

15. Jondal, M., Holm, G., and Wigzell, H. (1972) J. Exp. Med., 184:1232.

16. Perlmann, H., Perlmann, P., Pape, G.R., and Halldén, G. (1976) Scand. J. Immunol., suppl 5. 5:57.

17. Jonsdottir, I., Dillner-Centerlind, M-L., Perlmann, H., and Perlmann, P. (1979) Scand. J. Immunol., 10:525,

18. Troye, M., Perlmann, P., Larsson, Å., Blomgren, H., and Johansson, B. (1977) Int. J. Cancer., 20:188.

19. Hallberg, T., Gurner, B.W., and Coombs, R.R.A. (1973) Int. Arch Allergy Appl. Immunol., 44:500.

20. Trincheri, G., and Santoli, D. (1978) J. Exp. Med., 147:1314.

21. Einhorn, S., Blomgren, H. and Strander, H. (1980) Int. Arch Allergy Appl. Immunol., 118.

22. West, W.H., Cannon, G.B., Kay, H.D., Bonnard, G.D., and Herberman, R.B. (1977) J. Immunol., 118.

23. Herberman, R.B. and Holden, H.T. (1979) J. Natl. Cancer Inst., 62:441.

24. Vánky, F., Argov, S., Einhorn, S. and Klein, E. (1980) J. Exp. Med. 151:1151.

Mediation of Cellular Immunity in Cancer by Immune Modifiers, edited by M. A. Chirigos et al., Raven Press, New York © 1981.

Suppressor Mechanisms in Cellular Interrelationships in Cancer

Anthony C. Allison

International Laboratory for Research on Animal Diseases, Nairobi, Kenya

Although many tumors are antigenic, only too often they succeed in growing. Hence, immune responses to tumor cells may be ineffective, as when operational tolerance to allografts is established (10). One reason why immune responses are ineffective is because they are inhibited by suppressor mechanisms. During the past decade much has been learned about cellular interactions which augment or suppress immune responses. The purpose of this paper is to consider which suppressor mechanisms might be operative in cancer-bearing hosts. Information on this subject is at present scanty, but there are ways in which it might be made more precise. Understanding which supressor mechanisms are active in particular situations could lead to practical ways of reversing them in cancer therapy.

The main cell types to be considered are tumor cells, subsets of T- and B-lymphocytes (which are assumed to have surface membrane receptors for antigenic determinants on tumor cells) and mononuclear phagocytes. Interactions of these cell types provide a situation complex enough for discussion, which is not intended to exclude the participation of other cell types and mechanisms in the control of immune responses to tumors.

Some suppressor mechanisms are antigen specific, activated by a particular antigen and inhibiting selectively cellular or humoral responses to that antigen. Other suppressor mechanisms are nonspecific in their manifestations, although they may be initiated by specific immune responses. Such non-specific suppressor mechanisms may also inhibit responses of lymphocytes to mitogens and even the multiplication of tumor cells. Thus mechanisms nonspecifically suppressing immune responses (thereby reducing the probability of host survival) may also suppress tumor growth (thereby increasing the probabilty of host survival). This is a delicately balanced situation when possible effects of intervention must be considered carefully.

Suppressor mechanisms are complex, and only a few can be considered in this paper, which is not intended to be a comprehensive review. Moreover, each mechanism will be illustrated by only a few examples. Although attention is given in this paper to specific immune responses, these depend on and influence macrophages and interact with natural killer cells and antibody-dependent cytotoxic mechanisms. They are therefore relevant to the subject matter of this meeting. Thus, for antibody-dependent cytotoxic mechanisms to be effective, antibodies of the appropriate specificity and

subclasses must be formed. For T-lymphocytes to produce mediators a
specific immune response must be elicited.

Specific suppressor T-lymphocytes

An important advance in our understanding of the control of
immune responses has been the recognition that distinct subsets of
lymphocytes provide antigen-specific help to cellular and humoral
immune responses on the one hand and antigen-specific suppression
on the other. In the mouse helper T cells have the Lyt 1+ phenotype
whereas suppressor cells have the Lyt $2,3^+$ phenotype (4). Often
specific suppressor T-lymphocytes and their soluble mediators bear
determinants coded by the I-J subregion of the major histocompati-
bility complex (2).

An example of the role of suppressor T-lymphocytes in immunity
against tumors is provided by studies on the growth of a syngeneic
methylcholanthrene-induced fibrosarcoma in A/J mice (7,8). This
tumor elicits potent suppressor T-lymphocyte responses which inhibit
anti-tumor immunity. Administration of anti-I-J^K antiserum, which
selectively acts on the suppressor cells, decreases tumor growth in
these mice (11).

Analogous to the growth of an antigenic tumor is the maintenance
of operational tolerance to allografts. We have found that short-
term treatment with Cyclosporin A allows rabbits to accept indefi-
nitely renal allografts (10) and rats to accept bone marrow allografts (19,20). In the latter case both graft-versus-host and
host-versus-graft reactions following allogeneic bone marrow transplantation were prevented. This model is pertinent to the present
discussion because if allogeneic bone marrow transplantation were
feasible in humans it would provide an extension of major importance
to cancer therapy. Tutschka et al. (19,20) have found, in rats
bearing allogeneic bone marrow transplants, cells which suppress
mixed lymphocyte reactions between donor and recipient cells but
not third-party cells. These suppressor cells have the characteristics of specific suppressor T-lymphocytes. Moreover, Cyclosporin
A added to human mixed lymphocyte reactions allows the induction
of alloantigen-activated specific suppressor cells while preferentially inhibiting the induction of cytolytic effector lymphocytes
(12). The suppressor cells adhered to nylon wool columns, which
provides one way of eliminating them. The availability of antisera
selectively reacting with suppressor T-lymphocytes in man, as in
the mouse, provides another.

It would be of interest to establish whether specific suppressor
T-lymphocytes inhibit immune responses against tumor cells in man.
This could be investigated in patients bearing tumors that are
potentially highly antigenic such as choriocarcinomas bearing
alloantigens. Elimination of potential suppressor populations as
described above should reveal cytotoxic cells with specificity for
target cells bearing the same alloantigens.

If specific suppressors prove to be important in human tumors, their action might be inhibited in two ways. One is the use of drugs which act more or less selectively upon the suppressor population. For example, cyclophosphamide can be used under certain conditions to reduce T-cell-mediated suppressor effects (4). The development of drugs with more selective effects on suppressor cells would obviously be of interest. Second, antisera against the suppressor subpopulation of T-lymphocytes (17) might be used in vivo, in a manner analogous to that described in mice (11).

Role of macrophages in the activation of nonspecific suppressor T-lymphocytes.

Several studies using material from humans and experimental animals have demonstrated the presence of leukocytes able to suppress a variety of antigen-induced and mitogen-induced T- and B-lymphocyte functions. Suppressor effects have been ascribed predominantly to T-lymphocytes activated either by attachment of immune complexes to Fe receptors for IgG (Fcγ) (15) or by Concanavalin A. Suppression involving interactions between human T-lymphocyte subsets (17) or monocytes and lymphocytes (18) has also been postulated.

Since this meeting is concerned with interactions between mononuclear phagocytes (monocytes and macrophages) and other cell types, I shall focus attention on one model which appears to be of interest in cancer patients. This is based on the analysis of Durandy her colleagues (6) of nonspecific suppression induced by gammaglobulin therapy in children without severe immunodeficiency. Lymphocytes from such children failed to proliferate and to mature into plasma cells in culture after stimulation with pokeweed mitogen. The suppression could be generated in leukocytes from normal persons by incubation with gammaglobulin aggregates. Conversion to Fc (ab)'$_2$ fragments abolished suppression. Evidence was presented that the initial event was attachment of aggregated gammaglobulin to Fcγ receptors of monocytes, with subsequent production of prostaglandin E$_2$, which in turn activated nonspecific suppressor T-lymphocytes. Indomethacin or antiserum to prostaglandin E$_2$ inhibited the generation of suppression.

The relevance of this to cancer-bearing patients is that immune complexes could activate mononuclear phagocytes to produce prostaglandin E$_2$ which in turn may activate nonspecific suppressor T-lymphocytes. The role of PGE$_2$ in the nonspecific suppression frequently observed in Hodgkin's disease has been analysed (9).

Products of activated macrophages which can have immuno-suppressive effects.

Elsewhere I have reviewed products of activated macrophages with immunosuppressive effects (1). These include interferon, which, as discussed by several contributors to this meeting, when administered both in vivo and in vitro, can under different circumstances either increase or decrease specific and nonspecific immune

responses. The contrasting effects on specific immune responses
can perhaps be explained by postulating that interferon inhibits
cell proliferation and promotes differentation. When present soon
after antigenic stimulation, interferon could limit clonal proliferation and thereby suppress immune responses. When present after
clones have substantially expanded, interferon could promote
differentiation into antibody-forming or cytotoxic cells, thus
increasing immune responses assayed by these effects.

A second product of activated macrophages, argininase (14),
depletes arginine in cultures and thereby inhibits lymphocyte
proliferation. Whether this mechanism operates in vivo when arginine
is constantly being replenished is not known.

Another suppressor mechanism associated with macrophages
involves the enzyme polyamine oxidase. Amine oxidases are enzymes
which catalyse the oxidative deamination of amines with the formation
of stoichiometric amounts of aldehyde, hydrogen peroxide and ammonia
according to the equation: $RCH_2NH_2 + O_2 + H_2O \rightarrow RCHO + H_2O_2 + NH_3$.
The aldehydes produced can react with nucleic acids and other
groups, producing cytostatic or cytotoxic effects.

In mammals three polyamine oxidases able to metabolise spermine
and spermidine have been defined. The first to be described is the
polyamine oxidase of ruminant sera. This is present in fetal and
newborn calf sera which are used in many tissue culture media. The
enzyme has a molecular weight of 170,000 and converts spermine and
spermidine into N,N^1-bis(3-propionaldehyde-1,4-diaminobutane and
N-(4-aminobutyl)-3-aminopropionaldehyde respectively (see 16).
Byrd et al. (3) have shown that in the presence of polyamine oxidase
from bovine serum micromolar quantities of spermine and spermidine
inhibit the proliferative responses of immune spleen cells to
mitogens.

Another polyamine oxidase has been described in rat liver
(13). This has a molecular weight of 60,000 and converts spermine
and spermidine into 3-aminopropionaldehyde. We have found a
polyamine oxidase with properties so far indistinguishable from the
rat liver enzyme in mouse peritoneal and rabbit alveolar macrophages
(16). In macrophages taken from animals previously injected with
BCG polyamine oxidase activity was increased. The activity of the
enzyme in the spleen was considerably augmented in mice that had
been intravenously injected with BCG or Corynebacterium parvum. No
polyamine oxidase activity was found in the supernatants of cultures
of peritoneal macrophages, unless the cells were exposed to
lipopolysaccharide. The supernatants of LPS-treated cultures, or
of spleen cells taken from mice injected intravenously with C.
parvum, in the presence of spermine inhibited the proliferation of
mitogen-stimulated thymocytes.

Macrophages are present in tumors and are activated by

nonspecific stimulators of immunity, in which case they release the enzyme. In the pericellular medium the enzme could come into contact with spermine and spermidine, which are produced by and can be released from tumor cells. As a result products able to suppress the proliferation of lymphocytes could be generated.

Yet another polyamine oxidase is produced by the human placenta, is present in high concentrations in retroplacental fluid and is also demonstrable in late pregnancy serum. In the presence of this enzyme and spermidine products that inhibit lymphocyte transformation are formed. This mechanism may contribute to the failure of the mother to mount a cytoxic response against fetal antigens. Measurements of the activity of this enzyme in patients with choriocarcinoma might be of interest.

Macrophage polyamine oxidase in the presence of spermine has tumorostatic effects (15). High concentrations can kill tumor cells. This could be one mechanism by which macrophages inhibit tumor cell growth, as well as a mechanism suppressing immune responses.

Comment

Other suppressor mechanisms in cancer not immediately relevant to the present meeting, but potentially interesting, include anti-idiotypic responses. This is the second major development in understanding control of immune responses in recent years. Effects of agents modulating immune responses on these reactions are not at present understood. In general, the whole problem of control of immune responses to tumors is open to investigation. If as much were known about immune responses to tumors as is known about immune responses to sheep red blood cells, we would be in a better position to design immunotherapeutic procedures.

REFERENCES

1. Allison, A.C. (1978): Immunological Rev. 40:7-27.

2. Benacerraf, B. and Germain, R.N. (1978): Immunological Rev. 38:70-119.

3. Byrd, W. J., Jacobs, D.M. and Limoss, M.S. (1977): Nature, Lond. 267:621.

4. Cantor, H. and Boyse, E.A. (1976): Cold Spring Harbor Symp. Quant Biol. 41:23-32.

5. Debre, P. Waltenbaugh, C., Dorf, M.E. and Benacerraf, B. (1976): J. Exp. Med. 149:277-230.

6. Durandy, A., Fischer, A. and Griscelli, C. (1980): J. Clin. Invest. (in press).

7. Fujimoto, S., Greene, M.I. and Sehon, A.H. (1976): J. Immunol.

116:791-799.

8. Fujimoto, S., Greene, M.I. and Sehon, A.H. (1976): J. Immunol. 116:800-812.

9. Goodwin, J.S., Bankhurst, A.D. and Messner, R.P. (1977): J. Exp. Med. 146-1719-1732.

10. Green, C.J., Allison, A.C. and Precious, S. (1979): Lancet ii, 123-125.

11. Greene, M.I., Dorf, M.E., Pierres, M. and Benacerraf, B. (1977): Proc. Natl. Acad. Sci., USA 74:5118-5121.

12. Hess, A.D. and Tutschka, P.J. (1980): J. Immunol. 124:2601-2608.

13. Höltta, E. (1977): Biochemistry 16:91-100.

14. Kung, J.T., Brooks, S.B., Jakeway, J.B., Leonard, L.L. and Talmage, D.W. (1977): J. Exp. Med. 146:665-670.

15. Moretta, L., Webb, S.R., Grossi, C.E., Lydyard, P.M. and Cooper, M.D. (1977): J. Exp. Med. 146:184-200.

16. Morgan, D.M.L., Ferluga, J. and Allison, A.C. (1980): In Polyamines in Biomedical Research (ed. J.M. Gangas) New York, John Wiley, pp. 303-308.

17. Reinherz, E. and Schlossman, S.F. (1979): J. Immunol. 122:1335-1341.

18. Stobo, J.D. (1977): J. Immunol. 119:918-925.

19. Tutschka, P.J., Beschorner, W.E., Allison, A.C., Burns, W.H. and Santos, G.W. (1979): Nature, Lond. 280:5718-5720.

20. Tutschka, P.J., Beschorner, W.E. and Hess, A.D. (1980): Blut, Supplement 25, pp. 241-253.

Mediation of Cellular Immunity in Cancer by Immune Modifiers, edited by M. A. Chirigos et al., Raven Press, New York © 1981.

Activation of Macrophages for ADCC and Nonspecific Killing

Beth-Ellen Drysdale and Hyun S. Shin

Department of Microbiology, Johns Hopkins University School of Medicine, Baltimore, Maryland 21205

INTRODUCTION

For a number of years, efforts have been directed toward understanding the mechanism of antibody dependent suppression of tumor cell growth. Results of in vivo experiments done in our laboratory (4,10) have shown that macrophages cooperate quite effectively with antibody to suppress the growth of small tumors. However, as reported by many investigators (11), even in the presence of excess antibody, effector cells are markedly less efficient at inhibiting the growth of larger tumors. We have shown (5) that one factor which contributes to this problem is an apparent macrophage shortage at the tumor site. There are two possible explanations for this shortage; first, adequate numbers of effector cells may fail to accumulate, and second, the cells which do accumulate may not be optimally activated for cytotoxicity. In order to overcome the shortage, it is necessary to understand the biochemical basis of both chemotaxis and activation. We have first focused on the problem of activation, and our general approach has been to compare the biochemical basis of activation processes mediated by different agents. To do this an in vitro assay system has been used in which selective metabolic inhibitors can be tested for their effect on a particular activation process. A number of inhibitors have been tested, but to date, the most interesting has been the cyclooxygenase inhibitor, indomethacin. Results presented here show that there are two distinct activation pathways, one of which is sensitive to indomethacin and a second which is not.

MATERIALS AND METHODS

Media

Target cell lines were maintained in tissue culture medium consisting of RPMI 1640 supplemented with penicillin, streptomycin, glutamine, and fetal bovine serum (7). This same medium was used in all phases of the cytotoxicity assay except during activation. In this phase, supplemented phosphate buffered saline (SPBS) containing 100 U of penicillin/ml, 100 μg of streptomycin/ml, and 4% fetal bovine serum was used.

Tumor Cell Targets

In vitro lines of the C3H lymphosarcoma, 6C3HED, and the DBA mastocytoma, P815, have been used as targets. Cells were harvested from log
phase cultures by centrifugation, and the viability of the cells was at
least 95% by dye exclusion.

Macrophages

Seventy-two hr starch induced peritoneal exudate cells were obtained
from C3H/HeN mice as previously described (10) except that tissue culture medium was used for lavage. Differential counts done on stained
cytocentrifuge preparations showed that 70-80% of the cells were macrophages and monocytes.

Activating Agents

The endotoxin (LPS) used was produced commercially by the Westphal
method from *Escherichia coli* strain 0127:B8. Concentrated stock
solutions were prepared by dissolving the LPS in SPBS. The lymphokine
containing supernatants used in these experiments were prepared as
previously described (3) except that Concanavalin A (Con A) at a
concentration of 10 μg/ml was used to stimulate the lymph node cells.
Control supernatants were prepared by adding an equivalent amount of
Con A to supernatants from unstimulated lymph node cell cultures.
Syngeneic antibody directed against the 6C3HED target cells was produced in our laboratory by a procedure which has been described (5). In
some experiments, nonadherent peritoneal exudate cells were used as
activating agents. These nonadherent populations were isolated from the
starch induced exudates by sequential plating. Differential counts done
on stained cytocentrifuge preparations showed that the nonadherent cells
consisted of approximately 45% lymphocytes, 50% granulocytes, and 5%
monocytes.

Prostaglandins

Stock solutions of prostaglandins E_1, E_2, $F_1\alpha$ and $F_2\alpha$ at a concentration of 10 μg/ml were prepared in SPBS immediately before use.
Prostaglandin levels were measured for us by Dr. N. F. Adkinson using
a radioimmunoassay (1).

Inhibitors

Concentrated stock solutions of either indomethacin or acetylsalicylic acid were prepared immediately before use by first dissolving
the drug in 0.5 ml of 95% ethyl alcohol, and then adding 9.5 ml of SPBS.
These solutions were sterilized by filteration through a 0.2μ filter.
The final concentrations of the indomethacin and acetylsalicylic acid
stock solutions were 1.0 mg/ml (2.8×10^{-3}M) and 9.0 mg/ml (5×10^{-2}M)
respectively.

Cytotoxicity Assay

The peritoneal exudate cells were washed, counted, and diluted to a
final concentration of 1.5×10^6/ml. The suspension was aliquoted into

96 well microtiter plates at a volume of 0.1 ml per well. After allowing the cells to adhere for 2.5 hrs, the medium and nonadherent cells were aspirated, and the monolayers were washed twice with tissue culture medium. Differential counts done on stained monolayers showed that they were ≥97% macrophages. Lymphocytes and granulocytes were the predominant contaminants. Next, a 4 hr activation phase was initiated by adding an activating agent such as LPS to the monolayers. In addition, specific inhibitors can be added during this incubation. Following activation, the wells are again washed twice and to begin the 3rd phase of the assay, the effector phase, 1.25×10^4 tumor cell targets are added to the wells. At this point, inhibitors can also be added. After the addition of the target cells, the plates were incubated for 16 hr in a humidified 5% CO_2 environment. To study antibody dependent killing, the assay is done in a directly analogous way, except that nothing is added during the activation phase, and instead antibody coated tumor cells with or without inhibitors are added to the effector phase of the assay. These antibody coated cells serve simultaneously as activating agents and as targets.

Regardless of the procedure used to activate the macrophages, following the 16 hr incubation, the viability of the target cells was assessed by their ability to incorporate ^{125}I-5-iodo-2'-deoxyuridine ($^{125}IUDR$). The $^{125}IUDR$ (specific activity 5 Ci/mg), was diluted such that a 50 μl aliquot containing 0.05 μCi was added to each well. The plates were incubated for 2 hrs after which uptake was terminated by the addition of excess cold thymidine. Finally the contents of the wells were harvested and counted.

The suppression of target cell growth is expressed throughout as % cytotoxicity which is defined as follows:

$$\% \text{ cytotoxicity} = [1 - \frac{(\overline{CPM}_{TC+M\emptyset} - \overline{CPM}_{BKG})}{\overline{CPM}_{TC} - \overline{CPM}_{BKG}}] \times 100$$

Each test and all controls were done in triplicate and the counts were averaged. Mean counts incorporated by tumor cells in the presence of macrophages, $\overline{CPM}_{TC+M\emptyset}$, and in the absence of macrophages, $\overline{CPM}_{TC}$ (15,000-20,000 cpm) were corrected for background, $\overline{CPM}_{BKG}$ (150-200 cpm). The resulting quantities were divided, and % cytotoxicity was calculated as shown. Here, background refers to the counts obtained from wells containing only medium. However, this value is not statistically different from that obtained from wells containing macrophages alone.

RESULTS AND DISCUSSION

Dose response curves have been generated for all of the activating agents used in the assay system. The first figure shows a representative curve from an experiment in which LPS was used to activate the macrophages. When buffer alone with no LPS was added during the activation phase of the assay, little cytotoxicity was observed. However, as LPS, at concentrations ranging from 0.125 to 1.25 ng/ml was added, killing increased from 20-90% in a linear fashion. Treating the macrophages with higher doses of LPS resulted in nearly 100% cytotoxicity.

A number of different metabolic inhibitors have been tested in this

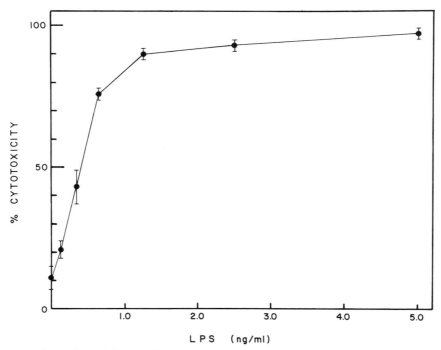

Figure 1. The effect of varying the dose of LPS on the activation of macrophages for tumor cell cytotoxicity. In this experiment, the target cells used were an <u>in vitro</u> line of 6C3HED. The values shown represent the means of triplicate determinations ± one standard deviation.

assay system. The one used in the experiments described here is indomethacin. We chose to test this drug to determine what role, if any, arachidonic acid metabolites might play in different activation processes. Figure 2 shows the results of adding indomethacin at a concentration of 10 μg/ml to the activation and/or effector phases of an assay in which LPS was used as the activating agent. Controls are shown in the first panel. As generally observed, unstimulated macrophages were marginally cytotoxic but when LPS was added (1.25 ng/ml) cytotoxicity increased to 90%. If indomethacin was added during the activation phase (2nd panel) or was present in both the activation and effector phases (4th panel) killing was inhibited nearly completely. However, if indomethacin was added to the effector phase alone, cytotoxicity was inhibited by only 30%. These results indicate that indomethacin acts primarily in the activation phase. As will be discussed, inhibition of cytotoxicity is dependent on the dose of indomethacin added during the activation phase over the range of 1.0 to 10 μg/ml.

These results are not limited to this particular assay system with respect to target cell type or with respect to the inhibitor used. In the experiments presented, the tumor cell targets were an <u>in vitro</u> line of the C3H lymphosarcoma, 6C3HED. However, directly analogous results were observed when cells from an <u>in vitro</u> line of the DBA mastocytoma, P815, were used as targets. In addition, if a second cyclooxygenase inhibitor, acetylsalicylic acid, at a concentration of 0.5 mM was added to the

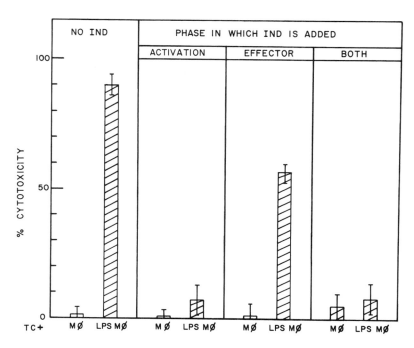

Figure 2. The effect of indomethacin on LPS mediated activation. The
tumor cell (TC) targets used in this experiment were 6C3HED. Controls
are shown in the first panel. Macrophages not treated with LPS (MØ)
exhibited little cytotoxic activity against either target, but addition
of LPS at a concentration of 0.625 ng/ml (LPS MØ) resulted in an
increase in cytotoxicity. The three remaining panels show the effect of
adding indomethacin (IND) at a concentration of 10 μg/ml to the activation and/or effector phases of the assay. The results are expressed as
the means of triplicate determinations ± one standard deviation.

activation and/or effector phases of the assay, the pattern of inhibition was comparable to that observed with indomethacin. The drug was most
effective in inhibiting cytotoxicity if it was added during activation.

One possible explanation for these results was that drug treatment
generally effected macrophage viability, even though they appeared
morphologically intact. In fact we have been able to show that this is
not the case. Since in a number of systems indomethacin had been shown
to be a reversible inhibitor, it seemed that if the drug were washed out
the macrophages should be able to be restimulated with LPS, provided no
permanent damage had occurred. The results of this experiment are shown
in Table I. If no LPS was added the macrophages were not cytotoxic,
but when LPS was present cytotoxicity increased, in this case, to 97%.
If indomethacin was added in the activation phase cytotoxicity was
inhibited by 50%. However, if LPS was added in the effector phase, to
monolayers which had been treated with both the drug and LPS during the
activation phase and then washed, cytotoxic activity was restored.

TABLE 1

Recovery of Cytotoxic Activity After Indomethacin Treatment [a]

Additions During

The Activation Phase	The Effector Phase	% Cytotoxicity
SPBS	SPBS	6 ± 6
LPS	SPBS	97 ± 2
LPS + Indomethacin	SPBS	47 ± 2
LPS + Indomethacin	LPS	98 ± 3

[a]
The concentrations of LPS and indomethacin used in this experiment were 1.25 ng/ml and 10 μg/ml respectively. The tumor cell targets used were an in vitro line of 6C3HED and the values shown are the means of triplicate determinations ± one standard deviation.

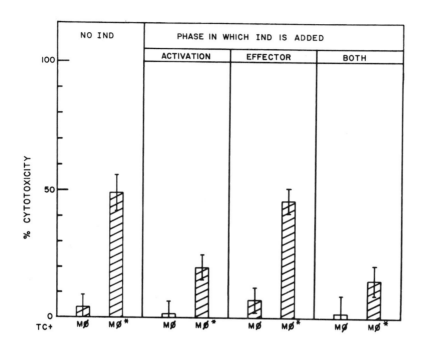

Figure 3. The effect of indomethacin on lymphokine mediated activation. The controls are shown in the first panel. Treatment of the macrophage monolayers with a 1:4 dilution of a Con A stimulated guinea pig lymph node cell supernatant (MØ*) resulted in 50 ± 7% cytotoxicity as tested on 6C3HED targets. However, treatment of the macrophages with supernatants from unstimulated guinea pig lymph node cell cultures to which a comparable amount of Con A had been added (MØ) produced little cytotoxicity, 4 ± 5%. The remaining three panels show the effect of adding indomethacin (IND) at a concentration of 10 μg/ml to the activation and/or effector phases of the assay. The values shown represent the means of triplicate determinations ± one standard deviation.

In attempts to compare various activation processes, lymphokine containing supernatants rather than LPS have been used as activating agents. Twenty-four hr Con A stimulated lymph node cell supernatants did contain MAF like activity and the cytotoxicity observed was dose dependent. Figure 3 shows the effect of adding indomethacin to the activation and/or effector phases of such an assay. The controls are shown in the first panel. Supernatants from unstimulated lymph node cells to which a comparable amount of Con A had been added were marginally cytotoxic with or without indomethacin. However, when a Con A supernatant containing MAF like activity was used as the activating agent cytotoxicity increased significantly to approximately 50%. If indomethacin was added to the activation phase (2nd panel) or to both the activation and effector phases (4th panel) approximately 2/3 of the cytotoxicity was inhibited. Adding indomethacin to the effector phase alone caused no decrease in cytotoxic activity.

LPS and lymphokine mediated cytotoxicity both exhibit similar inhibition patterns in the presence of indomethacin, but as shown in Table II antibody dependent cytotoxicity appears unaffected by the drug. The first four entries show the controls. The dose of LPS used here was high enough to cause virtually 100% cytotoxicity, but significant inhibition, 30%, was observed when indomethacin was present in both the activation and effector phases. As shown, the dilution of syngeneic antibody used, 1:1600, did cause significant cytotoxicity, approximately 60%, as compared to the controls. Even though the dose of antibody used was in the linear portion of the antibody dose response curve, the presence of indomethacin throughout the assay had no effect on cytotoxicity.

TABLE II

The Effect of Indomethacin on Antibody Dependent versus LPS

Mediated Macrophage Cytotoxicity [a]

Additions During

The Activation Phase	The Effector Phase	% Cytotoxicity
SPBS	SPBS	12 ± 3
LPS	SPBS	50 ± 5
LPS + Indomethacin	Indomethacin	20 ± 4
SPBS	Non-immune Ascites	10 ± 5
SPBS	Antibody	57 ± 2
Indomethacin	Antibody + Indomethacin	60 ± 6

The concentrations of LPS and Indomethacin used in this experiment were 0.312 ng/ml and 10 μg/ml respectively. The final dilution of both non-immune ascites and antibody was 1:1600. The values shown were calculated from triplicate determinations and represent the mean ± one standard deviation.

This antibody dependent process is not the only one which is unaffected by indomethacin. Results of several experiments indicated that the unfractionated peritoneal exudates contained non-adherent cells which were also able to activate macrophages. As normally prepared, the macrophage monolayers were substantially free of these cells, and after the 4 hr incubation in the absence of an activating agent and the subsequent washing procedure the macrophages were marginally cytotoxic. Interestingly, the addition of non-adherent populations consisting of approximately 45% lymphocytes, and 50% granulocytes to the activation phase of the assay caused an increase in cytotoxicity which was dependent on the number of cells added. This was not due to the presence of non-adherent cells alone since comparable or greater numbers of these cells were not cytotoxic. Indomethacin has been tested in this system, and as shown in figure 4, the addition of the drug over a range of 2.5 to 10 μg/ml had no effect on cytotoxicity induced

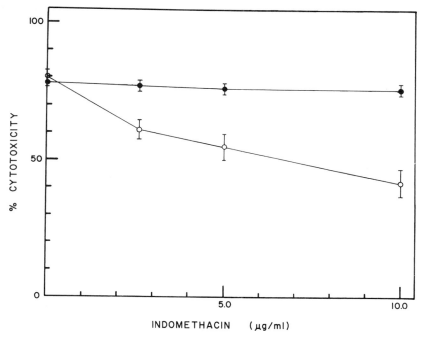

INDOMETHACIN (μg/ml)

Figure 4. The effect of indomethacin concentration on activation mediated by LPS versus activation mediated by a non-adherent cell population. The concentration of LPS used in this experiment was 0.625 ng/ml and the results are represented by o——o. In this experiment, the number of nonadherent cells added per well was 4.0×10^5, and the results are represented by ●——●. The values shown are the means of triplicate determinations ± one standard deviation.

by the added cells even though LPS mediated cytotoxicity was significantly inhibited. As already discussed, the two predominant cell types found in these nonadherent population were granulocytes and lymphocytes. Results of experiments using cells purified from the peritoneal exudates have shown that at least the lymphocytes are involved in this activation process. Therefore, our results suggest that there may actually be two ways in which lymphocytes can activate macrophages, one mediated by macrophage activating factor which is indomethacin sensitive and a second one on which the drug has no effect. Experiments are currently in progress to learn more about this last type of activation.

Collectively, the results presented thus far show that there are two distinct activation processes one of which is sensitive to indomethacin, and another which is not. At this point we had little information concerning precisely how the drug blocked cytotoxicity. While it is known that indomethacin inhibits cyclooxygenase activity and therefore can block macrophage prostaglandin production (9), it has also been reported that this drug inhibits at least 2 other enzymes involved in arachidonic acid metabolism, phospholipase A_2 (2) and a lipoxygenase pathway enzyme, fatty acid peroxidase (12,13). As a result, the identity of the arachidonic acid metabolite or metabolites involved in our system was unclear. In attempt to identify the participants, we decided to begin with prostaglandins and determine what role, if any, these compounds might play in LPS mediated activation. Shown in Table III are the results of an experiment in which both cytotoxicity and prostaglandin E_2 (PGE_2) production were measured as a function of indomethacin concentration. Here, 100% PGE_2 production corresponds to a concentration of approximately 1 nM. The dose response curves for both processes follow a similar trend, with increasing drug concentration, but they are not superimposable. The dose of indomethacin required to give half maximal inhibition of PGE_2 production was approximately 0.25 μg/ml while the corresponding value for cytotoxicity was between 1.0 and 5.0 μg/ml. It seemed possible that the difference in the dose response curves might be related to the fact that LPS activation for cytotoxicity is a complex process involving a number of steps only one of which is sensitive to indomethacin. Therefore, prostaglandins E_1, E_2, $F_1\alpha$, and $F_2\alpha$ were tested for their ability to serve either as activating agents or effector molecules, but none of these compounds at

TABLE III

The Effect of Indomethacin on LPS Mediated Macrophage

Cytotoxicity versus Prostaglandin E_2 Production[a]

Indomethacin μg/ml	% Cytotoxicity	% Prostaglandin E_2 Production
0	74 ± 4	100 ± 2.5
0.25	78 ± 5	49 ± 4.0
0.50	64 ± 1	22 ± 2.0
1.0	60 ± 5	≤13 ± 3.0
5.0	40 ± 6	"
10.0	40 ± 2	"

[a] In this experiment, the concentration of endotoxin used was 0.625 ng/ml. Percent cytoxicity was calculated as described in the text and the values shown are the means of triplicate determinations ± one standard deviation. Samples for prostaglandin E_2 analysis were prepared by carrying out the activation phase in a manner directly analogous to the cytotoxicity assay. After 4 hr the monolayers were washed twice as in the cytotoxicity assay, but instead of adding target cells or medium, 0.25 ml of SPBS was added to each well. Following an 18 hr incubation at 37°C in humidified 5% CO_2 environment, 0.20 ml of supernatant was removed from each well and the supernatants from triplicate wells were pooled and assayed for PGE_2. Here 100% represents the amount of PGE_2 produced (308.2 pg/ml) by monolayers treated only with LPS. Values shown are the means of duplicates ± one standard deviation.

concentrations ranging from 1.0 nM to 0.1 mM either activated the macrophages or effected target cell growth. One remaining possibility was that LPS mediated activation consisted of at least two steps, the first of which might be insensitive to indomethacin and a second which might be drug sensitive and require prostaglandin production. For this reason, we tested these four prostaglandins for their ability to reverse indomethacin inhibition of LPS mediated activation. To do this, the prostaglandins were added with the target cells to the effector phase of the assay. Shown in Table IV are the results of an experiment in which PGE_2 was used. The addition of indomethacin at a concentration of

TABLE IV

Enhancement of Cytotoxic Activity by Prostaglandin E_2[a]

Participants in

The Activation Phase	The Effector Phase Target Cells +	% Cytotoxicity
none	-	0 ± 2
none	$+ 10^{-7}M \ PGE_2$	0 ± 9
MØ	-	14 ± 3
MØ	$+ 10^{-7}M \ PGE_2$	14 ± 8
MØ + LPS	-	80 ± 2
MØ + LPS	$+ 10^{-7}M \ PGE_2$	100 ± 1
MØ + LPS + Indomethacin	-	50 ± 5
MØ + LPS + Indomethacin	$+ 10^{-9}M \ PGE_2$	74 ± 6
MØ + LPS + Indomethacin	$+ 10^{-8}M \ PGE_2$	77 ± 2
MØ + LPS + Indomethacin	$+ 10^{-7}M \ PGE_2$	94 ± 2

[a]
In this table the macrophages are designated as MØ. The target cells used were 6C3HED, and the concentrations of LPS and of indomethacin used were 0.625 ng/ml and 5.0 μg/ml respectively. The values shown represent the means of triplicate determinations $\pm$ one standard deviation.

5.0 μg/ml reduced the cytotoxic activity of the LPS activated macrophages from 80 to 50%. However, the addition of PGE_2 at a concentration as low as $10^{-9}M$ resulted in significant restoration of cytotoxic activity. This effect was dose dependent over the concentration range examined, 10^{-9} to $10^{-7}M$. When PGE_2 was added to macrophage monolayers treated with LPS alone during the activation phase, an increase in cytotoxicity was also observed. Again these effects were not the result of any direct action of the prostaglandins on either the macrophages or the target cells since as shown in the controls even at

the highest concentration used, $10^{-7}M$, PGE$_2$ did not activate the macrophages or effect target cell growth. Results of similar experiments
have shown that prostaglandins E$_1$ and E$_2$ restore cytotoxicity while
prostaglandins F$_1$α and F$_2$α do not.

Shown in figure 5 is our working model. On the left side is the LPS

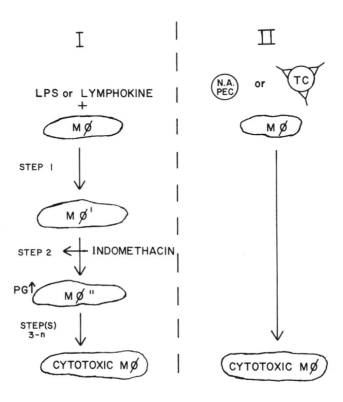

Figure 5. Activation pathways defined by indomethacin sensitivity. In
this diagram, the two steps which have been identified in LPS mediated
activation are designated as MØ' and MØ" respectively. PG↑ refers to
the production of E series prostaglandins.

and most likely the lymphokine activation pathway. It appears as
though these agents convert the macrophages via step one into cells
which are responsive to PG's. Step two involves the production of
prostaglandins which drive these cells through one or perhaps more
steps, 3 - n, to become fully cytotoxic. While we have represented
steps 1 and 2 as discrete steps based on the PG add back experiments it
is possible that in the absence of indomethacin they occur simultaneously. As shown in the right hand portion of this figure, antibody dependent or nonadherent cell induced cytotoxicity do not require the indomethacin sensitive step. At present, it is not clear whether these
different activation processes share any common steps, and it is for
this reason that the cytotoxic macrophages have been represented as
different.

These are the two pathways which have been identified in our assay system. However, these results are different from those reported by other investigators. Meltzer and Wahl (6) found that in their assay system, indomethacin had no affect on the cytotoxic activity of mouse peritoneal macrophages treated with lymphokines and LPS. Shaw and coworkers (9) have reported that while indomethacin inhibited prostaglandin synthesis by tumor associated, LPS activated macrophages, the drug did not affect cytolytic activity. In another study, Schultz et al. (8) have shown that the addition of exogeneous prostaglandin E_1 or E_2 inhibited the cytotoxic activity of interferon activated macrophages. The reason for the differences between our results and those reported by other investigators could be attributed to differences in the assay systems used. These include the source and/or mode of activation of the macrophages used, the target cell type, and the timecourse of the assays particularly with respect to the addition of the activating agents and/or drugs used. However, at present, it appears equally likely that once any experimental differences are resolved, there may be three activation pathways which differ in sensitivity to prostaglandins. The existence of more than one pathway of activation has been observed in other immunologically important systems such as the complement system. Therefore, it is not unexpected that cellular immune effectors, in this case macrophages, may be activated in more than one way.

SUMMARY

A comparison of macrophage activating agents in our assay system has shown that there are two distinct activation pathways; one of which is sensitive to indomethacin such as the LPS or lymphokine mediated process, and a second such as the antibody or lymphocyte mediated process which is insensitive to the drug. We have also shown that activation of macrophages by LPS requires at least two steps. At present, the first is biochemically undefined and is not blocked by indomethacin, but the second is inhibited by the drug and appears to require the production of E series prostaglandins. In a number of experiments presented here the dose of indomethacin used only partially blocked cytotoxicity, but virtually complete inhibition has been observed suggesting that both steps are required in order for LPS to activate the macrophages for cytotoxicity.

REFERENCES

1. Adkinson, N.F. (1977): *J. Lab. Clin. Med.* 90:1043-1053.

2. Flower, R.J., and Blackwell, G.J. (1976): *Biochem. Pharmacol.* 25: 285-291.

3. Gately, M.K., and Mayer, M.M. (1974): *J. Immunol.* 112:168-177.

4. Johnson, R.J., Pasternack, G.R., and Shin, H.S. (1977): *J. Immunol.* 118:489-493.

5. Johnson, R.J., Siliciano, R.S., and Shin, H.S. (1979): *J. Immunol.* 122:379-382.

6. Meltzer, M.S., and Wahl, L.M. (1978): *Fed. Proc. abst.* 3719. 38:933.

7. Pasternack, G.R., Johnson, R.J., and Shin, H.S. (1978): <u>J. Immunol.</u> 120:1560-1566.

8. Schultz, R.M., Pavalidis, N.A., Stylos, W.A., and Chirigos, M.A. (1978): <u>Science</u> 202:320-321.

9. Shaw, J.O., Russell, S.W., Printz, M.P., and Skidgel, R.A. (1979): <u>J. Immunol.</u> 123:50-54.

10. Shin, H.S., Hayden, M., Langley, S., Kaliss, N., and Smith, M.R. (1975): <u>J. Immunol.</u> 114:1255-1263.

11. Shin, H.S., Johnson, R.J., Pasternack, G.R., and Economou, J.S. (1978): <u>Prog. Allergy</u> 25:163-210.

12. Siegel, M.I., McConnell, R.T., and Cuatrecasas, P. (1979): <u>Proc. Natl. Acad. Sci.</u> 76:3774-3778.

13. Siegel, M.I., McConnell, R.T., Porter, N.A., and Cuatrecasas, P. (1980): <u>Proc. Natl. Acad. Sci.</u> 77:308-312.

Mediation of Cellular Immunity in Cancer by Immune Modifiers, edited by M. A. Chirigos et al., Raven Press, New York © 1981.

Cell–Cell Interactions Suppress ADCC to Tumor Targets

Sylvia B. Pollack and Sandra L. Emmons

Division of Tumor Immunology, Fred Hutchinson Cancer Research Center and the Department of Microbiology and Immunology, University of Washington, Seattle, Washington 98104

Three components are required for an antibody-dependent cellular cytotoxicity (ADCC) reaction: target cells, specific IgG antibody which reacts with target antigens, and effector cells which bind to and lyse the antibody-coated targets. Each of these components is a potential site of action of biological response modifiers. We have demonstrated the existence of a fourth component, suppressor cells, which can reduce cytotoxicity and which are themselves another potential site of action for biologically active drugs.

K cell mediated ADCC to tumor cell targets in both mice and humans can be inhibited by the addition of autologous lymphocytes (12,15). We postulated that this inhibition of cytotoxicity was due to a direct effect of suppressor cells on the K cells.

Previous experiments in murine models had demonstrated that putative suppressor cells obtained from lymph nodes did not adhere to erythrocyte-antibody monolayers, i.e. were not cells with high avidity Fc receptors (15). This suggested that inhibition of cytotoxicity was not due to competition between effector cells and suppressor cells for the antibody-coated targets. Suppressor cells did not adhere to either Sephadex G-10 or to nylon fibers. Thus, they did not appear to be adherent (macrophage?) suppressor cells such as have been reported to inhibit natural killer (NK) cells (4,11).

We present evidence in this report that the suppressors of ADCC in the murine system are, in fact, T cells, that their effect is not competitive but suppressive and that suppression is mediated via the cell-surface.

MATERIALS AND METHODS

Tumor

The SL-2 tumor, a T cell lymphoma of AKR origin, was obtained from Dr. Irwin Bernstein (Fred Hutchinson Cancer Research Center) and maintained in tissue culture at a cell density of approximately 10^6/ml in RPMI medium containing 10% heat inactivated fetal calf serum (FCS).

Antisera

Monoclonal anti-Thy 1.1 (IgG_2) which was used to induce ADCC to SL-2 cells (1,14) was a gift from Dr. I. Bernstein. Monoclonal anti-Thy 1.2 (IgM) (9) which was used to lyse T cells in the inhibitor LNC population was a gift of Dr. Edward Clark, University of Washington.

Mice

BALB/c, (BALB/c x C57B1/6J)F$_1$, and (BALB/c x C3H/HeJ)F$_1$ mice were bred and raised in our laboratory. The mice were maintained on pelleted chow and water ad libitum. BALB/c homozygous athymic nude mice and their heterozygote littermates were obtained from the FHCRC Central Animal Facility.

Spleen and Lymph Node Cells

Spleen cells (SC) and lymph node cells (LNC) were obtained from 6-12 week old mice unless otherwise stated. SC were teased from the splenic capsule with bent 18 gauge needles and filtered through a thin pad of glass wool to remove debris. Red blood cells were removed by hypotonic lysis. Lymph nodes were minced and pressed gently through a fine screen to obtain a single-cell suspension. Cells were suspended for use in RPMI-1640 media containing 5% heat-inactivated fetal calf serum, 10,000 units/ml pencillin, 10 mg/ml streptomycin, 4 mM L-glutamine, and 1 mM sodium pyruvate, pH 7.4 (5% RPMI).

ADCC Assay

5×10^6 SL-2 cells were suspended in 0.2 ml 10%-RPMI and mixed with 0.2 mCi Na$_2^{51}$Cr$_2$O$_4$ (New England Nuclear) in 0.1 ml. The mixture was incubated at 37°C for 45-60 min. The cells were then washed 3 times with PBS and resuspended in a 10^{-4} dilution of monoclonal IgG$_{2a}$ anti-Thy 1.1 serum in supplemented RPMI containing 10% FCS (10%-RPMI). The ^{51}Cr-labeled SL-2 cells were incubated on ice with the antibody for 45 min, then the antibody-coated cells were spun through 2 ml FCS to remove unbound antibody.

10^4 ^{51}Cr-labeled antibody-coated SL-2 target cells were mixed with normal B6 SC at various effector:target (E:T) ratios in Cooke round bottom microtest plates. The plates were centrifuged for 5 min at 700 rpm and incubated for 4 hr. at 37°C.

One hundred µl was then removed from each well for the assessment of ^{51}Cr-release into the supernatant. ADCC activity was measured according to the formula:

$$\% \text{ lysis} = 100 \times \frac{\text{experimental release - spontaneous release}}{\text{maximum release - spontaneous release}}$$

in which spontaneous release was the ^{51}Cr cpm released from target cells alone, and maximum release was the ^{51}Cr cpm released from target cells incubated in 0.05% Triton-X detergent.

Mixing Experiments to Determine Suppression

Increasing numbers of LNC were added to a fixed number of SC effector cells. The percentage ADCC in the presence of SC alone was compared with that obtained in the presence of SC and LNC. The significance of the difference between the values was tested with Student's t test.

Treatment of LNC with Anti-Thy 1.2 and C'

LNC were suspended at 2×10^7/ml in 5% RPMI. Newborn rabbit serum previously screened for lack of toxicity was diluted 1:10 in 5% RPMI and used as a C' source. Equal volumes of cells, C', and monoclonal anti-Thy 1.2 diluted to 1:10^5 were mixed together and incubated for 45 min at 37°. The cells were then washed with cold PBS and adjusted to 4×10^7 viable cells/ml for use in the assay. Recovery ranged from 28 - 40% (mean=33%; n=6).

EA Monolayers

Monolayers of sheep erythrocytes coated with the 7s fraction of antibody to sheep erythrocytes were prepared and used to deplete Fc receptor bearing LNC as described previously (16).

Kinetic Analysis

Previous studies from a number of laboratories have shown that cell-mediated cytotoxicity (T,K or NK-mediated) resembles an enzyme-substrate reaction (2,5,13,18,19). A rate equation can be derived and two kinetic parameters that characterize the reaction can be determined: K_{app}, analogous to the Michaelis-Menten constant and V_{max}, the maximal velocity of killing.

Varying numbers of antibody-coated ^{51}Cr-labeled SL-2 cells were mixed with a constant number of SC in the presence of increasing ratios of LNC. The ADCC assay was carried out as described above. The number of target cells killed in 4 hr. was estimated by multiplying the % lysis by the initial number of target cells and a velocity of lysis for each combination of cells was derived. The 4 hr. time point was used because measurable levels of cytotoxicity at high target cell numbers (i.e. low E:T) were not detectable prior to that time. Data were analyzed on a Wang 700 series advanced programming calculator using Wang program No. 1047 A/GS2 as reported previously (5,13) to obtain values for V_{max} and K_{app}.

The data are presented as Lineweaver-Burke plots, i.e. 1/target cell concentration versus 1/velocity.

Formalin Fixation

LNC were suspended at 5×10^6/ml in 0.2% formalin (HCOH) and fixed for 60 min at $4^{\circ}C$. The cells were washed three times with 5% RPMI prior to counting and use in the assay.

Trypsinization of LNC

2×10^7 LNC were sedimented, the medium removed, and the cells treated with 1 ml of trypsin for 15 min at $37^{\circ}C$; the trypsin concentrations are indicated in Results. Trypsinization was halted by the addition of 5 ml ice cold 10% RPMI. The cells were sedimented by centrifugation and resuspended at 4×10^7 cells/ml in 10% RPMI for use in the assay.

RESULTS

LNC Suppress ADCC to SL-2 Cells

The effects of autologous LNC on SC mediated ADCC to SL-2 were similar to those reported previously with EL-4 target cells. LNC, which did not themselves mediate ADCC, produced a dose-dependent decrease in the antibody-dependent killing of SL-2 by SC (Fig. 1).

T-Cell Dependence of Suppression

Treatment of LNC with monoclonal anti-Thy 1.2 and C' reduced or eliminated the ability of the LNC to suppress ADCC (Fig. 2). Control LNC treated with either the antibody or C' alone were suppressive.

In addition, LNC from BALB/c nu/nu mice did not suppress ADCC mediated by nu/nu SC, whereas LNC from their heterozogous nu/+ littermates were suppressive

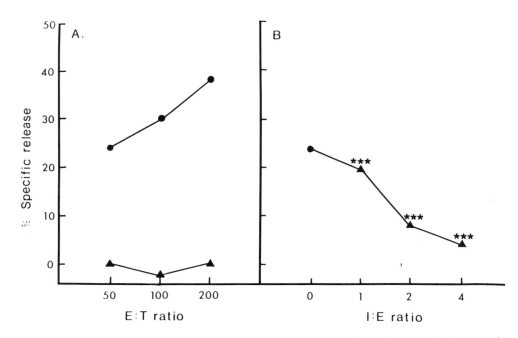

FIG. 1.   A.   Lysis of antibody-coated SL-2 cells by SC (●—●) and LNC (▲—▲) from 12 week old (BALB/c x C57B1/6)F_1 female mice. Effector to target ratios (E:T) were 50, 100 or 200 effectors to 1 target.   B.   Effect on ADCC of addition of increasing numbers of LNC to a constant number of SC (5 x 10^5).   Inhibitor LNC to effector SC ratios (I:E) were varied from 0 to 4:1.   *** p⟨ 0.001.

(Fig. 3). Nude LNC are highly efficient effectors of ADCC, however. In order to deplete this ADCC effector activity, nu/nu LNC were absorbed on EA-monolayers prior to testing in the mixing assay. LNC from nu/nu mice also were unable to suppress normal (+/+) SC (data not shown).

Kinetic Analysis of LNC-mediated Suppression of ADCC

To further investigate the mechanism of suppression the effect of LNC on the kinetic parameters of the ADCC reaction were measured. When inhibition is competitive, addition of the inhibitor to the reaction increases the K_{app}, but the V_{max} remains the same. If inhibition is not competitive, the V_{max} is decreased while the K_{app} remains the same.

A series of four experiments were done using varying concentrations of antibody-coated targets and a constant number of normal SC mixed with varying ratios of LNC. The data (Fig. 4) clearly demonstrated that LNC mediated suppression of ADCC was not competitive, i.e. addition of increasing numbers of LNC did not significantly affect the K_{app} (-1/x intercept) but did decrease the V_{max} (1/y intercept).

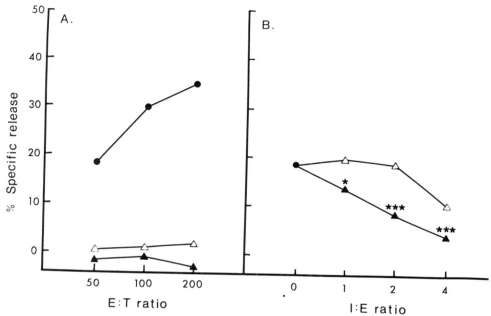

FIG. 2.   A.   Lysis of antibody-coated SL-2 cells by SC (● — ●),
LNC (▲ — ▲) and LNC treated with monoclonal anti-Thy 1.2 and C' to
remove T cells (△ — △).   Cells were obtained from 10 week old female (BALB/c x C57Bl/6)F$_1$ mice.   B.   Effect on ADCC of addition of
increasing numbers of viable control (▲ — ▲) or T-depleted (△ — △)
LNC to 5 x 10^5 SC (●).   * p ❬ 0.05; *** P ❬ 0.001.

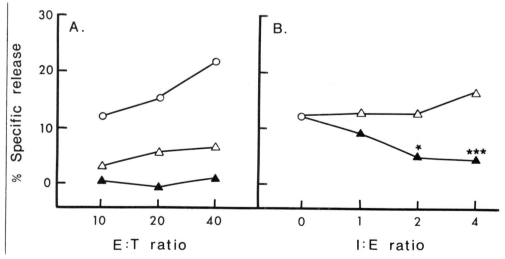

FIG. 3.   A.   Lysis of antibody-coated SL-2 cells by SC (○ — ○),
and LNC (△ — △) from a BALB/c nu/nu athymic mouse and by LNC
(▲ — ▲) from a heterogenous littermate.   LNC were EA monolayer absorbed.   B. Effect on ADCC of addition of increasing numbers of nu/nu
(△ — △) or nu/+ (▲ — ▲) LNC to 10^5 SC (○).   *p❬ 0.05: *** p❬ 0.001.

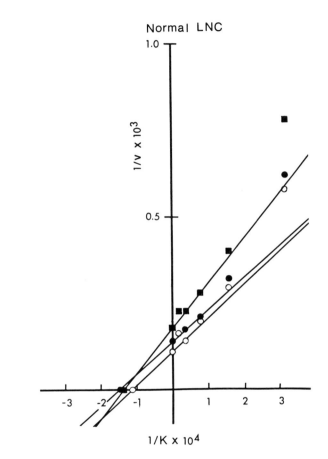

FIG. 4. A. Lineweaver-Burke plot of the inhibition obtained when increasing numbers of LNC were added to 5×10^5 SC. LNC and SC were from 8 week old (BALB/c x C57B1/6)F_1 male mice. Varying numbers of target cells were used. (O —O) SC only: $K_{app} = 0.9 \pm 0.3 \times 10^4$; $V_{max} = 8.9 \pm 1.0 \times 10^3$. (● —●) SC + 5×10^5 LNC: $K_{app} = 0.7 \pm 0.3 \times 10^4$; $V_{max} = 7.1 \pm 0.8 \times 10^3$. (■ —■) SC + 2×10^6 LNC: $K_{app} = 0.7 \pm 0.2 \times 10^4$; $V_{max} = 5.3 \pm 0.4 \times 10^3$.

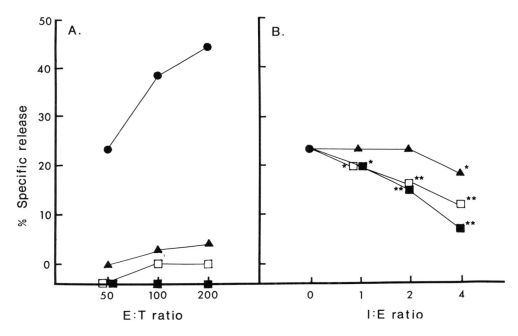

FIG. 5. A. Lysis of antibody-coated SL-2 cells by SC (● — ●), LNC (□ — □) and formalin-fixed LNC (■ — ■) from 5 week old female BALB/c nu/+ and formalin-fixed LNC (▲ — ▲) from 5 week old female BALB/c nu/nu. B. Effect of ADCC of addition of increasing numbers of LNC. * p < 0.05; ** p < 0.01.

Suppression of ADCC by Formalin-Fixed LNC

As one of a series of controls, the effect of formalin-fixed LNC on ADCC was tested. The fixed LNC were as suppressive as control LNC. The effect was not due to the fixative since fixed nu/nu LNC did not suppress ADCC at LNC:SC ratios at which fixed nu/+ LNC were significantly suppressive (Fig. 5). Kinetic analyses showed that the suppression by fixed, normal LNC was not competitive (Fig. 6), the same as suppression by unfixed LNC.

Trypsin Sensisitivity of Suppression

The experiments with formalin-fixed LNC suggested that a cell surface structure was involved in suppression of ADCC. To test this hypothesis, LNC were treated with 0.125 or 0.25 mg trypsin/ml versene buffer for 15 min at 37°C. Control LNC were either held on ice or incubated in versene at 37°C for 15 min. The LNC were then washed and tested for the ability to suppress ADCC. Trypsinization eliminated (0.25 mg/ml) or reduced (0.125 mg/ml) the ability of the LNC to inhibit ADCC (Fig. 7).

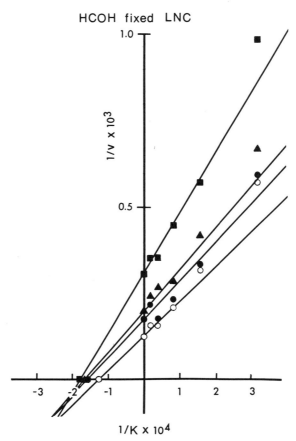

FIG. 6. Same conditions and cells as in Fig. 4 except that LNC were formalin-fixed prior to assay. (O—O) SC only; $K_{app} = 0.8 \pm 0.2 \times 10^4$, $V_{max} = 7.6 \pm 0.7 \times 10^3$; (●—●) SC + 5 x 10^5 fixed LNC: K_{app} $0.6 \pm 0.2 \times 10^4$, $V_{max} = 6.0 \pm 0.6 \times 10^3$; (▲—▲) SC + 10^6 fixed LNC: $K_{app} = 0.6 \pm 0.2 \times 10^4$, $V_{max} = 5.0 \pm 0.4 \times 10^3$; (■—■) SC + 2 x 10^6 fixed LNC: $K_{app} = 0.6 \pm 0.1 \times 10^4$, $V_{max} = 3.2 \pm 0.2 \times 10^3$.

DISCUSSION

Experiments reported here have demonstrated that LNC-mediated suppression of ADCC is T cell-dependent. Removal of Thy 1.2 bearing cells by treating LNC with a monoclonal anti-Thy 1.2 and C' removed the ability to suppress at low suppressor to effector ratios. Further, LNC from athymic nu/nu mice were not suppressive, whereas cells from their euthymic nu/+ litter mates were. Preliminary results with antisera to Lyt antigens suggest that the cell is not Lyt 1 or Lyt 2 positive. It should be noted that classical Lyt 2,3 positive suppressor cells act during the generation of cytotoxic T effector cells (3,8), not during the lytic phase as do the suppressors of ADCC.

Complete suppression of ADCC was not observed in these experiments, perhaps because mixed populations of cells were present. Similar degrees of lymphocyte-mediated inhibition have been reported in studies with murine NK cells and have

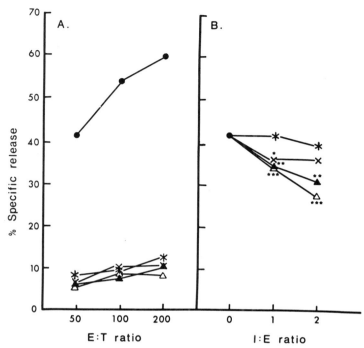

FIG. 7. A. Lysis of antibody-coated SL-2 cells by SC (O — O),
LNC (▲—▲), and LNC treated with 0.0 (△—△), 0.125 (X — X) or
0.25 (✶—✶) mg trypsin/ml for 15 min at 37°C. Cells were obtained
from 7 week old female (BALB/c x C3H/HeJ)F$_1$ mice. B. Effect on ADCC
of addition of increasing ratios of viable LNC to constant number of
SC. * p ⟨ 0.05; ** p ⟨ 0.01; *** p ⟨ 0.001.

been interpreted as due to supression rather than crowding or competition
(4,6,7,11,17). Using the kinetic model, one can distinguish between competitive
inhibition, such as would result, for example, from crowding, and noncompetitive
inhibition such as that resulting from suppression of cytotoxicity during the
effector phase.

The kinetic analysis presented here clearly showed that inhibition of antitumor
ADCC by LNC was not competitive. Addition of increasing numbers of LNC
significantly decreased the V_{max} of the reaction without significantly affecting
the K_{app}. This effect was observed also in three other similar experiments. These
data rule out the explanations that 1) the LNC were acting as cold targets and 2)
that the LNC were interacting with or occluding the F_c receptors of the K cells.

Based on the kinetic studies, several models for suppression can be proposed. It
is possible that the suppressor LNC interacts with the K cell-SL-2 complex,
thereby preventing lysis and effectively removing the K cell SL-2 complex from
the reaction. Another possibility is that the suppressor LNC directly interacts with
the K-cell at a site other than the FcR, thereby either preventing binding or, if
binding occurs, rendering the K cell-SL-2 complex inactive. The result, in either
case, is that lymph node T cells suppress the lytic phase of ADCC. Whether the
interaction affects recognition, the lethal hit step, or lysis itself remains to be
determined.

The most novel aspect of these results is that suppression is not mediated via a soluble interleukin but by a cell-bound suppressor structure (SS). Metabolically active cells were not required for suppression since formalin fixed LNC were as effective as unfixed LNC. The trypsin sensitivity of SS and its fixation by formaldehyde suggest that the SS may be a cell-surface component such as protein or lipoprotein.

SUMMARY

Murine lymph node cells (LNC) suppressed K-cell-mediated antibody-dependent cellular cytotoxicity (ADCC) to antibody-coated tumor cells. The experiments reported here demonstrated that suppression was T-cell dependent, was not competitive, and was mediated by the suppressor cell surface. Treatment of normal LNC with monoclonal anti-Thy 1.2 antibody and complement (C') depleted suppressor activity compared to untreated control LNC or LNC treated with either anti-Thy 1.2 or C' alone. LNC from homozygous athymic nude mice did not suppress ADCC whereas LNC from heterzyogous +/nu controls significantly suppressed ADCC. A kinetic analysis was used to determine whether the LNC were acting competitively or not. Lineweaver-Burke plots of the data indicated that inhibition of ADCC by LNC was not competitive. Noncompetitive inhibition was also demonstrated with formalin-fixed LNC. Trypsinization of the LNC, prior to use in the assay, decreased their ability to suppress ADCC. These results, plus those with formalin-fixed LNC, suggest that LNC surface structures were required for suppression. The data suggest that T-dependent LNC suppress K cell cytotoxicity by direct cell-cell interactions.

ACKNOWLEDGEMENT

The research described was supported by Grant CA 18647 from the National Cancer Institute.

Our thanks to Dr. Edward Clark for providing the monoclonal anti-Thy 1.2 serum for these studies, to Dr. Irwin Bernstein for the monoclonal anti-Thy 1.1 serum, to Kelly Thomas for technical assistance, to Linda Hallenbeck for preparing the figures and to Darlene Thomson for typing the manuscript.

REFERENCES

1. Bernstein, I.D., Tam, M.R., and Nowinski, R.C. (1980): Science, 207:68-71.

2. Callewaert, D.M., Johnson, D.F., and Kearney, J. (1978): J.Immunol., 121: 710-717.

3. Cantor, H. (1979): Ann. Rev. Med., 30:269-277.

4. Cudkowicz, G. and Hochman, P.S. (1979): Immunol. Rev. 44:13-41.

5. Herrick, M.V., and Pollack, S.B. (1978): J. Immunol., 121:1348-1352.

6. Hochman, P.S. and Cudkowicz, G. (1979): J. Immunol., 123:968-976.

7. Hochman, P.S., Cudkowicz, G., and Dausset, J. (1978): J. Natl. Cancer Inst., 61:265-268.

8. Kapp, J.A., Pierce, C.W., Theze, J., and Benacerraf, B. (1978): Fed. Proc., 37:2361-2364.

9. Lake, P., Clark, E.A., Khorshidi, M., and Sunshine, G. (1979): Eurp. J. Immunol., 9:875-886.

10. Lotzova, E. (1980): In: Natural Cell Mediated Immunity Against Tumors, edited by R.B. Herberman, pp. 735-752. Academic Press, New York.

11. Ojo, E., Haller, O., Kimura, A., and Wigzell, H. (1978): Int. J. Cancer, 21:444-452.

12. Pollack, S.B. and Emmons, S.L. (1979): J. Immunol., 122:718-722.

13. Pollack, S.B. and Emmons, S.L. (1979): J. Immunol., 123:160-165.

14. Pollack, S.B., Emmons, S.L., Hallenbeck, L.A., and Tam, M.R. (1980): In: Nautral Cell Medited Immunity Against Tumors, edited by R.B. Herberman, pp.139-150. Academic Press, New York.

15. Pollack, S.B., Emmons, S.L., and Herrick, M.V. (1980): Cell. Immunol., 49:250-259.

16. Pollack, S.B., and Herrick, M.V. (1977): J. Immunol., 119:2172-2178.

17. Savary, C.A. and Lotzova, E. (1978): J. Immunol., 120:239-243.

18. Thorn, R.M. and Henney, C.S. (1976): J. Immunol., 117:2213-2219.

19. Zeijlemaker, W.P., vanOers, R.H.J., deGoede, R.E.Y., and Schellekens, P. Th. A. (1977): J. Immunol., 119:1507-1514.

Mediation of Cellular Immunity in Cancer by Immune Modifiers, edited by M. A. Chirigos et al., Raven Press, New York © 1981.

In Vivo Activation of Monocyte and Alveolar Macrophage ADCC: A Rabbit Model

T. K. Huard, D. M. Garagiola, and A. F. LoBuglio

Simpson Memorial Research Institute, University of Michigan Medical Center, Ann Arbor, Michigan 48109

Peripheral blood monocytes are the circulating precursors of most tissue macrophages and represent the population which responds to chemotactic stimuli to produce macrophage infiltration at sites of inflammation or tumor. Our laboratory has been examining the cytotoxic potential of monocytes in vitro. We have characterized their ability to lyse tumor cell targets sensitized with either allogeneic (5), xenogeneic antisera (6), or erythrocyte targets sensitized with isoantibodies (7). We have compared their ability to function in antibody-dependent cellular cytotoxicity (ADCC) with Fc-receptor bearing lymphocytes and granulocytes (1,7). These studies have revealed that each effector cell population may exhibit several notable differences in the expression of Fc-receptor activity toward antibody displayed on the target cell surface. For example, all three cell types could carry out ADCC to CEM T-lymphoblast tumor cells sensitized with rabbit IgG. The granulocytes, however, required 10 to 100-fold more antibody/target cell in order to bind and lyse the tumor cells as compared to either lymphocyte or monocytes (1). In addition, lymphocytes were unable to bind or lyse sensitized erythrocyte targets if the isoantibody was distributed randomly on the target cell membrane, but could lyse sensitized red cells coated with the same number of IgG molecules distributed in a clustered arrangement. Monocytes, however, were able to lyse either red cell target regardless of the IgG distribution pattern (8,10). Thus, it would appear that these unique cell populations differ in regards to criteria for Fc-receptor interaction with antibody sensitized target cells.

In this study, we have examined whether two different stages of differentiation in the same cell lineage might exhibit differences in Fc-receptor activity toward antibody sensitized target cells. For these studies, we have utilized a rabbit model to examine the interaction of peripheral blood monocytes and tissue-bound macrophages (alveolar macrophages) with tumor cell targets sensitized with rabbit antibody. In addition, we have examined the in vivo effect of mycobacteria or their immunostimulatory components on monocyte and alveolar macrophage ADCC to tumor cells.

MATERIALS AND METHODS

Effector Cell Isolation

Peripheral blood monocytes were isolated from rabbit blood by a modification of methods, previously described for human monocytes (6). Briefly, peripheral blood was submitted to density gradient centrifugation on Ficoll-Hypaque at 1150 x g for 25'. The mononuclear cells were plated on 100 mm-petri dishes (Corning #25020) for 90' at $37^{\circ}C$. Plates were washed rigorously to remove non-adherent lymphocytes and the adherent monocytes were harvested by gentle scraping in cold 0.1% BSA-0.2% EDTA. Monocytes were $\geq$ 95% viable by trypan blue exclusion and $\geq$ 95% positive for the non-specific esterase. Rabbit alveolar macrophages were isolated by pulmonary lavage by the method of Myrvik et al. (4). These cells were also $\geq$ 95% viable and $\geq$ 92% non-specific esterase positive.

Target Cell Preparation

For ADCC assay, sensitized human tumor cells, CEM T-lymphoblasts, were used as targets (6). The tumor cells (10×10^6) were radiolabeled with 100 uCi of $Na_2^{51}CrO_4$ (New England Nuclear, Boston, MA) for 90' at $37^{\circ}C$. Nonbound ^{51}Cr was washed away and 2.5×10^6 labeled CEM were sensitized with 50 ul of undiluted, 1:8, 1:32, or 1:128 dilutions of rabbit anti-CEM antisera for 45' at $37^{\circ}C$. Unbound antibody was washed away and the cells were resuspended to 2×10^5/ml. These antisera dilutions produced a range of antibody densities on the tumor cell membranes of 400,000 IgG molecules/cell (undiluted antisera) to 25,000 IgG/cell (1:128 dilution) as measured by an ^{125}I-Staph protein A radioimmunoassay (10).

Antibody-Dependent Cellular Cytotoxicity (ADCC) Assay

The ability of rabbit monocytes and alveolar macrophages to lyse antibody sensitized tumor cells was determined in a 4 hr ^{51}Cr-release assay as previously described (6). Briefly, 2×10^4 sensitized CEM tumor cells in 0.1 ml were incubated with an equal volume of varying concentrations of isolated effector cells in 0.3 ml flat bottom-well microtiter plates (Costar, Cambridge, MA). The plates were incubated for 4 hr at $37^{\circ}C$ and 100 ul of supernatant was aspirated from each well to determine the amount of ^{51}Cr-released. Spontaneous release from tumor cell targets ranged from 6 to 15%.

In Vivo Activation

Normal NZW rabbits (Langshaw, Haslett, MI) were injected I.V. (via ear vein) with 1 ml of a 10% (V/V) solution of either complete Freund's adjuvant (CFA; Difco; 1 mg M. butyricum/ml), Bacillus-Calmette-Guerin (BCG; Connaught; 1 mg M. bovis/ml), or Muramyl dipeptide (MDP; Calbiochem.; 1 mg/ml) in Hank's balanced salt solution (HBSS). The BCG and MDP were reconstituted in either incomplete Freund's adjuvant (IFA) or normal saline prior to mixing with the HBSS. Three weeks (21 ± 2 days) past a single injection, the rabbits were bled for isolation of monocytes and sacrificed for alveolar macrophage isolation. The cells were then assayed for cytotoxic capacity and the results expressed as the mean ± 1 SD of at least 3 animals.

Effector Cell Binding of Target Cells

The binding of sensitized tumor cells to normal or activated
rabbit monocytes or alveolar macrophages was determined by a modification of a rosette-forming cell assay as previously described (9).
Briefly, isolated monocytes or alveolar macrophages were mixed with an
equal volume of optimally antibody sensitized tumor cells (undiluted
antisera) at an effector cell/target cell ratio (E/T) of 1:25. The
cell mixtures were sedimented to initiate cell-cell contact and incubated at ambient temperature for 15'. After incubation, the cells were
resuspended and the cell suspension was stained for the non-specific
esterase to differentiate the effector cells from the CEM T-lymphoblast
targets. The cell suspension was examined microscopically and effector
cells binding 0, 1-4, or > 4 sensitized tumor cells were enumerated.

RESULTS

Normal Monocyte and Alveolar Macrophage ADCC to Tumor Cell Targets

As seen in Table I, the alveolar macrophages were effective at ADCC
to the antibody sensitized tumor cell targets. The degree of target
cell lysis was directly related to the number of effector cells present
(E/T ratio), and to the amount of antibody used to sensitize the target
cells. Maximum lysis (28%) was observed when 4×10^5 macrophages (E/T
20:1) were incubated with target cells displaying 400,000 IgG/cell
(undiluted antisera). In contrast, the lysis of these same target cells
by peripheral blood monocytes was unimpressive with a maximum level of
2-3% (E/T 20:1). These same monocytes were effective at ADCC to sensitized RBC targets (data not shown).

Table I
Monocyte and Alv. Macrophage ADCC[a] to Tumor Cells[b]

E/T Ratio	Antiserum Dilutions			
	Neat	1:8	1:32	1:128
	Monocytes			
20:1	2 + 1	1 + 1	3 + 1	2 + 1
10:1	< 1	< 1	< 1	< 1
5:1	< 1	< 1	< 1	< 1
1:1	< 1	< 1	< 1	< 1
	Alv. Macrophages			
20:1	28 + 4	15 + 1	10 + 1	5 + 2
10:1	11 + 4	7 + 1	5 + 2	3 + 1
5:1	5 + 3	6 + 1	4 + 3	2 + 1
1:1	3 + 2	4 + 3	3 + 1	2 + 1

[a] Expressed as the mean ± SD % ADCC of ≥ 3 experiments.
[b] CEM T-lymphoblast tumor targets were sensitized with
50 ul/2.5×10^6 cells of varying dilutions of rabbit
anti-CEM antisera.

We next determined if the variant capacities of these two effector cell populations to carry out ADCC to CEM tumor target cells was related to initial Fc-receptor recognition and binding of the antibody sensitized targets. As seen in Table II, alveolar macrophages were effective at binding antibody sensitized tumor cells. Over 70% of the macrophages formed rosettes with at least 5 attached tumor cells. In contrast, at least 83% of the monocyte population failed to bind the tumor targets.

Table II
Monocyte and Alv. Macrophage Tumor Cell Binding

Effector Cells	Target Cells[a]	Number of Targets Bound[b]		
		0	1-4	> 4
Monocytes	TA	83 + 4	16 + 4	1 + 1
	T	98 + 2	2 + 2	0
Alv. Macrophages	TA	6 + 2	23 + 2	71 + 5
	T	92 + 4	7 + 3	1 + 1

[a] TA indicates CEM T-lymphoblast tumor cells sensitized with undiluted rabbit anti-CEM antisera; T indicates non-sensitized CEM tumor cells used as controls.

[b] Expressed as the per cent of effector cells binding the designated number of sensitized targets; results show the mean + SD of > 3 animals.

These results suggest that criteria for Fc-receptor interaction with antibody sensitized target cells can differ dramatically at different stages of differentiation in the monocyte-macrophage cell lineage. This may reflect different density, distribution or affinity of Fc-receptors on the effector cells. It may also result from changes in Fc-receptor requirements for antibody density, distribution, subclass or as yet undetermined factors which alter the Fc-receptor interaction with the Fc-portion of IgG displayed on cell surfaces.

Effects of In Vivo Activation on
Monocyte-Macrophage Fc-receptor Expression

We next examined whether administration of immunostimulants might modulate monocyte-macrophage Fc-receptor interaction with antibody sensitized tumor cells. As previously reported, rabbit alveolar macrophages, harvested 3 weeks after the I.V. injection of heat killed mycobacteria (100 ug) in oil, exhibited increased metabolic activity and Fc-receptor density (2,3). We chose this model to examine the effects of complete Freund's adjuvant (CFA) containing heat killed M. butyricum (100 ug), an equivalent weight (100 ug) of live Bacillus-Calmette-Guerin (BCG) suspended in oil (IFA) or in physiological saline, as well as 100 ug of muramyl dipeptide (MDP) in either oil or saline. Blood monocytes and alveolar macrophages were harvested three weeks after a single I.V. injection of stimulant. The animals appeared to exhibit no toxic effects during the three weeks of observation.

The effects of these agents on monocyte and alveolar macrophage ADCC to CEM tumor target cells are shown in Table III. CFA (heat killed mycobacteria in oil) caused a modest but significant increase in monocyte ADCC. The monocytes harvested from animals receiving live BCG

in either oil or saline had cytotoxicity comparable to or greater than
that seen with normal alveolar macrophages (refer to Table I). MDP,
the active immunopeptide of mycobacteria, elicited the greatest increase
in monocyte ADCC potential. Alveolar macrophage cytotoxicity was
enhanced 2-fold by all three stimulants.

Table III
Effect of In Vivo Activation on Monocyte/Macrophage
ADCC[a] to CEM Tumor Cells[c]

Activator[b]	Monocytes	Alv. Macrophages
None	2 + 1	28 + 4
CFA (100 ug)	13 + 3	47 + 10
BCG/IFA (100 ug)	28 + 3	52 + 5
BCG/Saline (100 ug)	25 + 10	48 + 4
MDP/IFA (100 ug)	43 + 4	51 + 7

[a] Expressed as mean + SD % ADCC of cells harvested
from at least 3 animals; E/T = 20:1.
[b] Cells were harvested 3 wks after a single intravenous
injection of immunostimulant.
[c] CEM T-lymphoblasts were sensitized with 50 ul/
2.5×10^6 cells of undiluted antisera.

We further characterized the effects of these agents by studying
cytotoxicity at various effector:target ratios and ADCC to target cells
sensitized with varying dilutions of antisera. As seen in Table IV-VI,
alveolar macrophages harvested from animals receiving CFA, BCG in saline
or MDP in oil had a striking activation of ADCC ability. At a 20:1 E/T
ratio and with optimally sensitized tumor cells (undiluted antisera),
the amount of cytotoxicity was increased 2-fold. Activated macrophages
at a 1:1 E/T ratio (20,000 macrophages) were able to lyse as many target cells as normal macrophages at a 20:1 E/T ratio (400,000 macrophages). In addition, target cells displaying only 25,000 IgG/target
cell were lysed by activated macrophages to a degree requiring at least
400,000 IgG/target cell by normal macrophages.

Surprisingly, the monocytes were also activated by these stimulii.
These cells have a $T\frac{1}{2}$ in the circulation of 5-7 days (possibly shorter
with inflammation) and yet three weeks after injection were still being
modulated to an activated state. The mycobacteria activation transformed the monocyte population from a non-cytotoxic state (Table I) to
a population which exceeded the cytotoxic activity of normal alveolar
macrophages (comparison of Table I and VI). The activation was reflected in enhanced cytotoxicity with fewer effector cells (low E/T
ratios) and increased recognition and lysis of target cells displaying
less IgG/cell.

Finally, we examined the ability of these activated effector cells
to bind the antibody sensitized tumor cells. As seen in Table VII, the
enhanced cytotoxic potential of blood monocytes following in vivo
stimulation correlated with an increase in monocyte Fc-receptor binding
of antibody sensitized tumor cell targets. Thus, it is clear that
mycobacteria or their products are capable of activating both blood
monocytes and alveolar macrophages as reflected in both greater cyto-

toxic capacity (increased lytic units) as well as increased capacity to recognize and lyse target cells with lower antibody density on their surface.

Table IV
In Vivo Effect of CFA[a] on Monocyte and Alv. Macrophage
ADCC[b] to Tumor Cell Targets[c]

E/T Ratio	Neat	1:8	1:32	1:128
		Antiserum Dilutions		
		Monocytes		
20:1	13 + 3	8 + 4	3 + 1	2 + 1
10:1	9 + 4	6 + 3	2 + 1	1 + 1
5:1	5 + 3	4 + 2	1 + 0	1
1:1	2 + 2	3 + 2	1	1
		Alv. Macrophages		
20:1	47 + 10	33 + 6	29 + 1	22 + 1
10:1	30 + 5	23 + 3	28 + 1	20 + 1
5:1	17 + 5	15 + 5	25 + 1	19 + 1
1:1	12 + 1	11 + 1	12 + 2	11 + 2

[a]CFA (100 ug of M. butyricum) was injected I.V. and effector cells harvested 3 weeks later.
[b]Expressed as the mean + SD % ADCC of at least 3 animals.
[c]CEM T-lymphoblasts were sensitized as in Table I.

Table V
In Vivo Effect of BCG[a] on Monocyte and Alv.
Macrophage ADCC[b] to CEM Targets[c]

E/T Ratio	Neat	1:8	1:32	1:128
		Antiserum Dilutions		
		Monocytes		
20:1	25 + 10	11 + 5	4 + 2	1 + 1
10:1	12 + 5	4 + 4	2 + 1	1 + 1
5:1	6 + 3	2 + 2	1 + 1	1
1:1	1 + 1	1 + 1	1 + 1	1
		Alv. Macrophages		
20:1	48 + 4	44 + 5	34 + 8	25 + 1
10:1	44 + 3	42 + 6	32 + 8	25 + 2
5:1	36 + 2	35 + 4	26 + 5	20 + 1
1:1	25 + 2	21 + 4	20 + 5	12 + 2

[a]100 ug of Connaught BCG in normal saline was injected I.V. and effector cells harvested 3 weeks later.
[b]Expressed as the mean + SD % ADCC of at least 3 animals.
[c]CEM targets identical to that in Table I.

Table VI

In Vivo Effect of MDP[a] on Monocyte and Alv.
Macrophage ADCC[b] to CEM Targets[c]

E/T Ratio	Neat	1:8	1:32	1:128
		Monocytes		
20:1	43 + 4	32 + 6	19 + 2	8 + 1
10:1	34 + 4	25 + 6	16 + 1	4 + 1
5:1	25 + 3	19 + 4	13 + 2	3 + 1
1:1	8 + 3	7 + 3	5 + 2	2 + 1
		Alv. Macrophages		
20:1	51 + 7	45 + 11	37 + 14	23 + 1
10:1	45 + 6	40 + 13	35 + 18	25 + 5
5:1	39 + 7	33 + 13	25 + 11	17 + 2
1:1	24 + 13	22 + 14	16 + 12	11 + 5

[a]100 ug muramyl dipeptide in IFA was injected I.V. and
effector cells harvested 3 wks later.
[b]Expressed as the mean + SD % ADCC of at least 3 animals.
[c]CEM targets same as in Table 2.

Table VII

Effect of In Vivo Activation on Monocyte
Tumor Cell[a] Binding

Activator	Number of Tumor Cells Bound[b]		
	0	1-4	> 4
None	83 + 4	16 + 4	1 + 1
CFA	44 + 6	52 + 3	4 + 2
BCG/IFA	22 + 4	55 + 3	23 + 4
BCG/Saline	34 + 8	35 + 7	31 + 10
MDP/IFA	12 + 3	60 + 3	28 + 4

[a]CEM T-lymphoblast tumor cell targets sensitized
with undiluted rabbit anti-CEM antisera.
[b]Expressed as the per cent of effector cells
binding the designated number of sensitized
targets; results show the mean + SD of > 3 animals.

ACKNOWLEDGEMENTS

This work was supported in part by the National Cancer Institute
Grant CA 25641-02. The authors wish to thank Ms. Helen Ilc for her
assistance in preparation of this manuscript.

REFERENCES

1. Levy, P.C., Shaw, G.M., and LoBuglio, A.F. (1979): J. Immunol., 123:594-599.
2. Montarosso, A.M., and Myrvik, Q.N. (1978): J. Reticuloendothel. Soc., 24:93-98.
3. Montarosso, A.M., and Myrvik, Q.N. (1979): J. Reticuloendothel. Soc., 25:559-574.
4. Myrvik, Q.N., Leake, E.S., and Fariss, B. (1961): J. Immunol., 86:128-135.
5. Shaw, G.M., Levy, P.C., and LoBuglio, A.F. (1978): J. Immunol., 121:573-578.
6. Shaw, G.M., Levy, P.C., and LoBuglio, A.F. (1978): J. Clin. Invest. 62:1172-1180.
7. Shaw, G.M., Levy, P.C., and LoBuglio, A.F. (1978): Cell. Immunol., 41:122-133.
8. Shaw, G.M., Levy, P.C., and LoBuglio, A.F. (1978): Blood, 52:696-705.
9. Shaw, G.M., Levy, P.C., and LoBuglio, A.F. (1979): Clin. Exp. Immunol. 36:496.
10. Shaw, G.M., Aminoff, D., Balcerzak, S.P., and LoBuglio, A.F. (1980): J. Immunol. 125:501-507.

Mediation of Cellular Immunity in Cancer by
Immune Modifiers, edited by M. A. Chirigos
et al., Raven Press, New York © 1981.

Effect of Cytosine Arabinoside on K Cells and Fc Receptors

J. Zighelboim and W. Shih

University of California at Los Angeles and the Department of Microbiology and Immunology, School of Medicine, The Center for the Health Sciences, Los Angeles, California 90024

ABSTRACT

Cytosine arabinoside (ara-c) an inhibitor of DNA polymerase can cause selective alteration in lymphocyte functions. Exposure of normal lymphocytes to ara-c in vitro (10-100 ug/ml) resulted in marked decrease in percent Fc-R cells and in antibody dependent cellular cytotoxicity while having no effect on receptors for SRBC or surface membrane immunoglobulin. These effects were dose and time dependent.

Inhibition of ADCC activity resulted from a) interference of effector cells binding to antibody coated targets and b) direct effect on cytolytic mechanism. This latter effect was only seen when the cells were exposed to the drug for $\leq$ 4 hours in vitro. By contrast using a similar protocol natural killer cells, ADCC effectors induced by exposure to PWM in vitro and allospecific CTL's were not influenced by ara-c.

INTRODUCTION

Cytotoxic drugs used for the treatment of neoplastic disorders can induce significant alterations of T and B lymphocyte functions (1,6,9). For the current studies the drug cytosine arabinoside (1-β-D-arabino-furanosylcytosine) a cytidine analog that inhibits the growth of a variety of cells in culture by inhibiting DNA synthesis was selected. The mechanism of action for this drug seems to involve inhibition of mammalian DNA polymerases in a manner that is competitive with the natural substrate cytidine 5' triphosphate (5). Ara-c has two main metabolic pathways - one which forms the active nucleotide and the other which converts the drug into an inactive compound (ara-u). In the activation pathway the drug is phosphorylated to ara-CTP by deoxycytidine kinase (10).

Ara-c has multiple effects on immune functions (6). Ara-c can inhibit antibody responses in mice (12) and humans while having no effects on delayed cutaneous hypersensitivity, allograft survival in rodents and dogs and development of graft versus host disease (8). By contrast, ara-c seems to have profound effects on Fc-R cells, antibody dependent and mitogen induced cellular cytotoxicity (ADCC and MICC respectively).

Patients with acute myelogenous leukemia (AML) in remission receiving monthly courses of ara-c demonstrate marked reduction of Fc-R cells, ADCC and MICC (18).

The present study was undertaken to directly investigate the mechanism(s) whereby ara-c influences ADCC activity and Fc-R cells.

MATERIALS AND METHODS

Peripheral Blood Lymphocytes (PBL's)

Lymphocytes were obtained from heparinized peripheral blood of normal healthy donors by Ficoll-Hypaque gradient centrifugation (2) and carbonyl iron-magnet treatment (4). After purification, the samples contained 99% lymphocytes with better than 95% viability.

Ara-c treatment
PBL's were resuspended to 5×10^6 cells/ml in complete medium (RPMI 1640 supplemented with 10% heat inactivated fetal calf serum {Grand Island Biological Co., Grand Island, N.Y.} 10mM glutamine, 100 μ/ml of penicillin G, and 100 μ/ml of streptomycin) with or without ara-c (1-D-arabinofuranosylcytosine, Upjohn Company, Kalamazoo, Michigan). After incubation at $37^{\circ}C$ in 5% CO_2 for various periods of time (see results), the cells were washed three times with phosphate-buffered saline (PBS). In some experiments, the washed cells were resuspended in complete medium and cultured for additional periods of time before further testing.

Detection of lymphocyte cell surface markers
T cells and Fc receptor bearing (Fc-R) cells were enumerated by their ability to form rosettes with sheep red blood cells (E-RFC), or antibody coated SRBC (EA-RFC) respectively. B cells bearing surface Ig (sMIg) were detected by using fluorescein-conjugated goat anti-human immunoglobulin (3).

ADCC and NK activity: A human B lymphoblastoid cell line (Raji) and myeloid leukemia cell line (K562) were used as target cells for measuring ADCC and NK activity respectively. The ^{51}Cr-labeled targets were resuspended to 1×10^5/ml in complete medium. For the ADCC assay, 100 μl of ^{51}Cr-labeled Raji cells, 100μl of effectors, and 50 μl of diluted rabbit anti-Raji serum were added to each well of a V bottom microtiter plate (Dynatech Lab., Inc., Inc., Alexandria, VA) in triplicates. To measure NK activity 100 μl of ^{51}Cr-labeled K562 were mixed with 100 μl of effector cells in each well. Most experiments were performed using an effector:target (E:T) ratio of 20:1. The plates were incubated at $37^{\circ}C$ in 5% CO_2 for 3h and the assay terminated by centrifuging the plates for 10 min at 500xg. One hundred μl of supernatant was collected from each well and the amount of ^{51}Cr release was measured in a gamma counter (Nuclear Chicago Corp.). Percent specific lysis was calculated using the following formula:

$$\frac{\text{Experimental cpm - control cpm}}{\text{Detergent releasable cpm - control cpm}} \times 100$$

Control cultures for ADCC assay contained effectors and targets with no antiserum while for the NK assay controls consisted of just targets. Treatment of targets with 1% Triton released approximately 80% of total incorporated counts.

Single cell ADCC assay

Percent lymphocytes forming conjugates with antibody coated targets and causing target cell lysis were measured using the single cell cytotoxic assay as described by Neville et. al. (13). In brief, P815 targets (a mouse mastocytoma tumor cell line) were incubated with a 10^{-2} final dilution of rabbit anti-P815 or normal rabbit serum (NRS) for 10 min at $37^{O}C$ and then washed 2x with PBS. Purified lymphocytes (usually at $1x10^{5}/0.1$ ml) were mixed with equal number of antibody coated targets in a total volume of 200 µl, the cell suspension centrifuged at 400xg for 5 min and the cell pellets vigorously resuspended with a pasteur pipette. To each tube, 0.4 ml of liquified (warmed to 39-40C) 1% agarose (Sigma type 1, St. Louis, MO) was added, and then vigorously vortexed for 5 sec. Subsequently 0.2 ml of the suspension was transfered into a ½ of a 3" x 1" x 1.2 mm glass slide previously coated with a 1% agar-water solution. The gel was allowed to solidify for about 30 sec (at room temperature) and immediately thereafter submerged in complete medium for 1 hr at $37^{O}C$, in a 5% CO_2 atmosphere. After completing the incubation, the slides were stained with 1% trypan blue for 1 min, cleared of the dye by washings with normal saline and fixed in 5% formaldehyde for 2 min. The gels were desalted by 2 washes in distilled water and dehydrated on a warm hot plate. A drop of water and coverslip were placed on each slide and read using direct illuminating microscope at 400X magnification. To determine % conjugated targets the number of lymphocyte-target conjugates per 400 lymphocytes was counted and the percent calculated. To determine % killer cells the number of lymphocytes bound to dead targets per 400 lymphocytes was counted and the percent calculated. To calculate the proportion of killers among conjugating lymphocytes the following formula was used:

$$\text{Proportion of Killers} = \frac{\%\ \text{killers}}{\%\ \text{conjugates}} \times 100$$

Interferon treatment

PBL's ($2.5x10^{6}$ cells/ml) were incubated in complete medium with or without interferon (IF, human leukocyte interferon, National Institute of Allergy and Infectious Diseases, HEW, Rockville, MD) at $37^{O}C$ in 5% CO_2. After 1 h incubation, the cells were washed three times with PBS and their function measured using the single cell conjugate assay.

RESULTS

The administration of cytosine arabinoside alone or in combination with 6 thioguanine to patients with AML in remission resulted in marked decreases in their % Fc-R cells and ability to mediate ADCC (Table 1). After each cycle of chemotherapy (with either ara-c alone or in combination with 6 tg) further suppression of these parameters was seen with a peak effect measured between 14 and 21 days (18). In patients in whom chemotherapy was delayed $\geq$ 35 days (secondary to non-hematologic drug induced toxicity) a complete restoration of % Fc-R cells and ADCC activity was seen indicating that the derangement described above were drug induced. To better ascertain the mechanisms whereby ara-c causes these derangements in vivo we investigated its effects on these and other immune parameters in vitro.

TABLE 1. ADCC effector cell function in patients with AML
          in bone marrow and clinical remission

Studies were performed prior to the administration of the
first course of maintenance chemotherapy

Subjects	N	ADCC (% specific lysis)		MICC	Lymphocytes
		Heterologous[a]	Homologous[b]		
AML (remission)	15	24.8±14.8[c,d]	13.6±7.1[d]	13.8±4.3	1.0±0.3[e]
Control[f]	40	42.3±15.6	34.5±9.3	22.3±6.5	1.8±0.4

[a]Target cells coated with rabbit antiserum

[b]Target cells coated with human (anti-HLA) serum

[c]Mean ± S.D.

[d]$p < 0.001$

[e]$p < 0.01$

[f]Caucasian population composed of individuals healthy enough to
work and between the ages of 21 and 70

Effects of Ara-c on Fc-R Cells In Vitro

PBL's from normal donors were exposed to 1, 10, and 100 μg/ml of
ara-c in vitro for 24 hours. Figure 1 shows a profound decrease in the
% of cells forming rosettes with antibody coated SRBC, while the % of
E rosette forming T cells or the numbers of surface membrane Ig bearing B cells was unchanged. The changes in EA rosette formation could
not be explained on the basis of poor viability or cell recovery.
After exposure to the drug for 24 hours viability was usually better
than 80% in all groups and recovery ranged between 60-90% in either
control or treated groups (data not shown). Moreover, polymorphonuclear
cells (PMN's) exposed to ara-C (10-100 μg/ml) under identical conditions
showed minimal or no change in their ability to rosette with antibody
coated SRBC's (data not shown). Thus exposure to $\geq$ 10 μg/ml of ara-C
in vitro selectively decrease the number of Fc receptor bearing
lymphocytes.

This effect was not only dose dependent (as shown in Fig. 1) but
also time dependent. It required between 14-24 h exposure to the drug
for the effect to be readily seen (Fig. 2). No changes were detected
during the first 8 h of exposure. However, by 14 h the % #A-RFC was
reduced by over 40% and by 24 h the reduction was over 90% of control
values. Irrespective of dose (1-500 μg/ml) changes in EA-RFC were
never noticed during the initial 14 hours following exposure to the
drug.

FIG. 1.

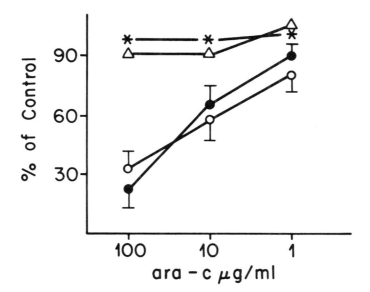

Effect of ara-c on percentages of T,B,and
Fc-R cells and ADCC function. PBL's were
cultured with ara-c for 24 hours. The
percentages of E-rosetting T cells (△),
smIg-bearing B cells (*), and EA-rosetting
Fc-R cells (●) were determined. ADCC
function (O) was assayed by ^{51}Cr-release
of antibody coated Raji cells at E:T
ratio of 20:1. The data were expressed
as percent activity relative to the
control culture incubated for the same
length of time without ara-c. Means
and standard deviation of duplicate
cultures were plotted.

FIG. 2.

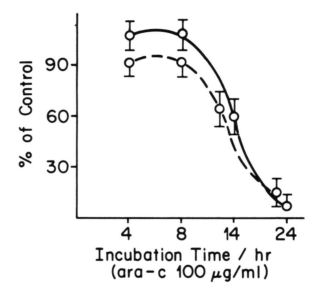

Effects of ara-c on percent Fc-R cells and ADCC
function as a function of time. PBLs were
exposed to 100 μg/ml of ara-c for the indicated
length of time, washed twice and assayed for %
Fc-R cells (-) and ADCC function (-----) as
described in the legend of Figure 1.

To determine the minimal time required for the effect of ara-c on Fc-R cells to be evident, PBL's were first cultured with 100 µg/ml of ara-c for variable times, extensively washed and then maintained in culture for a total period of 24 h before testing. As demonstrated in Figure 3, over 50% inhibition of % Fc-R cells was seen when lymphocytes were exposed to ara-C (100 µg/ml) for as short as 0.5 h. Thus, despite the delay in the onset of the effect, the cells required to be in contact with the drug for only short periods of time.

FIG. 3.

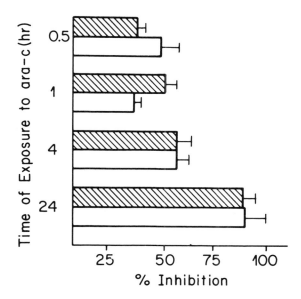

Effect of ara-c pulsing on percent Fc-R cells. PBL's were pulsed with 100 (open bar) or 50 (hatched bar) µg/ml of ara-c for various periods of time. Cells were washed twice with PBS and recultured in complete medium for a total culturing time of 24 hours before further testing.

Culturing ara-c treated cells in vitro for 24-48h after drug exposure resulted in partial recovery of EA rosette forming cells. After 48h in culture however, the treated cells exhibited poor viability thus hampering our efforts to evaluate whether EA rosette formation was fully reversible or not.

Exposure of purified T cells to ara-c markedly reduced the % of T γ cells as well as the % T cells capable of binding B lymphoblastoid cell lines (Table 2). The latter receptor is expressed in >80% of E (+) T cells and therefore the profound reduction in the % of cells expressing this receptor suggests that ara-c selectively influenced a surface marker on T cells (i.e. receptor for B-LCL) without affecting the expression or function of a different receptor on the same cell (I.E. receptor for SRBC).

TABLE 2. Effects of ara-c on T cell[1] markers

Drug	% E	% Fc-R	% B-LCL
MEM	85	12	74
Ara-C (1 h)	82 (-3)	8 (-33)	64 (-14)
Ara-C (24h)	84 (-1)	5 (-59)	24 (-68)
MEM	ND	18	55
Ara-C (24h)	ND	02 (-89)	16 (-71)

[1]T cells purified by centrifugation on ficoll hypaque after rosetting with SRBC's

Effects of ara-c on ADCC activity

PBL's treated with ara-c according to the protocol described before exhibited a marked decrease in ADCC activity (Fig. 1,2, and 4). This effect depended both on the dose and time of exposure to the drug. As seen in Fig. 1, the effects of ara-c on ADCC activity was maximal when using 100 μg/ml and declined progressively when the dose was decreased. Similar to the effect exerted on % Fc-R cells, the reduction of ADCC function was first detected ≥ 14 h following initial exposure to the drug. Brief (0.5 h) exposure, however, followed by 23.5 h incubation in vitro resulted in more than 50% of reduction in ADCC activity (Fig. 4). Similar degrees of inhibition were observed when lymphocytes were exposed to the drug for 0.5, 1, or 4 hours. Only when the drug was present during the entire 24 h of in vitro culture, was maximal reduction in ADCC seen.

Although the effector cells for NK and ADCC activities share many similarities, and may even belong to the same subpopulation exposure to ara-c had minimal or no effect on NK activity (Fig. 5).

Mechanism(s) of ara-c inhibition of ADCC function

To determine more precisely the mechanism(s) whereby ara-c causes decreased ADCC effector function, we employed the single cell conjugate and cytotoxicity assay. The frequency of effector cells binding to antibody coated targets and their killing capacity were evaluated in PBL's treated with 100 μg/ml of ara-c for 24h (Table 3). Exposure to ara-c reduced the number of cells capable of forming conjugates with targets by more than 65%. Additionally, the frequency of killers among the ara-c treated population was 11% compared to 27% in the controls. Clearly, exposure to ara-c for 24 h decreased the numbers of available effector cells as well as the cytolytic potential of the

remaining cells. The inhibition of cytolysis was not due to direct
toxic effects of ara-c on PBL's. Addition of ara-c during conjugate
formation had no effect on either binding or cytolytic activity of the
effector cells.

FIG. 4.

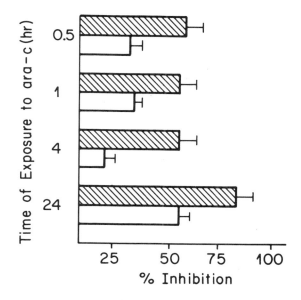

Effect of ara-c pulsing on ADCC activity.
Cells were treated with ara-c as described
in legend of Figure 3. ADCC activity was
measured by ^{51}Cr-release assay using a
E:T ratio of 20=1.

FIG. 5.

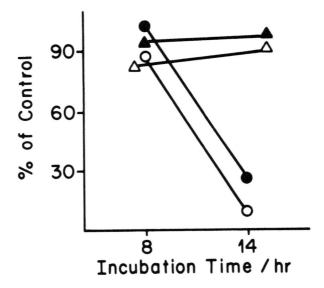

Effect of ara-c on ADCC and NK functions. PBL's were cultured with ara-c at 10 or 100 µg/ml for 8 or 14 hours. Cells were washed twice with PBS and assayed for NK and ADCC using the ^{51}Cr release assay. ADCC functions of cultures exposed to 10 (●) or 100 (o) µg/ml of ara-c and NK function of cultures exposed to 10 (Δ) or 100 (▲) µg/ml of the drug were plotted (as % of control culture).

TABLE 3. Changes in % conjugates and killers after treatment of PBL with ara-c for 24 hours in vitro

Effector Cells	% Conjugates	Incubation Time	% Killer[o] Cells T.C.	Proportion of Killers Among Conjugating PBL's
PBL+MEM	10	0	0.5	5
PBL+ARA-C 100μg/ml	3.5	0	0.3	10
PBL+MEM	11	1 hr	3.0	27
PBL+ARA-C 100μg/ml	2.8	1 hr	0.3	11
PBL+MEM	12.5	1 hr	4.5	36
PBL*+MEM+ARA-C 100μg/ml	13.0	1 hr	4.0	30

* ARA-C added at the time the conjugates were being formed
[o] % killer cells = % PBL attached to a dead target

TABLE 4. Effect of short term exposure to ara-c on binding and cytotoxic potential of K cells

Effector	Time Inc.	% Conj	% Killer* Cells	Proportion[Δ] Killers
PBL+MEM	–	10.4	1.8	18
+ARA-C[o]	10'	12.0	0.3	3
+ARA-C	60'	14.0	1.0	7
+ARA-C	240'	13.0	0.8	6
PBL+ARA-C[•]	10'	10.2	1.6	16
PBL+ARA	60'	10.8	0.6	5
PBL+ARA	240'	8.8	0.6	6

* % killer cells = % PBL attached to a dead target Cell
[Δ] Proportion killers = % killer cells among conjugating PBL's
[o] ARA-C 100 μg/ml
[•] ARA-C 10 μg/ml

These observations suggested that ara-c may be directly affecting the cytolytic potential of effector cells. To investigate this we exposed PBL's to ara-c for short periods of time (10-240 min.), following which the cells were kept in culture for a total of 24h before testing. As shown in Table 4 a marked decrease in the proportion of killers was detected under conditions where % conjugates was unaffected. This indicates that ara-c can influence ADCC by directly affecting the cytolytic event(s).

To explore whether the lytic capability of ara-c treated cells can be augmented by interferon, PBL's were first exposed to ara-c for 24h, and followed by 1 hour of incubation with IF (Table 5). Exposure to IF resulted in an increase in the frequency of conjugates capable of killing bound targets, while the % of conjugates was not altered. The % of killers after 20U of IF treatment was comparable in ara-c treated and control groups. Similar results were seen when exposing the cells to ara-c for only 4 h (data not shown). Thus the frequency of pre-NK cells or the lytic mechanism(s) influenced by IF were not affected by ara-c.

TABLE 5. Effects of interferon on killer cells activity of cells exposed to ara-c (100µg/ml for 24 hours

Effectors		% Conj.	% Killer Cells	Proportion of Killers
PBL+MEM	–	9.8	1.6	16
PBL+MEM[o]	IF 10U/ml	8.6	2.6	30
PBL+MEM[o]	IF 20U/ml	8.4	1.8	21
PBL+ARA-C*	–	2.6	0	0
PBL+ARA[o]	IF 10U	3.4	0.2	05
PBL+ARA[o]	IF 20U	2.8	0.8	28

*Ara-c 100µg/ml for 24 hours

[o]Cells exposed to IF for 60' before used in assay.

DISCUSSION

This study demonstrates that cytosine arabinoside at a dosage ≥10 µg/ml disrupts K cell function. The experimental evidence suggest that the mechanism's for the interference are a) alterations in the expression or function of Fc receptors (leading to decreased number of cells capable of binding antibody coated targets) and/or b) alteration in the cytolytic capacity of the cells that do bind. The data presented, demonstrates that ara-c has selective effects i.e. it affects certain cells or cell functions preferentially. Clearly, exposure to ara-c caused marked decrease (>50%) in the % of cells rosetting with antibody coated SRBC's while it did not alter the percentage of cells rosetting with SRBC's or the number of SmIG bearing lymphocytes. From the experiments reported here we cannot discern whether the decrease in EA-RFC was due to a loss of Fc receptors or to their functional disruption.

Ara-c did not affect all Fc receptors bearing cells equally. In fact, PMN's exposed to ara-c for 24 hours did not demonstrate a substantial decrease in their ability to bind EA. This data suggests that Fc receptor susceptibility might vary between cells (lymphocytes and neutrophils) or that ara-c effects on Fc receptors is associated with cells that actively divide. Winfield et. al. (17) described three discreet types of Fc-R cells. Fc receptors of the three types of cells differed in their sensitivity to trypsin and in their absolute or localized density on the cell surface. It is possible therefore that Fc-R cells not affected by ara-c belong to one of these discreet lymphocyte subpopulations. Studies are currently underway to investigate this intriguing possibility.

The decrease in expression or activity of Fc receptors partly explains the decrease in ADCC activity reported i.e. disruption of Fc-R from K cells reduces their ability to bind antibody coated targets. Furthermore, when these cells are exposed to ara-c for short periods of time (4 hours) a selective effect on the cytolytic component of ADCC was demonstrated with no alteration of the binding component (i.e. percent conjugates remained unchanged). These results clearly suggest that ara-c influences ADCC activity via 2 independent mechanisms 1) by altering binding and 2) by altering effector cells cytolytic potential. The exact mechanism of ADCC is unknown. Clearly, contact between antibody coated targets and effector cells is required but not sufficient (14). For the initiation of lysis, effector cells must be alive and metabolically active. Protein synthesis may be required (16) but DNA synthesis is not. Despite the fact that there is no good evidence that soluble factors released by activated lymphocytes are responsible for the cytolytic event (11) it is quite possible that the cytolytic event is mediated by lytic molecules released once effector cells bind the antibody coated targets. Although highly speculative, the results reported here raise the possibility that the production or release of such lytic molecules may be suppressed by ara-c. The lag period seen between initial contact with drug and suppression of ADCC suggests that K cells may have a reservoir of lytic molecules which are either discharged or inactivated (if not used). A similar reasoning can be used to interpret the changes in Fc receptor activity. To date no studies measuring turnover of Fc receptors have been reported. Recently Di San Secondo et. al. (15) reported on studies of the turnover of complement receptors on normal and lymphoblastoid cell lines. They reported an active turnover with a half-life of about 3-4 hr. If Fc-R have similar or comparable turnover rates their expression on the cell surface would be highly influenced by ara-c and other drugs capable of inhibiting protein synthesis.

Interferon in a dose of 20 U/ml was able to increase K cell activity of PBL exposed to ara-c for 24 hours confirming previous reports on the ability of IF to enhance ADCC (7). The results obtained with the single cell conjugate assay revealed that the proportion of killer cells among ADCC effectors bound to the antibody coated targets was increased. Evidently, interferon activated Fc-R cells that had not yet expressed their cytolytic capacity. The effects of ara-c in vitro on cytotoxic mechanisms was selective in the sense that NK cells were mildly or not affected at all. Similarly, exposure of PBL's to ara-c for 4 hours (followed by incubation in vitro for another 20 hours) did not decrease the generation of alloreactive cytotoxic T cells.

Our previous in vivo studies revealed that patients with AML in remission exhibit decreased K cell activity and % Fc-Receptor cells (18). These alterations were detected at times when the WBC and platelet counts were within normal limits. The in vitro results suggest that rather then absent, K cells might be present in a non-functional state.

In summary, ara-c selectively modulates the function, and/or structural constitutents of lymphoid cells. The data presented, suggests that the drug could effectively and selectively influence K cells in situations where the activity of such cells would be undesirable. We are currently investigating the effects of in vivo ara-c in patients with multiple sclerosis, a disorder in which antibodies to myelin basic protein are found and in which ADCC may be involved in the causation of the neural damage.

REFERENCES

1. Bach: J.F. (1975): In: The Mode of Action of Immunosuppressive Agents, edited by Amsterdam: North Holland Publishing Co.

2. Boyum, A. (1968): Scand. J. Clin. Lab. Invest., 21 (Suppl. 92): 77-89.

3. Elhilali, M.M., Britton, S., Brosman, S., and Fahey, J.L. (1976): Cancer Res., 36:132-137.

4. Gale, R.P., Zighelboim, J., Ossorio, R.C., and Fahey, J.L. (1975): Clin. Immunol. Immunopathol.,3:377-384.

5. Graham, F.L., Whitamore, G.F. (1970): Cancer Res.,30:2636.

6. Heppner, G.H., and Calabresi, P.(1976): Annu. Rev. Pharmacol., 16:367-379.

7. Herberman, R.B., Djeu, J.Y., Ortaldo, J.R., Holden, H.T., West, W.H., Bonnard, G.D. (1978): Cancer Treat. Rep., 62(11):1893-1896.

8. Hersch, E.M. (1974): In: Antineoplastic and Immunosuppressive Agents, edited by A.C. Sartorelli and D.G. Johns, pp. 577-612. Springer-Verlag, Berlin.

9. Kaplan, S.R., Calabresi, P. (1973): N. Engl. J. Med., 289-952-955.

10. Kessel, D. (1968): J. Biol. Chem.,243:4739.

11. MacLennan, I.C.M. (1972): Transpl. Rev., 13:67-90.

12. Mitchell, M.S., Wade, M.E., DeConte, R.C., Bertino, J.R. and Calabresi, P. (1969): Ann. Intern. Med., 70:535-547.

13. Neville, M.E., Grimm, E., Bonavida, B. J. Immunol. Methods, (in press).

14. Perlmann, P., Perlmann, H. (1970): Cell. Immunol., 1:300-315.

15. Rosso di San Secondo, V.E.M., Meroni, P.L., Fortis, C., Tedexo, F. (1979): J. Immunol., 122:1658-1662.

16. Strom, T.B., Garovoy, M.R., Bear, R.A., Bribik, M., Carpenter, C.B. (1975): Cell. Immunol.,20:247-256.

17. Winfield, J.B., Lobo, P.I., Hamilton, M.E. (1977): J. Immunol., 119:1778-1784.

18. Zighelboim, J. (1979): Cancer Res., 39:3357-3362.

Mediation of Cellular Immunity in Cancer by
Immune Modifiers, edited by M. A. Chirigos
et al., Raven Press, New York © 1981.

Overview of Role of Macrophages, Natural Killer Cells, and Antibody-Dependent Cellular Cytotoxicity as Mediators of Biological Response Modification

Ronald B. Herberman

Laboratory of Immunodiagnosis, National Cancer Institute, National Institutes of Health, Bethesda, Maryland 20205

The large amount of interesting information presented at this meeting can be discussed on two levels: First, there has been considerable basic information presented about the characteristics of cytotoxicity against tumor cells by macrophages, natural killer cells (NK cells) and antibody-dependent cellular cytotoxicity (ADCC). In addition, the presentations made at this meeting have important implications for the possible role of these effector cell mechanisms as mediators of biological response modification.

In regard to the discussions on macrophage cytotoxicity, several rather new pieces of basic information were presented. Carlton Stewart showed that all of his clones of macrophages that developed in culture could develop cytolytic activity upon appropriate stimulation. This suggests that the heterogeneity of macrophages may be attributable to different states of activation or differentiation as opposed to the alternative possibility of subpopulations of macrophages with varying activity, as has been shown with other cell types. However, it should be noted that these clones may have been selected in some way or the heterogeneity in macrophage cell populations may arise subsequent to the proliferation of the stem cells involved in the cloning procedure. The information presented by Joost Oppenheim regarding the ability to stimulate Ia negative macrophages to develop this antigen again supports the concept that the heterogeneity of macrophages may be attributable to different stages of differentiation. Furthermore, considerable information was presented during the course of the meeting which indicated that the activation of macrophages is a multi-step process. Monte Meltzer and Stephen Russell both presented considerable information to support the concept of multi-step activation of macrophages for cytolysis. However, it should be noted that this information has been developed entirely in studies with mouse macrohages, where lipopolysaccharide (LPS) has played a key role as a second signal. For activation of mouse macrophages by macrophage activation factor (MAF) at least, there appeared to be general agreement that the presence of LPS, if not requisite, was at least needed for even close to optimal activation, especially by relatively low concentrations of MAF. However, an important issue which was discussed briefly was how much one can generalize from this information. Even in the mouse, as Howard Holden briefly discussed, it does not appear that a second signal by LPS is required or even particularly helpful for activation of macrophages by interferon (IFN) or IFN-inducers. This is of particular relevance to this meeting since at least the majority of biological response modifiers under consideration would be expected to activate macrophages via this pathway and not via the MAF pathway. Another aspect related to this issue is how well the data from mouse studies on the requirement for LPS can be translated into human, clinical situations. Alberto Mantovani and Albert LoBuglio stated that they found no evidence for an important role of LPS in activation of human monocytes and if so, one can seriously question the wisdom of relying on the mouse as a model, at least in regard to strategies involving activation by lymphokines. It also should be noted that these investigators, working with human monocytes, have failed to note the problem of in vitro lability of cytolytic activity that has been characteristic of mouse macrophages. It will be of interest to determine whether multi-step activation processes occur with human macrohages or monocytes, even though the LPS signal may not be an important second signal.

We heard considerable discussion regarding the possible mechanisms for suppressor activity by macrophages. James Bennett focused on the important role of prostaglandins of the E type (PGE), showing their ability to inhibit the generation of cytotoxic T cells. Anthony Allison further showed that PGE could lead to the activation of suppressor T cells. Stephen Russell and Richard Schultz also presented evidence that PGE could inhibit the activation of macrophages or the maintenance of the activated state. It is also noteworthy that PGE can inhibit cytotoxicity by NK cells and it seems quite possible that the suppression of NK activity by macrophages may be mediated by this mechanism. However, it does not appear that PGE fully accounts for the suppressor activity by macrophages. As Luigi Varesio from my laboratory noted earlier in the meeting, PGE does not appear to fully account for the suppression by macrophages of lymphokine production. Furthermore, to further complicate the situation, Beth Ellen Drysdale and Hyun Shin presented evidence for augmentation of macrophage activity by PGE.

Another possible mechanism by which soluble mediators may be involved in suppressor activity by macrophages was raised by Allison. He suggested the involvement of polyamine oxidases and it would be of considerable interest to look for direct evidence for involvement of such a system in situations where macrophages are acting as suppressor cells.

It should be noted that during the course of the meeting we heard relatively little about the mechanisms for cytotoxicity by macrophages. John Hibbs presented some evidence for deranged oxygen metabolism but since this was similar in target cells with either a lytic or nonlytic phenotype, it is not clear how these effects are directly related to lysis. Alternative possiblilities for the mechanism of cytotoxicity by macrophages would include the effects of oxygen radicals, proteases, or C3a as previously suggested by Allison.

In regard to the presentations on NK cells, it seems clear that there have been considerable advances in our basic understanding of these cells and in the technical ability to characterize these cells. One important achievement has been the demonstration of a strong association of human and rat NK and K cells with large granular lymphocytes (LGL), and the ability to highly purify these cells by density gradient centrifugation and rosetting with sheep erythrocytes. A further opportunity for detailed studies has come from the apparant ability to expand the NK cell populations with supernatants from mitogen-stimulated lymphocytes and then to obtain clones of these effector cells. Another major technical advance for the characterization of human NK cells has been related to the growing availability of monoclonal antibodies to various lymphoid cell populations. This has presented new opportunities to characterize in detail the surface phenotype of NK cells and to relate this information to that associated with other lymphoid cell types. Yet another area of rapid advancing information is related to the regulation of NK activity. On the one hand it has been clearly demonstrated that IFN plays a major role in the activation in NK cells or in their augmentation. On the other hand, Gustavo Cudkowicz and Sylvia Pollack presented considerable evidence for the negative regulation of NK activity by suppressor cells.

Despite the appreciable activity in this field and the rapid accumulation of information, there still remain a number of areas of considerable uncertainty or controversy. One such issue is the specificity of NK cells and whether they are a clonally heterogeneous population. Detailed studies with the cultures of NK cells, that are now possible with supernatants containing T cell growth factor, should be very helpful to resolve this important question. Another major and unsettled issue relates to the possible cell lineage of NK cells. In particular it remains uncertain whether NK cells are related to T cells or to macrophages or whether they represent a separate cell lineage. Again, now we should obtain substantial help from the studies with the cultured effector cells. For example, it will be important to document whether NK cells in fact can grow in response to purified T cell growth factor rather than other lymphokines that are present in mitogen-stimulated supernatants, and to carefully examine the changes in differentiation and in phenotype of the cells during growth in vitro. It will also be quite important to determine whether typical T cell functions can be associated with NK cells, e.g. their ability to respond to T cell mitogens or to recognize specific antigens and act as helpers or suppressor cells.

The most important practical question to be answered regarding NK cells is their possible in vivo relevance to resistance against tumor growth. It should now be possible to study purified populations of LGL and to determine whether they can transfer in vivo reactivity against tumor growth. The use of LGL will also be a valuable approach to determine whether such cells can differentiate in vivo into T cells or whether transfer of thymocytes can lead to the development of LGL.

In regard to ADCC, it seems quite clear that there was substantial overlap with information related to the other areas in this meeting since the same cell populations appear to be able to directly lyse targets and also to mediate ADCC. However, some differences were reported regarding the properties for activation or inhibition of ADCC as opposed to direct cytotoxicity. This was particularly true for the different effector activities of macrophages. It remains uncertain whether the very same subpopulations of macrophages, or macrophages at the same state of activation, are in fact responsible for both types of cytotoxic activity. It is intriguing that there has also been a strong overlap between NK activity and ADCC, and it appears likely that the same cells can have both activities. This has been supported by recent indications that clones of mouse cultured effector cells can mediate both types of activity. However, it should be noted that this intimate association has not been invariably seen. The clones of Gunther Dennert have been positive for NK activity but have lacked ADCC activity. Other dissociations between these two activities have also been noted. For example, Gert Riethmuller has commented on a patient with T cell chronic lymphocytic leukemia that had NK activity but was negative for ADCC. Conversely, Franco Pandolfi from my laboratory has recently reported, in Blood, on another patient with chronic T cell lymphocytic leukemia, in which the leukemic cells had strong ADCC activity but lacked NK activity. Thomas Herd and Albert LoBuglio also presented evidence for heterogeneity among the effectors for ADCC. A quite important but unanswered question is whether the mechanisms of killing for NK and ADCC is the same and whether the main differences are related to the receptors involved in causing close binding of effector cells and targets.

During the course of the meeting, considerable attention was devoted to the major role of soluble mediators in biological response modification. Soluble mediators may be involved in both positive and negative regulation of effector cell activities and may play a key role in facilitating the interactions among various cell types. IFN, which provided much of the impetus for the organization of the Biological Response Modifiers Program, continues to appear to be a very important positive regulator of various host effector functions. In addition to the rather well known effects of IFN, i.e. the ability to augment NK activity, macrophage cytolytic activity and ADCC, we also heard about some newer aspects of IFN action on effector cell function. Oppenheim described the role of IFN in the differentiation of macrophages, and as suggested by Allison, the primary effect of IFN may be to alter states of differentiation of various cells and this may provide a useful unifying concept for explaining the apparently contradictory effects of IFN on various immune functions. Julie Djeu presented new and potentially quite important information about the ability of NK-enriched populations to produce IFN, in addition to their abililty to respond to this mediator.

A major remaining question is whether IFN is the only physiologic positive regulatory mechanism for activation of NK cells or macrophages. As suggested by Howard Holden, some agents appear to be able to augment NK cells or macrophages in the absence of IFN induction and there may in fact be other lymphokines involved. However, this point needs to be documented and the other putative mediators identified.

Some important current technical problems were also raised in regard to the soluble mediators. It is often rather difficult, in studies with supernatants of lymphocytes, to determine what effects are related to interferon, MAF, or other lymphokines. One approach has been to use antibodies directed against one or another factor. However, this approach is limited by the lack of documented monospecificity of such reagents. The coming availability of clonal production of IFN, MAF, and other lymphokines and the anticipated availability of mono-clonal antibodies against such materials should be extremely valuable to resolve most of these current problems.

While these above points and many others that I have neglected to summarize are very interesting and intellectually gratifying, workers in this field are clearly faced with the challenge of moving from such basic research information, which is clearly complex and often apparently conflicting or contradictory, to practical attempts at biological response modification, particularly at the clinical level. One major problem, as summarized by our chairmen, Michael Chirigos, is that many or most of the currently available biological response modifying agents are pleiotropic, affecting more than one of these and other effector mechanisms. It certainly would be very desirable and important to identify more agents or protocols which could selectively affect only one of the possibly relevant parameters. At the moment, with most of the agents, we are faced with the difficult decision of determining which parameter or effector function to concentrate on. The central question is which of the various effector mechanisms is important and particularly which is most likely to be involved in mediating in vivo resistance against tumor growth. This issue has not been extensively covered during the course of the meeting, perhaps in fact because it's so difficult and because so little solid information is available. However, we will soon have to directly face this issue since the strategies for biological response modification will probably vary appreciably even with the same agent, depending on the effector cell function to be focused on. It also seems fair to say that most interest is now centered on one or more of the functions that have been discussed at this meeting, since the role of immune T cells and of direct anti-tumor effects by antibodies now seem less likely to play central roles in host resistance or in immune surveillance. The possible in vivo anti-tumor role of macrophages has been actively considered for the longest period of time. However, the current situation is rather confusing, in that some data point towards protection against various tumors but other data point towards the possibility for activated macrophages to actually stimulate tumor growth. It should be noted that most of the available data on tumor protection has been obtained with transplatable cell lines and very little information exists on the effect of activated macrophages in primary tumor systems. Also, it has been very difficult to distinguish between possible direct effects by macrophages and their ability to provide accessory function for NK activity or to mediate ADCC. It would seem important to set up more studies in which there might be selective expression of macrophage activities without a possible role of NK cells or K cells. For example, one might examine the role of activated macrophages in mice that have been pretreated with asialo GM1, estradiol, or in beige mice, where NK activity and ADCC appears to be selectively depressed. Regarding the demonstrations of stimulatory effects of macrophages on tumor growth, it would seem important to determine the possible mechanism for such effects. This might in part be related to the ability of activated macrophages to function as suppressors of immune responses as well as to function as effector cells. The challenge then would be to identify means to induce cytotoxic, preferably cytolytic macrophages without inducing suppressor activity. Some clues have been mentioned at this meeting in this regard. It would appear that the stimuli needed for activation of macrophages for cytolytic activity and for PGE production might be different. Along this line, the possibility exists for giving various stimuli in association with indomethacin or other inhibitors of PGE synthesis, since the majority of speakers, e.g. Russell and Schultz, provided evidence for decreased activation or maintenance of activity of macrophages by PGE. However, it again must be noted that Drysdale presented evidence in the opposite direction.

Regarding NK cells, there has been increasing evidence for an in vivo role of these effector cells. Much of this information has been presented during this meeting. It seems quite possible that NK cells play an important role not only in resistance against tumors but also, as discussed by Cudkowicz, in natural resistance against bone marrow transplants and possibly even in regulation of normal differentiation. There also are increasing suggestions that NK cells may be important in protection against virus infections, as Carlos Lopez has recently reported for resistance against herpes simplex type I infections. It should be noted that my inthusiam for a possible important in vivo role of NK cells may be related at least in part to my direct involvement in this area of research. In any event, with the availability of purified cell populations and of knowledge of some situations with selective depression of NK activity, it should be possible during the next couple of years to abtain more clear cut evidence for or against this hypothesis. There don't appear to be the same problems with NK cells as with macrophages regarding possibly opposing effects on tumor growth. Here the challenge is more as to whether the data gathered with a few selective, highly sensitive targets, can be easily extrapolated to activity against autologous tumors, which in most cases are clearly more resistant to lyses by NK cells and may also be affected by discrete subpopulations of NK cells. However, Joyce Zarling and Alberto Mantovani have both shown here that some primary tumor cells are sensitive to NK activity, especially when tested in an overnight cytotoxicity assay or when the effector cells have been pretreated with IFN. Mantovani has demonstrated that not only allogeneic primary tumor cells but also autologous tumor cells may be sensitive to lysis by NK cells.

Regarding the possible in vivo role of ADCC, some quite interesting possibilities exist. However, as summarized by Hillel Koren, there still is very little evidence for such a role of ADCC in vivo. This may be in large part related to the difficulties to distinguish between the direct cytotoxic effects of various effector cells and the possible involvement of such cells in ADCC. As with macrophages or NK cells, there is virtually no information regarding the possible in vivo role of ADCC in primary tumor systems. In some respects, the distinction between direct cytotoxic effects versus collaboration of effector cells with circulating antibodies may turn out to be an academic issue since it appears that both macrophages and NK cells can participate in ADCC and factors which augment the direct cytolytic activity of each of these cell populations also usually augment their ADCC activities.

Although it is very difficult, if not impossible, at this moment to adequately choose between the various possible effector mechanisms, I think this in part must be done in order to develop rational strategies for biological response modification. One possibility might be to set and compare alternative protocols e.g. one to optimize augmentation of macrophage cytolytic activity and another to optimize augmentation of NK activity, and perhaps a third to optimally augment ADCC activity. Then one might try to determine which of these protocols has the greatest therapeutic efficacy against various tumors. In each case the concern will be to use a protocol to optimally augment the cell function and to keep it up as high and as long as possible, and to avoid or at least to minimize any inhibitory influences on this parameter. In this context, it should be noted that there is little reason to believe that more of a particular agent will be better. The relevant principles here are likely to be quite different from those that have been developed for treatment with chemotherapeutic agents, where the highest possible dose is given. I feel that the primary concern in a phase I trial with a putative biological response modifying agent would be to carefully monitor for the effects of the agent at various doses and schedules of administration. This would appear to be an obvious and straightforward approach. However, in fact, this has tended not to be the case with agents that have been brought to the clinical level so far. We have heard at this meeting of attempts to evaluate the effects of IFN on NK activity in cancer patients or in other patients and there have been apparent contradictory results. Stefan Einhorn has observed prolonged augmentation of NK activity whereas Riethmuller has noted only transient augmentation. These differences may be due to variations in the schedule of administration, or the type of IFN used. It is possible that the doses of IFN used by Riethmuller and by others in the United States may be too high or too frequent and therefore lead to refractoriness after a transient period of augmentation. Careful dose response studies are needed to settle this issue. Another technical issue to be raised in regard to the monitoring of the effects of various agents on effector activity is the problem of substantial spontaneous fluctuation in the cytotoxicity assays, especially when cells from cancer patients are tested. There is a real need to carefully control the monitoring. The experience in my own laboratory has been that it is important to serially monitor concomitant untreated patients and also to obtain more than one baseline, pretreatment value.

In general, despite the problems, I am encouraged and optimistic about the prospects for an important role of biological response modification in the treatment of cancer. There is a wealth of recent information regarding effector mechanisms and it is pleasing that this conference has focused in so much detail on many of the fundamental aspects of activation in these systems. The challenge now is to translate this information into practical reality. My main caution is that this will be a quite difficult task and will probably take a prolonged period of time. The experience with immunotherapy over the last 5-10 years has amply demonstrated that successful immunotherapy by a range of various modalities will not come easily or from empiricism.

Subject Index